TOP TRAILS

Yellowstone & Grand Teton National Parks

46 MUST-DO HIKES FOR EVERYONE

Written by

Andrew Dean Nystrom & Bradley Mayhew

 WILDERNESS PRESS . . . *on the tráil since 1967*

Top Trails Yellowstone & Grand Teton National Parks: 46 Must-Do Hikes for Everyone
1st edition 2005
2nd edition 2009
3rd edition 2017

Copyright © 2017 by Andrew Dean Nystrom and Bradley Mayhew

Interior photos: © Andrew Dean Nystrom, except where noted
Maps: Scott McGrew, Anthony Hertzel, and Thomas Hertzel
Cover design: Frances Baca Design and Scott McGrew
Text design: Frances Baca

Cataloging-in-Publication Data is available from the Library of Congress

ISBN: 978-0-89997-797-3; eISBN: 978-0-89997-798-0

Manufactured in the United States of America

Published by: **WILDERNESS PRESS**
An imprint of AdventureKEEN
2204 First Ave. S., Suite 102
Birmingham, AL 35233
800-443-7227, fax 205-326-1012

Visit our website for a complete listing of our books and for ordering information. Contact us at our website, at facebook.com/wildernesspress1967, or at twitter.com/wilderness1967 with questions or comments. To find out more about who we are and what we're doing, visit blog.wildernesspress.com.

Distributed by Publishers Group West

Cover photo: Cascade Canyon (see Trail 36) © Dezso Matyas/Shutterstock

SAFETY NOTICE: Although Wilderness Press and the authors have made every attempt to ensure that the information in this book is accurate at press time, they are not responsible for any loss, damage, injury, or inconvenience that may occur to anyone while using this book. You are responsible for your own safety and health while in the wilderness. The fact that a trail is described in this book does not mean that it will be safe for you. Be aware that trail conditions can change from day to day. Always check local conditions, know your own limitations, and consult a map.

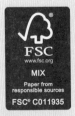

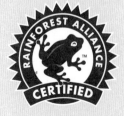

The Top Trails Series

Wilderness Press

When Wilderness Press published *Sierra North* in 1967, no other trail guide like it existed for the Sierra backcountry. The first print run sold out in less than two months, and its success heralded the beginning of Wilderness Press. In the past 50 years, we have expanded our territories to cover California, Alaska, Hawaii, the Southwest, the Pacific Northwest, New England, Canada, and Baja California.

Wilderness Press continues to publish comprehensive, accurate, and readable outdoor books. Hikers, backpackers, kayakers, skiers, snowshoers, climbers, cyclists, and trail runners rely on Wilderness Press for accurate outdoor adventure information.

Top Trails

In its Top Trails guides, Wilderness Press has paid special attention to organization so that you can find the perfect hike each and every time. Whether you're looking for a steep trail to test yourself on or a walk in the park, a romantic waterfall, or a city view, Top Trails will lead you there.

Each Top Trails guide contains trails for everyone. The trails selected provide a sampling of the best the region has to offer. These are the "must-do" hikes, walks, runs and bike rides, with every feature of the area represented.

Every book in the Top Trails series offers:
- The Wilderness Press commitment to accuracy and reliability
- Ratings and rankings for each trail
- Distances and approximate times
- Easy-to-follow trail notes
- Maps and permit information

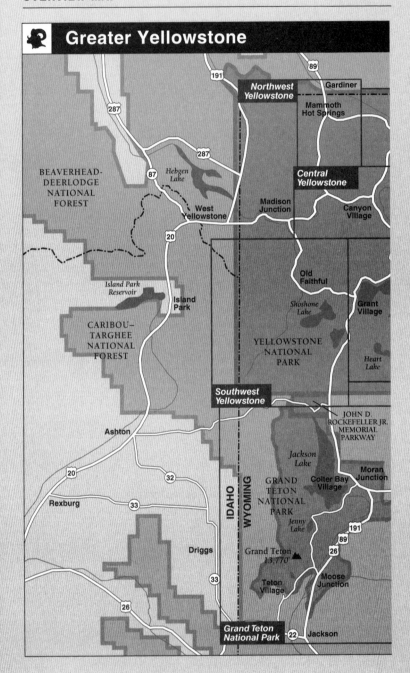

Greater Yellowstone

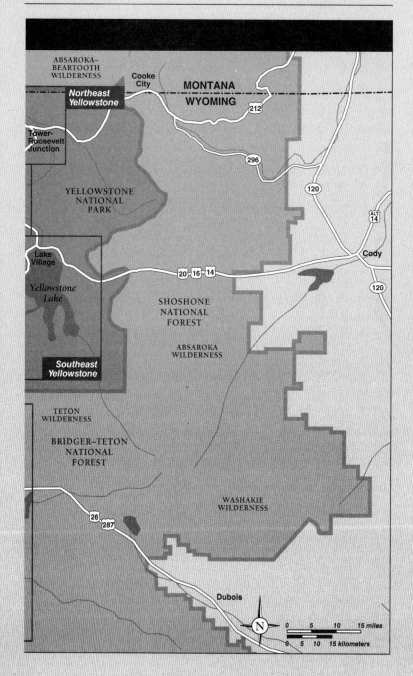

TRAIL FEATURES TABLE

Yellowstone & Grand Teton Trails

TRAIL NUMBER AND NAME	Page	Difficulty -12345+	Length in Miles	Type	Hiking	Bicycling	Horses	Backpacking	Child-Friendly	Wheelchair Access	Permit
1. Northwest Yellowstone: Mammoth/Gallatin Country											
1 Beaver Ponds Loop	39	3	5.5	Loop	Hiking				Child-Friendly		
2 Boiling River	45	1	1.0	Out-and-back	Hiking				Child-Friendly	Wheelchair	
3 Bunsen Peak	51	4/5	4.2/7.0	Out-and-back	Hiking						
4 Cache Lake and Electric Peak	57	5	11.2/21.5	Out-and-back	Hiking			Backpacking			Permit
5 Gallatin Sky Rim Trail	63	5	16.3/18.4	Loop	Hiking						
6 Howard Eaton Trail	70	3/4	4.0/6.6	Point-to-point	Hiking						
7 Mammoth Hot Springs	74	1	1.0	Loop	Hiking				Child-Friendly	Wheelchair	
8 Osprey Falls	80	5	10.2	Out-and-back	Hiking	Bicycling					
2. Northeast Yellowstone: Tower/Roosevelt Country											
9 Black Canyon of the Yellowstone	92	5	18.5	Point-to-point	Hiking		Horses	Backpacking			Permit
10 Fossil Forest	101	4	3.0	Out-and-back	Hiking						
11 Trout Lake	107	1	1.8	Out-and-back	Hiking				Child-Friendly		
12 Yellowstone River Picnic Area Overlook	111	2	4.0	Out-and-back	Hiking				Child-Friendly		
3. Central Yellowstone: Norris/Canyon Country											
13 Artists Paint Pots	126	1	1.2	Loop	Hiking				Child-Friendly		
14 Grand Canyon of the Yellowstone: North Rim	130	2	3.8	Point-to-point	Hiking				Child-Friendly	Wheelchair	
15 Grand Canyon of the Yellowstone: South Rim	136	2	3.0	Point-to-point	Hiking				Child-Friendly	Wheelchair	
16 Hayden Valley: Mary Mountain East	141	4	10.0	Out-and-back	Hiking						
17 Monument Geyser Basin	146	3	3.0	Out-and-back	Hiking						
18 Mount Washburn	151	4	6.0	Out-and-back	Hiking	Bicycling					
19 Norris Geyser Basin: Porcelain and Back Basins	157	2	2.0	Loop	Hiking				Child-Friendly	Wheelchair	

USES & ACCESS	TYPE	TERRAIN	FLORA & FAUNA	OTHER
🚶 Day Hiking	🔄 Loop	🔲 Canyon	Autumn Colors	▲ Camping
🚴 Bicycling	✒ Out-and-back	⛰ Mountain	✳ Wildflowers	≈ Swimming
🐴 Horses	↘ Point-to-point	△ Summit	🦌 Birds	🏠 Historic/Secluded
🎒 Backpacking		▤ Lake	🐂 Wildlife	Geologic Interest
👫 Child-Friendly	DIFFICULTY	🔲 Stream	EXPOSURE	Geothermal
♿ Wheelchair Access	-12345+	▮ Waterfall	🌲 Cool & Shady	☽ Moonlight
✅ Permit	less more		⛰ Great Views	Steep
			📷 Photo Opportunity	

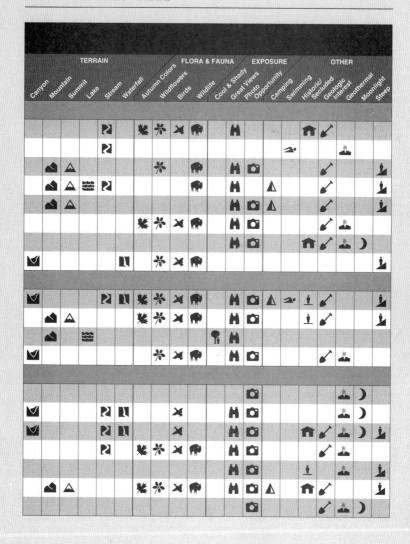

TRAIL FEATURES TABLE

Yellowstone & Grand Teton Trails

TRAIL NUMBER AND NAME	Page	Difficulty 1-2-3-4-5+	Length in Miles	Type	Hiking	Bicycling	Horses	Backpacking	Child-Friendly	Wheelchair Access	Permit
4. Southeast Yellowstone: Lake Country											
20 Avalanche Peak	172	4	4.0	↗	🚶						
21 Elephant Back Mountain	176	3	3.5	↻	🚶				👫		
22 Heart Lake and Mount Sheridan	179	5	15.0	↗	🚶			🎒			✓
23 Pelican Valley	183	4	15.3	↻	🚶		🐎				
24 West Thumb Geyser Basin	188	1	0.6	↻	🚶				👫	♿	
5. Southwest Yellowstone: Cascade and Geyser Country											
25 Bechler River	204	5	29.7	↘	🚶		🐎	🎒			✓
26 Cave Falls and Bechler Falls	215	3	7.3	↻	🚶		🐎		👫		
27 Dunanda Falls and Silver Scarf Falls	220	5	16.4	↗	🚶		🐎	🎒			✓
28 Fairy Falls and Imperial Geyser	226	3	6.8	↗	🚶	🚲		🎒	👫		
29 Lone Star Geyser	233	2	5.0	↗	🚶	🚲		🎒	👫	♿	
30 Mystic Falls	239	3	4.0	↻	🚶				👫		
31 Old Faithful and Observation Point	243	2	2.4	↻	🚶				👫	♿	
32 Shoshone Lake and Shoshone Geyser Basin	251	5	17.0	↗	🚶			🎒			✓
33 Terraced Falls	258	2	3.6	↗	🚶				👫		
34 Union Falls and Mountain Ash Creek	263	5	15.8	↗	🚶		🐎	🎒			✓
6. Grand Teton National Park											
35 Bradley and Taggart Lakes	281	3	5.8	↻	🚶		🐎		👫		
36 Cascade Canyon	286	4	9.1	↗	🚶		🐎	🎒			
37 Hermitage Point	293	4	9.4	↻	🚶		🐎	🎒	👫		
38 Jenny Lake and Moose Ponds	298	3	7.0	↻	🚶		🐎		👫	♿	
39 Laurance S. Rockefeller Preserve	305	2	3.0	↻	🚶				👫		
40 Leigh, Bearpaw, and Trapper Lakes	311	2/3	2.2/8.4	↗	🚶		🐎	🎒	👫		
41 Phelps Lake	316	2	4.0	↗	🚶		🐎	🎒	👫		
42 Rendezvous Mountain to Granite Canyon	320	4	12.4	↻	🚶		🐎	🎒			
43 String Lake	328	2	3.4	↻	🚶		🐎		👫	♿	
44 Surprise and Amphitheater Lakes	332	5	9.6	↗	🚶			🎒			
45 Table Mountain	338	4	14.0	↗	🚶						
46 Two Ocean Lake	343	3	6.4	↻	🚶		🐎				

TRAIL FEATURES TABLE

	TERRAIN						FLORA & FAUNA					EXPOSURE		OTHER							
Canyon	Mountain	Summit	Lake	Stream	Waterfall	Autumn Colors	Wildflowers	Birds	Wildlife	Cool & Shady	Great Views	Photo Opportunity	Camping	Swimming	Historic/	Secluded	Geologic Interest	Geothermal	Moonlight	Steep
	●	●					●				●	●			●					●
	●	●				●	●		●	●	●	●								●
	●	●	●	●				●	●		●	●	●					●		
				●			●	●	●		●	●		●				●		
			●						●		●	●						●	●	
●	●			●	●	●	●	●	●	●	●	●	●	●	●			●		
				●	●	●			●	●		●		●						
				●	●	●			●			●	●	●	●			●		
					●		●	●		●	●	●	●	●				●		
				●					●	●		●	●					●	●	
●				●	●	●					●	●						●		●
											●	●						●	●	●
			●	●		●	●	●	●		●	●	●					●		
●				●	●	●					●	●			●	●				
●				●	●	●						●	●	●	●	●				
			●			●	●	●	●		●					●				
●			●	●	●	●	●		●	●	●		●			●				●
			●				●	●	●	●	●	●	●							
			●		●	●		●	●	●	●	●				●				
			●	●		●	●	●	●	●	●	●		●	●					
			●			●	●	●	●		●	●				●				
			●	●		●	●	●	●	●	●	●		●		●				
●	●	●		●		●	●	●	●		●	●	●			●				●
			●	●		●	●	●	●	●	●	●		●		●				
●	●		●			●	●	●	●		●	●	●			●				●
	●	●		●			●				●									●
		●	●			●	●	●	●		●	●			●	●				

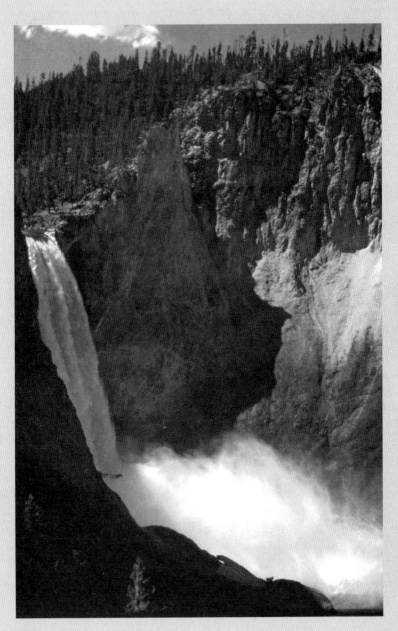

Yellowstone's *Lower Falls* (Trail 15)

Contents

CHAPTER 5

Southwest Yellowstone: Cascade and Geyser Country   195

CHAPTER 6

Grand Teton National Park   271

Map Legend

Featured trail	Amphitheater	One-way (road)
Alternate trail	Bicycle trail	Parking
Boardwalk	Birds	Peak
Freeway	Boat launch	Photo opportunity
Highway	Cabin	Picnic area
Road	Campground	Primitive campsite
Unpaved road	Feature	Radio tower
Ski lift	Fire/lookout tower	Ranger station/park office
Borderline	Footbridge	Restroom
Forest/park	Gate	Scenic view
Water body	Gelogic interest	Spring
River/stream	Glacier	Swimming access
	Lodging	Trailhead
	Marina	Waterfall
	Marsh	Wildlife
	Motorbike access	

Using Top Trails

Organization of Top Trails

The Top Trails series is designed to make identifying the perfect trail easy and enjoyable, and to make every outing a success and a pleasure. With this book you'll find it's a snap to select the right trail, whether you're planning a major hike or just a sociable stroll with friends.

The Region

Top Trails begins with the Greater Yellowstone map (pages iv–v), displaying the entire region covered by the guide and providing a geographic overview. The map is clearly marked to show which area is covered by which chapter.

After the regional map comes the Yellowstone and Grand Teton Trails table (pages vi–ix), which lists every trail covered in the guide, along with attributes for each one. A quick reading of the regional map and the trail table will give you a good overview of the region covered by this book.

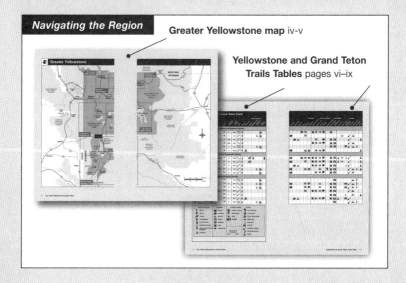

Navigating the Region

Greater Yellowstone map iv-v

Yellowstone and Grand Teton Trails Tables pages vi–ix

The Areas

The region covered by this book is divided into areas, with each chapter corresponding to one area in the region.

Each area chapter starts with information to help you choose and enjoy a trail each time you go out. Use the table of contents or the regional map to identify an area of interest, and then turn to the area chapter to find the following:

- An area overview, including maps and permits
- An area map, with all trails clearly marked
- A trail feature table, providing trail-by-trail details
- Trail summaries, written in a lively, accessible style

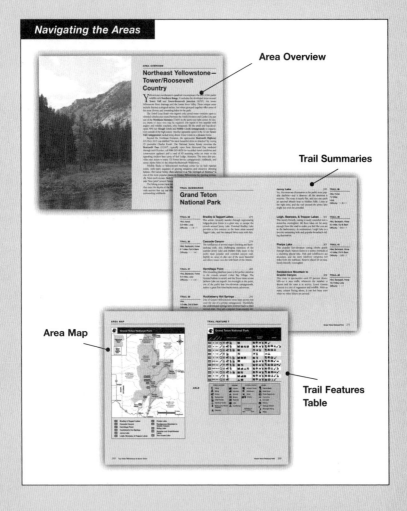

The Trails

The basic building block of the Top Trails guide is the trail entry. Each one is arranged to make finding and following the trail as simple as possible, with all pertinent information presented in an easy-to-follow format:

- A trail map
- Trail descriptors covering difficulty, length, and other essential data
- Narrative trail text
- Trail milestones, providing turn-by-turn trail directions

Some trail descriptions offer additional information, such as:

- An elevation profile
- Trail options
- Trail highlights
- Trail teasers

In the margins of the trail entries, look for icons that point out notable features at specific points along the trail.

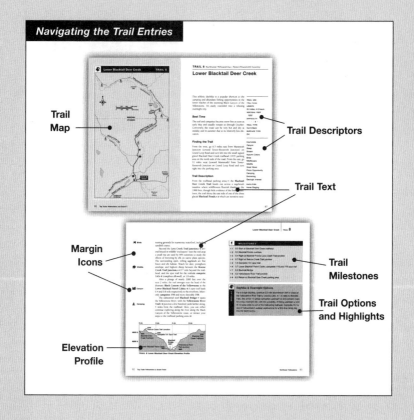

Choosing a Trail

Top Trails provides several ways of choosing a trail, presented in easy-to-read tables, charts, and maps.

Location

If you know in general where you want to go, Top Trails makes it easy to find the right trail in the right place. Each chapter begins with a large-scale map showing the starting point of every trail in that area.

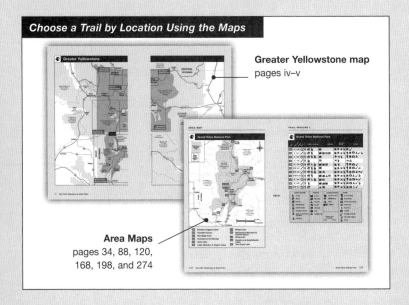

Choose a Trail by Location Using the Maps

Greater Yellowstone map
pages iv–v

Area Maps
pages 34, 88, 120,
168, 198, and 274

Features

This guide describes the top trails of Yellowstone and Grand Teton National Parks, and each trail is chosen because it offers one or more features that make it appealing. Using the trail descriptors, summaries, and tables, you can quickly examine all the trails for the features they offer or seek a particular feature among the list of trails.

Season and Condition

Time of year and current conditions can be important factors in selecting the best trail. For example, an exposed, low-elevation trail may be a riot of color in early spring but an oven-baked taste of hell in midsummer. Wherever relevant, Top Trails identifies the best and worst conditions for the trails.

Difficulty

The overall difficulty of each trail is rated on a scale of 1–5, which considers length, elevation change, exposure, and trail quality to establish one (admittedly subjective) rating. The ratings assume you are an able-bodied adult who is in reasonably good shape and using the trail for hiking. The ratings also assume normal weather conditions—clear and dry. Make an honest assessment of your own abilities, and adjust time estimates accordingly. Rain, snow, heat, wind, and poor visibility can also affect your pace on even the easiest of trails.

Choose a Trail by Length, Difficulty, or Features Using the Tables

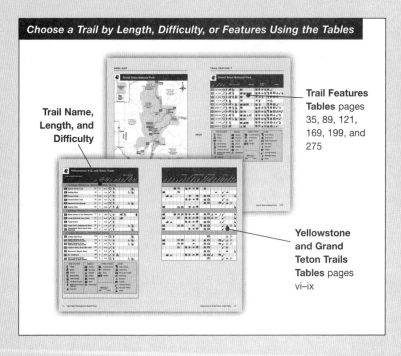

Trail Name, Length, and Difficulty

Trail Features Tables pages 35, 89, 121, 169, 199, and 275

Yellowstone and Grand Teton Trails Tables pages vi–ix

Vertical Feet

Every trail description contains the approximate trail length and the overall elevation gain and loss over the course of the trail. It's important to use both figures when considering a hike; on average, plan one hour for every 2 miles, and add an hour for every 1,000 feet you climb.

This important measurement is often underestimated by hikers when gauging the difficulty of a trail. The Top Trails measurement accounts for all elevation change, not simply the difference between the highest and lowest points, so you can identify rolling terrain with lots of ups and downs.

The calculation of vertical feet in the Top Trails series is accomplished by a combination of trail measurement and computer-aided estimation. For routes that begin and end at the same spot—such as loop or out-and-back—the vertical gain exactly matches the vertical descent. With a point-to-point route, the vertical gain and loss will most likely differ, and both figures will be provided in the text.

Finally, all trail entries with more than 1,000 feet of elevation gain include an elevation profile—an easy means of visualizing the topography of the route. These profiles graphically depict the elevation over the length of the trail.

Surface Type

Each trail entry describes the surface of the trail. This information is useful in determining what type of footwear is appropriate. Surface type should also be considered when checking the weather—on a rainy day early or late in the hiking season, a dirt surface can be a muddy slog; a boardwalk jaunt or gravel surface might be a better choice.

 Top Trails Difficulty Ratings

1. A short trail, generally level, that can be completed in one hour or less.

2. A route of 1 to 3 miles, with some up and down, that can be completed in one to two hours.

3. A longer route, up to 5 miles, with uphill and/or downhill sections.

4. A long or steep route, perhaps more than 5 miles, or with climbs of more than 1,000 vertical feet.

5. The most severe route, both long and steep, more than 5 miles long, with climbs of more than 1,000 vertical feet.

Introduction to Yellowstone and Grand Teton National Parks

Yellowstone and Grand Teton National Parks compose the core of the Greater Yellowstone Ecosystem, the world's largest intact temperate-zone crucible of raw, wild nature. The Greater Yellowstone concept originated in the early 1970s, based on a pioneering study of grizzly bear population dynamics directed by brothers John and Frank Craighead. After 12 years of field research, they calculated that the year-round range of the region's bears exceeded 5 million acres, an area larger than Connecticut.

Jazz lovers may beg to differ, but many have called our national park system "the best idea America ever had." Yellowstone was set aside as the world's first national park in 1872 and named a United Nations World Biosphere Reserve in 1976. The establishment of National Elk Refuge near Jackson in 1912 opened public access to the region's southern flank. Much of the area eventually set aside as Grand Teton National Park in 1929 was part of a 1918 proposed enlargement to Yellowstone.

These two world-famous parks are surrounded by a buffer zone consisting of six national forests, six wilderness areas, three national wildlife refuges, 125,000 acres of Bureau of Land Management rangeland, and more than 1 million acres of private property and tribal lands.

All told, this vast complex of wild lands encompasses 28,000 square miles, about the size of West Virginia. Yellowstone alone protects 2.22 million acres (3,468 square miles), roughly the same size as Puerto Rico, or Delaware and Rhode Island combined. In contrast, Grand Teton's wilderness punch is concentrated in a mere 311,000 acres.

To give you a better idea of just how big the region is, Yellowstone's seasonal Thorofare patrol cabin in the park's bottom right corner is around 30 trail miles from the nearest road—a long day's horseback ride—making it the most remote inhabited wilderness outpost and the farthest spot from a road in the Lower 48.

Long-range planning for holistic management of the buffer zone, home to a rapidly growing human population of well over 200,000 residents, is

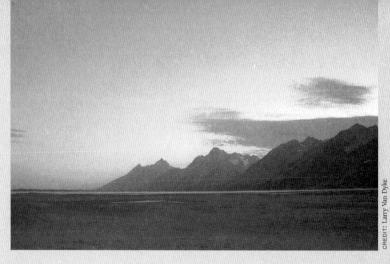

CREDIT: Larry Van Dyke

Teton Range *and Jackson Hole*

increasingly seen as the key to preserving this unique region, which is often described as "Island Yellowstone" or "an island of mountains in the high, dry plains."

Geography and Topography

The topography of Greater Yellowstone is the result of an underlying magmatic hot spot and millions of years of volcanic influence. The massif of high, moist plateaus, peaks, and valleys is surrounded by arid plains.

The region contains the headwaters of many of the continent's grandest waterways: two of the three forks of the Missouri; the headwaters of the Snake River, which flows into the Columbia and eventually into the Pacific Ocean; and the Yellowstone River, the United States' longest free-flowing river, which runs north and drains approximately 70,000 square miles.

The Continental Divide, the crest of the North American continent, zigzags across the southwest corner of Yellowstone. The region's landforms channel westerly storm systems onto Yellowstone's Central Plateau, where most of the park's snow drops. The Tetons' topographic extremes create their own semiarid microclimate, with most storms approaching from the southwest. Here, snowfall averages 190-plus inches, but annual rainfall hovers around just 10 inches.

The majority of Yellowstone consists of broad volcanic plateaus scored by deep river canyons, with an average elevation of 8,000 feet. There are 370 miles of paved roads and more than 1,000 miles of maintained hiking trails. Yellowstone is covered 5% by water, 15% by grassland, and 80% by lodgepole pine forest. The highest point is the seldom-scaled Eagle Peak (11,358 feet), near the park's remote southeast corner. The lowest point is near the

North Entrance at Reese Creek (5,282 feet), just north of the prominent Electric Peak (10,992 feet).

Grand Teton's centerpiece is the 40-mile-long Teton Range, an active fault-block mountain front. Twelve peaks exceeding 12,000 feet tower over the Snake River Plain and the valley known as Jackson Hole, which averages 6,800 feet in elevation and tilts subtly southward toward the gateway town of Jackson. In addition to the string of morainal piedmont lakes at the base of the range, the park is home to more than 100 alluring tarns (steep-banked glacial lakes). In Yellowstone, more than 600 lakes and ponds cover approximately 107,000 surface acres, 94% of which can be attributed to Yellowstone, Lewis, Shoshone, and Heart Lakes. Some 1,000 rivers and streams account for more than 2,000 miles of running water.

Geology and Hydrothermal Activity

Glaciers and supervolcanoes are the primary influences in Greater Yellowstone's dynamic landscape. In the past 2.1 million years, three cataclysmic eruptions have rocked the region. The most recent massive volcanic explosion, which occurred around 640,000 years ago, created the gigantic Yellowstone Caldera, a vast, collapsed crater that defines the park's Central Plateau.

Since 2001, the Yellowstone Volcano Observatory has tracked the uplift of the dome beneath Yellowstone Lake resulting from the pressure exerted by superplumes of near-surface magma in what it calls the "largest volcanic system in North America." Multiple earthquakes are registered daily, but a swarm of 400 temblors centered in the park's northwest sector in 2004 sparked renewed speculation about the possibility of another gigantic volcanic event and the possible resulting global climate disruption. Volcanologists downplay the possibility of such an event in our lifetime. However, some say its likelihood is 5 to 10 times greater than that of a globally destructive asteroid impact.

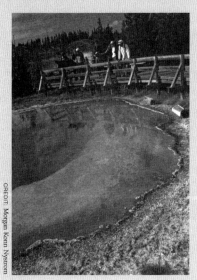

CREDIT: Morgan Konn Nystrom

Also related to the hot spot are Yellowstone's unique, superheated hydrothermal features. A recent inventory conducted by the

Boardwalks *provide close access to many frontcountry hot springs.*

Yellowstone Center for Resources estimates that the park is home to more than 18,000 distinct geothermal features. The most common surface expressions of the park's extensive subterranean plumbing network are hot springs, where colorful thermophiles (heat-loving microorganisms, also known as extremophiles) and cyanobacteria (single-celled photosynthetic bacteria) thrive in pools of geothermally heated water. These springs are often linked to geysers (from the Icelandic word *geysir,* which means "to gush or rage"), where highly pressurized water rockets toward the surface and often flashes to steam. Fumaroles are dry, hissing vents that issue hydrogen sulfide (the source of that "rotten egg" odor), hydrochloric acid, and other gases. A solfatara is a sulfur-emitting fumarole. Mud pots (also known as paint pots when tinted by minerals) form in thermal areas where precipitation mixes with fine volcanic soils to create a bubbling, viscous—and often very acidic—slurry, sometimes forming mud volcanoes.

For hikers, this ancient ice sculpting and geothermal hyperactivity translates into many unusual geologic features to explore, including multilayered fossil forests, lava flows, dramatic U-shaped canyons, glacial boulder fields, and black mountains of obsidian. These varied and dramatic landscapes form numerous ecological niches that support an amazing diversity of wildlife and plants, many of them reachable only on foot.

Flora

Some 1,100 native species of flowering plants are found in Yellowstone alone, but only three species are endemic: the Yellowstone sand verbena, the Yellowstone sulfur wild buckwheat, and Ross's bentgrass. There are more than 200 nonnative species, some of which are starting to invade the backcountry. An additional 600 species of fungi, lichens, mosses, and liverworts have been cataloged. It's legal to collect small quantities of edible plants and berries for personal consumption, but keep it to a minimum to maintain your good bear karma.

Elevation has the most influence over which plant species flourish where. Though the vegetation varies significantly throughout the ecosystem, it's mostly typical of the Rocky Mountains. The observant hiker may notice elements of seven distinct biomes from the surrounding deserts, plains, montane forests, and arctic tundra.

Thanks to their shallow root systems, vast tracts of drought-tolerant lodgepole pines dominate the nutrient-poor, volcanic soils within the Yellowstone Caldera. In sharp contrast, the clayey glacial lake beds beyond the caldera encourage a much more diverse flora.

Botanists group Rocky Mountain vegetation into five zones: foothills, riparian, montane, subalpine, and alpine. These zones overlap considerably and are not strictly defined. The altitude and width of each zone increase progressively as you move from north to south. Fall colors peak around the autumnal equinox (third week in September) in the Tetons, a bit later on Yellowstone's relatively low-lying Northern Range.

Most of Yellowstone's lower-elevation hikes begin in sagebrush-blanketed foothills (5,500–6,500 feet). A prime example of this type of habitat is the arid Northern Range, where the annual precipitation hovers around 20 inches. The lower elevations here make the region a preferred spring and fall hiking destination. Unique species found here include cacti and Rocky Mountain juniper. In the absence of foothills in the Tetons, most trails begin near Jackson Hole and the Snake River Plain, where porous soils support sagebrush, grasses, and numerous wildflowers.

Riparian or wetland communities prosper near year-round streams. Typical moisture-loving plants in this zone include rushes; sedges; colorful deciduous trees such as cottonwoods; and shrubs such as willow, quaking aspen, dogwood, mountain ash, and Rocky Mountain maple. These lush but narrow areas are often home to rare, water-loving wildflowers and provide a transition between aquatic and upland steppe environments. North-facing slopes, which receive less sunlight and thus retain more moisture, are favored by most plants. Several rare aquatic plants thrive in Yellowstone's hydrothermal areas, such as the Shoshone Geyser Basin.

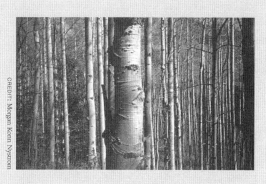

CREDIT: Morgan Konn Nystrom

Aspen grove *near Taggart Lake (Trail 35)*

Semiarid steppe vegetation is primarily scrubby and is dotted by lots of fragrant Big Mountain sagebrush, open woodlands, and more than a hundred species of sparse grasses. Prime, wildlife-rich examples of this habitat occur in Yellowstone's Hayden Valley, Pelican Valley, and Swan Lake Flats. Conspicuous blooms of wildflowers such as the pungent yellow arrowleaf balsamroot; snow-white, mat-forming phlox; flaming scarlet-orange Indian paintbrush; and pastel lupines and penstemons festoon hillsides in late June and early July.

Sagebrush-interspersed meadows mark the transition between rolling prairies and the forested montane zone (6,000–9,500 feet). Snow persists at higher elevations until July or August around the highest passes. The resulting short, cool growing season limits the number of plant species. Snowmelt on

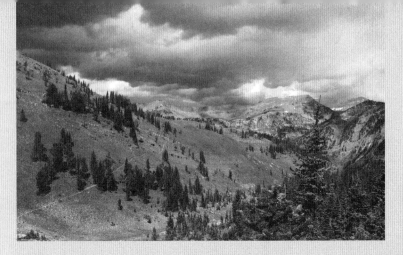

Subalpine habitat *below Rendezvous Mountain in the Teton Range (Trail 42)*

warmer, south-facing slopes waters hearty conifer (cone-bearing) species, such as Douglas-fir; Englemann spruce, which dominates older forests; and the higher-ranging subalpine fir. Shrubs and berries dominate the damp understory. If there is a prolonged absence of fire, spruce–fir forests should begin to succeed the currently dominant lodgepole stands.

Beyond the upper montane zone, the wild subalpine zone (7,500–10,000 feet) continues up to timberline. Isolated spruce–fir stands dominate where snow lingers longest. Short-lived wildflower displays can be fantastic after the spring snowmelt. At higher elevations, such as around Mount Washburn, the nuts of whitebark pine (which is sometimes confused with limber pine) are a favored but erratic source of prehibernation nutrition for ravenous grizzly bears.

Above timberline, the alpine zone (above 9,000–10,000 feet) is reserved for the most robust species of both plants and humans. The exposed meadows and rocky outcrops host bountiful but short-lived wildflower shows in late July and August. Wind-stunted Krummholz trees abide in sheltered areas of southern exposure. More than 200 plant species have been cataloged just beyond Yellowstone's Northeast Entrance on the untamed Beartooth Plateau, one of the largest swaths of alpine tundra in the Lower 48.

Fauna

Let's face it: geyser gazing and rambling around alpine peaks aside, a trip to Yellowstone and the Tetons isn't complete without spotting—and photographing—a root-grubbing bear with her cute yearling cub, a bugling eight-point elk, a drooling moose, or, at the very least, a wallowing bison.

Besides the iconic thermal features that earned Yellowstone its early nickname "Wonderland," the park's photogenic wildlife is the main draw for most visitors. Thanks to the successful wolf-reintroduction effort (see page 10), Greater Yellowstone now supports all of the 61 native mammal species it has historically hosted. With such an incredible concentration of charismatic megafauna, these parks are easily among the world's foremost wildlife-watching hot spots.

The comparison frequently drawn between Yellowstone's Lamar Valley and the Serengeti Plains in northern Tanzania isn't frivolous. Both parks grapple with similar issues: managing large, migrating wildlife herds, reducing the spread of disease, curbing invasive species, and coping with ranching and human development in their shrinking buffer zones.

If Greater Yellowstone has a totem species, it's the great grizzly bear (known as the brown bear, bruin, or Kodiak bear in Alaska). Yellowstone constitutes the heart of its range, which is estimated to have expanded by as much as 40% since 1975, when the 136 remaining animals in the region were listed as threatened under the Endangered Species Act. The rise in grizzly numbers has been a major conservation success story. Current estimates of the park's population hover around 150, with 717 bruins inhabiting the Greater Yellowstone region in 2016. The region in northwestern Montana around Glacier National Park (the Northern Continental Divide) harbors the only other major grizzly population in the Lower 48, with around 1,000 bears, though there are a handful of grizzlies in Montana's Cabinet-Yaak region and Washington's Cascade Mountains. That said, grizzlies currently occupy less than 4% of their original range, and numbers are down from a historical population of 50,000.

Since 2007, the U.S. Fish and Wildlife Service has been trying to delist the grizzly (remove it from the list of endangered species), claiming that the Yellowstone region has reached its capacity. The delisting process has been wrapped up

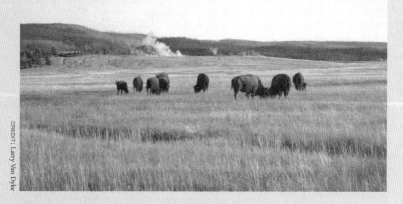

CREDIT: Larry Van Dyke

Bison *graze in Fountain Flats in the Midway Geyser Basin.*

in legal proceedings for the last decade, but the grizzly is expected to be delisted in 2017 and management passed to individual states, with the likelihood that grizzlies will then be hunted for sport in Montana, Wyoming, and Idaho (but not within Yellowstone or Grand Teton National Parks). Critics of delisting say that the long-term genetic health of the grizzly has not yet been secured because bear populations survive only in isolated pockets, separated from each other.

Besides poaching near park boundaries, current threats to grizzlies include a decline in cutthroat trout caused by the so-called whirling disease and illegally introduced lake trout, as well as the blister rust fungus and spread of bark beetles that have been decimating the supply of whitebark pine nuts, a prime source of late-season sustenance for grizzlies. Researchers have found that wolf reintroduction has actually increased the bears' food supply: since 2000, all wolf-killed ungulate (hooved mammal) carcasses in the Pelican Valley have ultimately been taken over by grizzlies.

Each year, most of the bear sightings typically reported in Yellowstone are in the vicinity of Tower–Roosevelt Junction. Other areas with frequent sightings include Bridge Bay, and from Fishing Bridge to Yellowstone's East Entrance. Less frequent sightings occur around dawn and dusk near Mammoth, on the north slopes of Mount Washburn, and in the Hayden and Lamar Valleys. In recent years, grizzly sightings have become more common than black bear sightings.

Yellowstone's abundant, omnivorous black bear, with an estimated population of 500–650, exists primarily in niches not filled by territorial grizzlies. Sightings (and resulting roadside "bear jams") are common around Tower

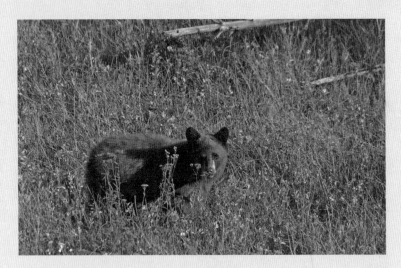

Black bear cubs *never stray far from their mothers.*

Bear Safety Guidelines

Restrictions in Yellowstone's 16 **Bear Management Areas** include seasonal closures, recommendations on minimum party size, and off-trail travel and camping prohibitions. Several trails in this book pass through these areas. No matter where you hike, it's always wise to take the following precautions:

- Ask at a ranger station or visitor center about recent bear activity before heading out.
- Do not travel alone or at night, when most bear feeding occurs. Parties of three or more are ideal.
- Stay alert for bear signs. Make noise and stay on marked trails; half of all attacks occur off-trail.
- Avoid carcasses, and do not carry smelly food.
- Never leave your pack unattended on the trail.
- Follow NPS guidelines for proper camping and food-storage techniques, as outlined in free hiking and backcountry camping brochures available at ranger stations and backcountry offices.
- Always carry bear spray, have it accessible at all times, and know how to use it. Reliable brands are Counter Assault and UDAP. You can't fly with bear spray, so buy it at outdoors stores in gateway towns or at visitor center bookstores. You can also rent bear spray by the day or week at a booth outside Canyon Visitor Center.
- Report any incidents to park rangers.

Even if you follow all of these guidelines, it's still quite possible that you will encounter a bear, especially if visiting the backcountry. If you see a bear before it sees you, keep out of sight and backtrack the way you came, or detour downwind as far as possible. There are various schools of thought about what to do in case of an encounter. Here's an executive summary of what the NPS recommends:

- Stay calm. Do not run or make sudden movements—you cannot outrun a bear!
- Back away slowly. Do not drop your pack.
- Talk quietly to the bear, do not shout. Avoid looking directly at the bear.
- Only climb a tree if it's nearby and you can climb at least 15–20 feet.

If you are charged, the NPS recommends standing still (easier said than done!) since most charges are bluff charges. If the bear makes physical contact, drop to the ground, face down with your hands behind your neck. In the case of a nighttime attack on a tent (these are extremely rare), you should fight back aggressively and use pepper spray.

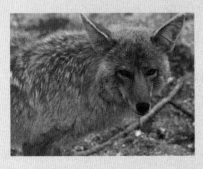

Coyote populations *have halved since wolves were reintroduced in 1995.*

and Mammoth. Despite their name, their coloration actually ranges from black to cinnamon. Both black bears and grizzlies start denning around mid-November, emerging from hibernation starting in April.

In both Yellowstone and Grand Teton, black bears have become quite pesky in seeking food from garbage cans, dumpsters, and campgrounds. However, the majority of bears you might see in the backcountry remain timid and are wary of humans. See the Bear Safety Guidelines on page 9 for advice on avoiding or managing encounters with bears and other wildlife.

In 1995, 31 Canadian gray wolves were reintroduced to Yellowstone, marking the beginning of an unprecedented effort to restore them to their historical range in the Northern Rockies. Wolves now live throughout Yellowstone and increasingly around the fringes of Grand Teton. In the initial phase of the reintroduction, wolf numbers grew rapidly to around 170, but numbers have since leveled off to around 100 inside Yellowstone, in 10 shifting packs. It is estimated that there are 500 of the primo predators in 50 packs in Greater Yellowstone, with 1,700 individuals in 282 packs (including 95 breeding pairs) in the whole of Montana, Idaho, and Wyoming.

Since 2008, battles have raged in the courts over plans to remove the gray wolf's endangered-species status. Since 2011, control of wolf numbers has shifted to state authorities in Montana and Idaho, where several hundred wolves a year are now killed by hunters. Wolves once again enjoy federal protection in Wyoming, but several of Yellowstone National Park's most iconic wolves were killed outside the park when the species was temporarily delisted in Wyoming between 2012 and 2014.

Outside of sunny winter days, the best times to spot wolves are at dawn and dusk. The most reliable method of finding them? Scan roadside turnouts for an array of high-powered binoculars and spotting scopes, telephoto lenses mounted on camouflage tripods, and CB radio antennas on the roofs of expedition-equipped four-wheel-drive vehicles. Then stop and ask if you can take a look; devoted wolf-watchers are usually quite happy to share their knowledge and passion with passersby.

The highly adaptable, omnivorous coyote is often seen loping across meadows, fields, and other open grasslands. The coyote population has decreased by as much as 50% in Yellowstone since wolf reintroduction, which has been

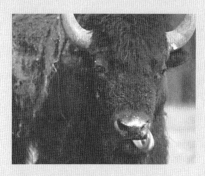

Stay clear *of bull bison like this fellow in Pelican Valley (Trail 23)*

shown conclusively to have relegated coyotes to a scavenger role. However, the nighttime chorus of yelps (sometimes mistaken for wolf howls) still reverberates through backcountry campsites.

Estimates of the numbers of the seven species of native ungulates vary as widely as the large animals' migratory range. Counts of Yellowstone's bugling Rocky Mountain elk (also known as wapiti) vary seasonally from 10,000 to 20,000 in summer to 5,000 in winter, in seven distinct herds. Over 100,000 elk inhabit Greater Yellowstone. In summer, you can hardly toss a bison chip without hitting a member of the largest elk herd in North America: look around Gibbon Meadows or the Lamar Valley. During the autumn rut (mating season), elk take over the lawns around Mammoth Hot Springs and flock to meadows around Norris Geyser Basin. In Jackson Hole, Timbered Island becomes a no-go zone during the rut. In winter, they migrate south to the National Elk Refuge, or north and east to Gardiner and West Yellowstone, where hunters await just beyond the park boundaries.

Yellowstone's population of persistent bison (often used interchangeably with buffalo), the largest land animal in North America, is estimated at between 2,300 and 5,000. Watch year-round for what remains of the United States' largest free-roaming herd in the Hayden and Lamar Valleys, in summer in open meadows and grasslands, and in winter in thermal areas and along the Madison River. In Grand Teton, smaller herds roam the sagelands around Mormon Row. In 2016, President Obama signed legislation designating the bison as the national mammal of the United States.

Common, floppy-eared mule deer prefer open forests and grassy meadows, where they munch on leaves, shrubs, and sedges. Watch for them browsing around dusk near forest edges. The furtive, less common white-tailed deer is only occasionally spotted near waterways in Yellowstone's Northern Range.

A declining population of moody, drooling moose lurk in willow thickets in riparian zones, mainly in marshy meadows, near lakeshores, and along rivers. In Yellowstone, they are most frequently seen browsing in the Bechler region and in the Soda Butte Creek, Pelican Creek, Lewis River, and Gallatin River drainages. They are more common in Grand Teton, wherever willows colonize marshes and ponds. Appearances are deceptive: they are superb swimmers and can—and will—charge at up to 35 miles per hour, so give them wide berth.

A population of 350–400 fleet-footed pronghorn are more closely related to goats and are not true antelopes. They are found in summer in sage flats and grasslands in the Lamar Valley, in Jackson Hole, and near Yellowstone's North Entrance. Their numbers declined by 50% in Yellowstone between 1991 and 1995; for context, the pre-European American settlement population is estimated at 35 million. The population has since stabilized, but large-scale energy developments outside Grand Teton jeopardize their long-distance winter migration routes around the park.

Numbering up to 300, Rocky Mountain bighorn sheep are often spotted scampering along cliffs and roaming Yellowstone's alpine meadows. In summer, they are most easily found on the slopes of Mount Washburn, and year-round in Gardner Canyon between Mammoth and the North Entrance. Also watch for their silhouettes on cliff tops along the Yellowstone River, and above Soda Butte in the Lamar Valley.

Invasive, nonnative mountain goats are increasingly common and thought to be colonizing rocky slopes in Yellowstone's northern reaches.

The population of the seldom-seen American cougar (also known as the mountain lion) is estimated at 26–42, making it Yellowstone's most common cat species. Primarily nocturnal, cougars have been called "the ghosts of the Rockies."

The similarly nocturnal and reclusive bobcat is poorly studied but thought to be widespread. You're more likely to hear its bloodcurdling scream at night while snuggled inside your sleeping bag than to see it from the trail. Most reports are from the northern half of Yellowstone in sagebrush and conifer forests.

Other common small mammals include the wily, weasellike marten, found in coniferous forests; the playful river otter, found in rivers, lakes, and ponds; and two species of weasel (also known as ermine), widespread in both willows and spruce–fir forests. Beavers dam watercourses and cobble together lodges adjacent to trails in both parks.

Animals rarely seen by hikers include the sagebrush-loving badger and the red fox, found in the Lamar Valley and around Canyon Village at the edges of forest and sagelands. A recent three-year study confirmed the presence and reproduction of the wide-ranging Canadian lynx, which hides out in remote subalpine forests, on Yellowstone's eastern flank. Other rare mammals include the relatively scarce raccoon; the carnivorous, forest-dwelling fisher; the weasel-like mink, occasionally seen in riparian forests; the striped skunk, seen flitting between the forest and riparian zones; and the fierce, elusive wolverine, the largest land member of the weasel family. Researchers live-trapped and released a wolverine in March 2006 just north of Yellowstone park—pretty impressive given the animal's 350- to 500-mile range.

Three territorial species of chipmunk are common in conifer forests. Four squirrel species are common around rocky outcroppings in forests. The yellow-bellied marmot is commonly seen, or at least its high-pitched whistle is heard, where trails traverse rocky slopes. The bleating, round-eared pika is also common in this kind of landscape. Other rodents often spotted scurrying about the forest understory include gophers, mice, several species of voles, shrews, muskrats, bushy-tailed wood rats, and porcupines.

At last count, 322 bird species were winging around the skies above Greater Yellowstone, with 148 of those observed nesting. Early morning in spring (from mid-May through early July) is the best time for birding. While hiking around lakes and waterways, keep your eyes peeled for big raptors such as the threatened but recovering bald eagle and trout-loving osprey swooping around hunting for prey. Majestic but imperiled trumpeter swans range between Montana's Paradise Valley and the Madison River. The reintroduced peregrine falcon, which preys on songbirds and waterfowl, nests in Yellowstone and is well on its way to recovery but is rarely seen.

Other common species that exhibit entertaining antics include the boisterous Clark's nutcracker, the diminutive mountain chickadee, the mountain bluebird, and Steller's jay, a bold scavenger. Other monitored species of special concern include the American white pelican, common loon, harlequin duck, osprey, colonial nesting bird, and great gray owl.

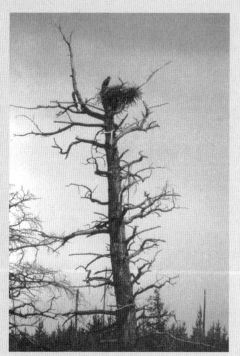

Bald eagle nest: *Eagles are often found fishing for trout around Heart Lake (Trail 22).*

Yellowstone contains one of the most significant aquatic ecosystems in the United States. It's home to 16 fish species: 11 native and 5 nonnative. Since 2001, regulations have required the release of all native sport fishes hooked in park waters. The fishing season runs from Memorial Day weekend through the first Sunday of November.

The three subspecies of native cutthroat trout are an essential but increasingly threatened source of grizzly sustenance. They are being eaten out of house and home by the proliferation of illegally introduced, nonnative lake trout, also known as mackinaws. Other native sport fish are the rare, protected Arctic grayling and the slender, silver mountain whitefish. Introduced sport fish include brook trout, brown trout, rainbow trout, and lake chub.

Six species of reptiles (prairie rattlesnake, bull snake, valley garter snake, wandering garter snake, rubber boa, and sagebrush lizard) and four decreasingly common species of amphibians (boreal toad, chorus frog, spotted frog, and tiger salamander) are found in Yellowstone. Encountering a poisonous prairie rattlesnake in Yellowstone's low-lying Northern Range is unlikely but possible.

More than 12,000 insects, including 128 species of butterflies, provide fodder for many quick-tongued predators. Of greatest concern to hikers are mosquitoes (see Trail Safety, page 19).

When to Go

As two of North America's most popular summer destinations, both parks have the unfortunate reputation of being overcrowded, especially Yellowstone. This certainly can be true on major holiday weekends, on heavily trafficked roads, and at campgrounds and must-see attractions, but solitude is not hard to come by—if you know where to look.

Both parks are four-season recreation destinations. Less than 5% of Yellowstone's visitors arrive between November and April. Likewise, in Grand Teton 80% of visitors arrive between June and September. Annual Yellowstone visitor numbers have risen noticeably in the past 15 years to almost 4 million (most coming via the West Entrance), while Grand Teton averages around 3 million.

Thankfully, even in summer, escaping the crowds is reasonably easy, especially in Yellowstone. To find solitude, head for the backcountry. Surveys by the Park Service found that less than 1.5% of visitors apply for a backcountry permit in Yellowstone; only half of 1% do so in Grand Teton.

To avoid crowds, especially in the frontcountry, the usual rules of thumb apply: visit midweek instead of on weekends, and during spring and fall shoulder periods. Some of the finest hiking conditions coincide with diminishing crowds after Labor Day weekend and the peak of fall-foliage colors. The last week of August is a good time to come, for its combination of summer weather and slightly lighter crowds.

Accommodation in Yellowstone is a different matter. During the peak months of July and August you need to have booked your park accommodation at least six months in advance (some rooms sell out a year in advance). Even the reservable Xanterra campsites are often booked up a month in advance in summer. Unreservable park campgrounds are generally full by noon, with many campgrounds full by 9 a.m. Reservations are essential in Yellowstone. There's more room to move in Grand Teton, since most of the campgrounds are nonreservable, but you'd be wise to book RV sites in advance and make your lodge reservations at least six months ahead.

Weather and Seasons

Throughout Greater Yellowstone, conversations (and tall tales told by the fireplace over a posthike pint) are peppered with anecdotes about the region's famously mercurial weather. Snowfall has been recorded every single day of the year here, so the best advice is to always come prepared for the possibility of extreme conditions and four seasons in a single day. Locals claim there are nine months of winter and three months of relatives. This isn't that far from the truth. Perhaps the most reliable climate-related axiom is, "If you don't like the weather, just wait five minutes." In any case, on any given day, Yellowstone is often the coldest spot on a US weather map.

Always be ready for afternoon thundershowers (locally called "rollers") and to beat a hasty retreat from the higher elevations when lightning threatens. Because conditions on the trails change as quickly as the weather, it's best to check in with a ranger station before hitting the trail, even if you're only going for a day hike.

Given the right disposition, conditions, and over-snow travel gear, winter can be the ideal season to explore the parks in relative tranquility. During winter, the mercury hovers around 0°F during the short daylight hours, with occasional highs in the 20s. Subzero overnight lows are the norm. Infrequent warm "chinook" winds push daytime highs into the 40s. Annual snowfall averages 150 inches in most of Yellowstone, with 200 to 400 inches routinely recorded at higher elevations.

Yellowstone's winter tourism plan has been in flux for the last decade, as the park tries to balance the demands of local communities while limiting the number of snowmobiles through the park each day. As of winter 2016–2017, Yellowstone National Park allows a maximum of 110 daily "transportation events" (defined as one snow coach or group of snowmobiles) to enter the park. Only half of these "events" can be snowmobiles. The plan also allows one noncommercially guided group of up to five snowmobiles to enter through each park entrance every day. Noncommercial guides must get a noncommercial snowmobile access permit, which is awarded by lottery at recreation.gov starting September 1. Leftover permits are available on a first-come, first-served basis starting in November. Permits cost $40 per day, plus a $6 application fee. Each snowmobile driver must have completed a free online certification training course. Snowmobilers can drive their own machines or rent them at park gateway towns, as long as they meet or exceed available technology standards. In addition, a dozen operators offer increasingly popular guided tours by snow

Yellowstone and Grand Teton National Parks Spring Bicycling Period

Weather permitting (after the winter snowmobiling season ends in mid- to late March and before the park opens to wheeled vehicles, typically the third Friday in April), there's a glorious opportunity for bicyclists, hikers, joggers, in-line skaters, roller skiers, and the like to explore Yellowstone between the West Entrance and Mammoth Hot Springs, via the nearly auto-free **Grand Loop Road.** Call 307-344-2109 to confirm the **Spring Bicycling Period** schedule. There's no in-park lodging open (Mammoth Campground is open year-round, or you can stay in nearby gateway towns). The 6 miles between the East Entrance and the east end of Sylvan Pass and the South Entrance road to West Thumb Junction also some- times has limited access. The road from Madison Junction to Old Faithful typically does not open.

In Grand Teton, the beautiful 15-mile section of Teton Park Road between Taggart Lake Parking Area and Signal Mountain Lodge is similarly open to nonmotorized use in the month of April.

coach (vehicles such as vans or buses that have been adapted to travel over snow). Skiers and snowshoers don't need a guide, and the parks have many groomed and ungroomed trails to choose from.

Though February sees some frosty but crystal-clear days of sunshine, snow blankets most of both parks well after the vernal equinox (March 21). The appearance of migrating mountain bluebirds and the emergence of Uinta ground squirrels are reliable indicators of the arrival of spring, usually in the second half of March. Depending on snow conditions, nonmotorized explora- tion (including hiking, bicycling, jogging, in-line skates, and roller skis) is per- mitted in Yellowstone between the West Entrance and Mammoth Hot Springs from mid-March through the third week in April.

The spring hiking season begins as snow starts to melt from the lowest-lying trails (as early as May on Yellowstone's Northern Range, a bit later around Jackson Hole) and after trail maintenance crews clear winter deadfall. Early-season hiking coincides with the reemergence of ravenous bears and their newborn cubs from their dens as they prowl for elk calves. Many of the Yellowstone trails that pass through Bear Management Areas are off-limits from May into June. Hiking can be superb before crowds begin to arrive for Memorial Day, when both parks are a hive of calving, nesting, spawning, and blooming activity. River fords are most

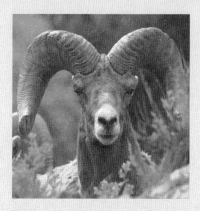

Mature bighorn rams *with horns in full curl are often seen around Bunsen Peak (Trail 3).*

dangerous in May and June, when snowmelt-fed waterfalls are also the most spectacular. Daytime temperatures average in the 40s and 50s in May. By June they reach the 60s and 70s, but nighttime lows still occasionally dip below freezing. The most precipitation (an average of around 2 inches per month) falls during May and the "June monsoon."

The prime summer hiking and backpacking season starts as the snow line progressively retreats up mountainsides until the highest passes are clear—typically by late July in Yellowstone, and early August around the highest Teton passes. Elk and bison continue to drop calves until the summer solstice (June 21), the longest day of the year. The opening of Yellowstone's fishing season (the first Saturday of Memorial Day weekend) coincides with the start of the stonefly hatch—when mosquitoes and biting flies really hit their stride. Wildflower-watching heats up soon after snowmelt and peaks around mid-July in most of Yellowstone, a bit later at higher elevations and in the Tetons. Midsummer, daytime temperatures are typically in the 70s (and 80s at lower elevations). Nights remain cool, in the 40s and 30s, with the odd frosty spell.

The courting and mating season (the rut) begins as early as late July. During this period, it's especially important to give elk and bison a wide berth on trails. Mosquitoes and other biting pests finally die down in August; that's also when berries are ripe for the picking in riparian zones. July and August are the driest months, but afternoon showers are still fairly common. Blooming goldenrod and gentians are reliable indicators of the coming of autumn.

Fall colors start to appear in the riparian zone by mid-August and peak around the autumnal equinox (September 21), with slight variations according to elevation. Vibrant yellows, reds, and oranges persist on Yellowstone's Northern Range until early October, when the first significant snowfall usually occurs. Temperatures can remain surprisingly pleasant through October, but nighttime lows often plunge into the teens. Squirrels, chipmunks, and other rodents frantically preparing winter seed caches are a sure sign of another impending long winter.

Trail Selection

Three criteria were used in selecting trails for this guide. Only the premier day hikes and overnight backpacking trips are included, based on beautiful scenery, ease of access, and diversity of experience. Many of the trails are very popular, while several others see infrequent use. If you are fortunate enough to be able to complete all the trips in this book, you will gain a comprehensive appreciation for the complex beauty of one of the world's most scenic and intact temperate-zone ecosystems.

Nearly half of the trails included in this guide are out-and-back trips, requiring you to retrace your steps back to the trailhead. Forty percent of the routes are full or partial loop trips, with the remaining six routes being point-to-point trips that are worthy of the required vehicle shuttle. For these, you'll have to travel with friends or family who don't mind picking you up at the end of the day, or arrange a commercial shuttle service for longer trips. It's fairly common for people to hitchhike short distances through the parks to get to the trailhead before hiking back to their car.

Key Features

Top Trails books contain information about the features of each trail. Yellowstone and the Tetons are blessed with diverse terrain—no matter what your interests, you're sure to find a trail to match them.

Water lovers and anglers will find plenty of pristine lakes, rivers, and streams, while peak-baggers will be spoiled by the choice of world-class alpine panoramas. The abundant open meadows are graced with riotous wildflower displays, and aspen groves provide plenty of fall color. All these features combine to make Greater Yellowstone a photographer's paradise. With a bit of planning, the opportunities for camping, fishing, boating, swimming, and wildlife-watching are endless.

Multiple Uses

All the trails described in this guide are suitable for hiking. Although all the trails are equally legal for jogging, the vast majority are not suited for it, as running can incite predatory behavior in some wildlife. The only exceptions are the few gravel and paved roads in more developed areas that also allow bicycling, notably the road to Lone Geyser in Yellowstone. Where applicable, trail descriptions note where routes receive heavy stock use by horse packers and llama outfitters. Kayaking and canoeing are increasingly popular ways to reach some of both parks' more secluded backcountry campsites—for example, Shoshone Lake in Yellowstone and Leigh Lake in Grand Teton. Fishing is superb in both parks too. As in most national parks, pets and mountain biking are prohibited. Winter use is limited but growing in both parks, with cross-country skiing, snowshoeing, and snow-coach tours becoming more popular as snowmobiling is increasingly restricted.

Trail Safety

Dramatic elevation changes pose a possible danger to visitors arriving from near sea level. Signs of altitude sickness include headache, fatigue, loss of appetite, shortness of breath, nausea, vomiting, drowsiness, dizziness, memory loss, and diminished mental acuity. A rapid descent generally alleviates any symptoms. The best advice is to eat lots of carbohydrates prior to the trip, acclimatize slowly, avoid alcohol and heavy foods, and drink plenty of fluids.

Burns from thermal features are a common cause of death and serious injury in Yellowstone. Follow posted regulations about off-trail travel, don't traverse thermal areas after dark, and don't bathe in thermal waters that aren't National Park Service–approved (see "Bathers Beware" on page 20).

Ticks are a nuisance from mid-March through mid-July in the lowest-lying areas. Wear insect repellent, tuck your shirt and pant legs in, and check your body often. Depending on elevation and the rate at which the previous winter's snowpack melts, the peak of the mosquito season hits the backcountry in June and July and abates in mid-August. Repellent, netting, and protective clothing are your best forms of protection.

Most of Yellowstone's backcountry river crossings intentionally lack bridges, and many fords are dangerous (over thigh-deep) until at least July. Check current conditions during trip planning, and when in doubt, pick another route, or turn back.

Dehydration is a concern on longer trails where water is lacking. The presence of *Giardia* means that all water should be boiled, filtered, or otherwise treated before drinking. Keep your hands clean to avoid transmitting nasty microbes to your hiking companions.

Sunburn is a concern, especially at higher altitudes. Sun protection, sunglasses, and a good wide-brimmed hat are essential. Due to the possibility of rapid weather changes, hypothermia is a concern year-round. Most hypothermia cases happen when air temperatures are between 30°F and 50°F. Always check the weather forecast before heading out, and carry extra warm and waterproof gear. It's not uncommon to experience four seasons during a midsummer hike.

Cell phone coverage is sketchy at best throughout both parks, though it has improved greatly in recent years and is available at most junctions in Yellowstone. In general Verizon offers the best coverage. That said, you

Bathers Beware

Soaking directly in thermal waters is not officially allowed in Yellowstone, so as to protect both bathers' skin and the park's unique thermophilic microbiological resources. Swimming *is* allowed in a few places where thermal runoff mixes with cold-water sources, such as the Boiling River (Trail 2, page 45) and the Firehole River Canyon near Madison Junction.

In 2016 a parasitic amoeba was found in Kelly Warm Springs and Huckleberry and Polecat Springs in Grand Teton National Park. Dubbed the "brain-eating bacteria," the amoeba can enter the body through nasal cavities and cause fatal meningitis-like symptoms. The park has closed all springs to the public.

See page 49 for the full list of our favorite Greater Yellowstone hot springs where soaking is allowed.

---

should not count on your phone as a reliable means of communication in an emergency, especially in the backcountry.

Free Wi-Fi is available in Yellowstone at Mammoth's Albright Visitor Center and in Grand Teton at Craig Thomas Visitor Center in Moose, Colter Bay Village, Signal Mountain gas station, Jenny Lake Lodge, and Jackson Lake Lodge. Paid Wi-Fi is available ($5 per hour) at several of Yellowstone's lodges, including the Old Faithful Snow Lodge, Lake Hotel, Grant Village lodges, and Canyon bar.

Park Entrance Fees

The park entrance fee ($30 per car, $25 per motorcycle/snowmobile, $15 per hiker or bicyclist) is valid for seven days' admission to either Yellowstone or Grand Teton National Park. A seven-day pass to both parks is also available ($50 per car, $40 per motorcycle, $20 per hiker or bicyclist). The annual National Parks & Federal Recreational Lands Pass ($80, $10 for US citizens ages 62 and older, free with proof of permanent disability) grants entrance to federal recreation sites for one year from the date of purchase. Yearlong, park-specific passes ($60) allow entrance to a single park, so you are better off with a federal pass if visiting both parks.

Camping

Myriad camping opportunities exist throughout the Greater Yellowstone region. The challenge can be securing a spot, as the most popular campgrounds fill to capacity early in the day during the summer, especially on weekends. Where available, reservations are strongly advised between Memorial Day and Labor Day weekends.

In Yellowstone, the National Park Service runs seven first-come, first-served campgrounds ($15–$20 per night). Call 307-344-2114 for details. The concessionaire Xanterra manages four reservable campgrounds ($23.50–$28 plus tax per night) and the Fishing Bridge RV Park ($50 plus tax), which can be booked online. Call 307-344-7311 or visit yellowstonenationalparklodges. com for details. With the exception of Slough Creek, all campgrounds have a few first-come, first-served hiker/biker sites ($4), which camp hosts might offer to car campers late in the day. The National Park Service sites are much smaller and less developed, most with basic vault toilets and prohibitions against generators. The more developed sites allow generators and have flush toilets, dump stations, and showers and laundry nearby. Campgrounds at Canyon and Grant Villages include two hot showers in their site fees. There is a 14-day limit on camping June 15–September 15 everywhere except Fishing Bridge, and a 30-day limit the rest of the year.

In Grand Teton, there are five first-come, first-served frontcountry campgrounds ($24–$25 per night) with hiker/biker sites ($10–$11 per night). There are also concessionaire-operated "trailer villages" (reservable RV parks with showers, laundry, and full hookups) at Colter Bay Village and at Flagg Ranch, between Grand Teton and Yellowstone. Download the Backcountry Trip Planner at tinyurl.com/yellowstonebackcountry for details on current reservation procedures.

Beyond these two parks, plenty of private campgrounds afford ample opportunity for primitive and dispersed camping in the nearby national forests and wilderness areas.

Signs at the entrances to both parks will tell you which campgrounds have spaces. Check nps.gov/yell/planyourvisit/campgrounds.htm for live information on which campgrounds are open and at what time they filled, and plan your arrival accordingly. For Grand Teton campground status, visit gtlc.com /camping.

Backcountry Permits

Permits are required for all overnight stays in the backcountry of Yellowstone and Grand Teton. Backpackers can stay only in fixed campsites in the backcountry. Fees are also charged for mandatory boating and fishing permits. Permits are not required for day hikes in either park.

In Yellowstone, advance reservations for the more than 300 backcountry campsites are accepted (for a $25 fee) only by mail or fax or in person, starting April 1. Fortunately, several backcountry sites in each area of the park

Family-Friendly Overnight Backpacking Favorites

Yellowstone has more easily accessible family-friendly backcountry overnight camping options, thanks to sheer size and topography, but Grand Teton has its fair share of alluring options—if you can score a reservation. Here are our personal favorites; advance reservations are highly recommended for all these sites.

Only 1.7 flat miles from the trailhead, campsite OD1 en route to **Fairy Falls** (Trail 28, page 226) is tucked away off the main trail in a mature stand of lodgepole pines that survived the 1988 fires. Drawbacks include no easy water access and little shade, but it's only a mile from Fairy Falls, and you can even bicycle the first mile from the trailhead. Nearby site OD5 at **Goose Lake** is even more accessible as a disabled-access site. Rangers release the site to the able-bodied public after 4 p.m. on the day of use.

Just under 3 miles from the trailhead near **Lone Star Geyser** (Trail 29, page 233), campsite OA1 also includes the option to cycle the majority of the way to a pleasant overnight setting. To avoid the possibility of sharing the site with stock parties, you can head nearly 0.5 mile farther along the lovely Upper Firehole River to hiker-only campsite OA2.

If you're really looking to escape the frontcountry hubbub and see what Yellowstone looked like before the 1988 fires, head for

are left open for in-person reservations, which can be made not more than 48 hours before the first date of the trip. For a full rundown of the extensive regulations, contact Yellowstone's Backcountry Office at 307-344-2160 to request a free Backcountry Trip Planner, or download a copy at tinyurl.com /yellowstonebackcountry.

Backcountry Use Permits are available at most ranger stations and dedicated backcountry offices. Permits cost $3 per person per night, up to a maximum fee of $25 per year. Popular backcountry sites at Heart Lake, the Black Canyon of the Yellowstone, and Shoshone Lake book up quickly, so make reservations or come with a flexible itinerary. You will need to watch a video on backcountry safety. Part of your permit goes in the car you park at the trailhead, while the main permit goes with you in your pack or on your tent. Contact the main backcountry office and consult the Backcountry Trip Planner (see above) for updates.

In Yellowstone, trailheads are sometimes referred to on maps (and in this book, where applicable) by an alphanumeric naming system, such as "Lone

Cascade Corner and Bechler Meadows. Boy Scout troops have long recognized the beauty of the region, so you won't be alone, but you will be surrounded by beautiful, lush country at hiker-only campsite 9B1, 3.4 flat miles from the trailhead. This route gets you into the heart of the wildlife-rich meadows while avoiding tricky stream crossings. If your family is up for a longer two-night loop, equally appealing campsite 9C1 is only 0.5 mile farther along.

In Grand Teton, a series of three campsites fronting the east shore of **Leigh Lake** (Trail 40, page 311) is about 3 flat miles in from the String Lake Picnic Area trailhead. Swimming is a joy after the water temperatures rise a bit in July, and boating is popular.

The **Hermitage Point Loop** (Trail 37, page 293) features Grand Teton's next most accessible, low-elevation backcountry campsite. It's 4.5 nearly flat miles from the trailhead in Colter Bay via the most direct route, or 4.9 miles via a more scenic route heading west along the lakeshore, for a total of 9.4 miles for the full loop. It can get windy, but the Teton views are fantastic. It's technically a group site, but rangers at Colter Bay will book it for nongroups.

Unfortunately, the campsite fronting the north shore of **Bradley Lake** (Trail 35, page 281) is available only to backpackers doing multiday loop trips. Nearby, the rustic bunks at the Grand Teton Climbers' Ranch (see page 276) could be a fun way to rough it without fully camping out.

Star (OK1)"; a complete list of these trailhead names appears in the Backcountry Trip Planner.

Grand Teton has a similar backcountry permit system but has fewer specific numbered sites, using instead camping zones in the alpine canyons, where backpackers can choose a site within their designated zone. One-third of sites can be reserved January 1–May 15 by mail or fax, or online in real time at recreation.gov. The remaining sites are available to walk-ins no more than a day in advance. Permits cost $25 each ($35 for an advance reservation), regardless of the number of people or nights. You must pick up your permit by 10 a.m. on the day of departure. Backcountry offices at both Yellowstone and Grand Teton accept debit and credit cards, as well as cash.

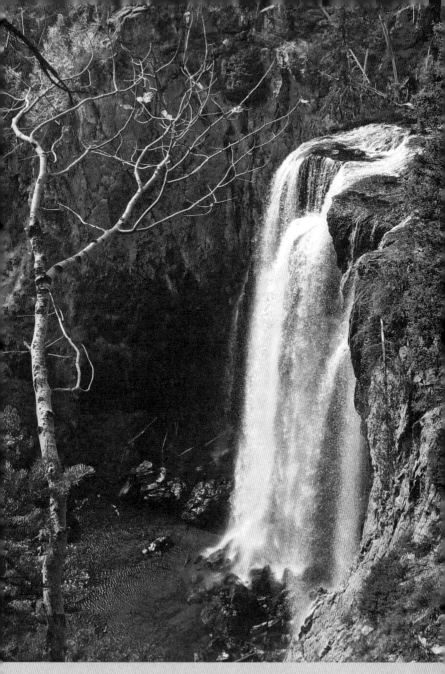

Dunanda Falls (*Trail 27*)

CREDIT: Bradley Mayhew

On the Trail

Every outing should begin with proper preparation, which usually takes only a few minutes. Even the easiest trail can turn up unexpected surprises. People seldom think about getting lost or injured, but unexpected things can and do happen. Simple precautions can make the difference between a good story and a miserable outcome.

Use the Top Trails ratings and descriptions to determine if a particular trail is a good match with your fitness and energy level, given current conditions and time of year.

Have a Plan

Choose Wisely The first step to enjoying any trail, no matter the activity or the degree of difficulty, is to match the trail to your abilities. It's no use overestimating your fitness or experience—know your abilities and limitations, and use the Top Trails difficulty rating that accompanies each trail.

Leave Word About Your Plans The most basic of precautions is leaving word of your intentions with friends or family. Many people will hike the backcountry their entire lives without ever relying on this safety net, but establishing this simple habit is free insurance.

It's best to leave specific information—location, trail name, intended time of travel—with a responsible person. However, if this is not possible or if plans change at the last minute, you should still leave word. If there is a registration process available, use it. If there is a ranger station, trail register, or visitor center, check in.

Prepare and Plan

- Know your abilities and your limitations.
- Leave word about your plans.
- Know the area and the route.

Review the Route Before embarking on any hike, read the entire description, and study the map. It isn't necessary to memorize every detail, but it is worthwhile to have a clear mental picture of the trail and general area.

If the trail or terrain is complex, augment the trail guide with a topographic map. Maps and current weather and trail-condition information are available from local ranger stations and backcountry offices, so use these resources (see Appendix, page 348).

Carry the Essentials

Proper preparation for any type of trail use includes gathering the essential items you will carry. The checklist will vary tremendously by trail and conditions.

Clothing When the weather is good, light, comfortable clothes are the obvious choice. It's easy to believe that little in the way of spare clothing is needed, but a prepared hiker has something tucked away for the unexpected, ranging from a surprise shower to an emergency overnight in more remote areas.

Clothing includes proper footwear—essential for hiking and backpacking. Running shoes are fine for shorter trails, but if you will be carrying substantial weight or encountering sustained rugged terrain, step up to hiking boots.

In hot, sunny weather, proper clothing includes a hat, sunglasses, a long-sleeved shirt, and sunscreen. In cooler weather, particularly when it's wet, carry waterproof outer garments and quick-drying undergarments (avoid cotton). As a general rule, whatever the conditions, bring layers that can be combined or removed to provide comfort and protection from the elements in a wide and unpredictable variety of conditions.

Water Never set out on a trail without water. At all times, but particularly in warm weather, adequate water is of key importance. Experts recommend at least 2 quarts of water per day. When hiking in heat, a gallon or more may be appropriate. At the extreme, dehydration can be life-threatening. More commonly, inadequate water causes fatigue and muscle aches.

For most outings, unless the day is very hot or the trail very long, you should plan to carry sufficient water for the entire trail. Unfortunately in North America, natural water sources are questionable, often contaminated with bacteria, viruses, and fertilizers.

Trail Essentials

- Dress to keep cool, but be ready for cold.
- Carry plenty of water.
- Have adequate food (plus a little extra).

Water Treatment If you have to use trailside water, you should filter or treat it. There are three methods: boiling, chemical treatment, and filtering. Boiling is best, but it's often impractical because it requires a heat source, a pot, and time. Chemical treatments, readily available in outdoor stores, handle some problems—including the troublesome *Giardia* parasite—but they will not combat many of the chemical pollutants. The preferred method is filtration. A good filter system removes *Giardia* and other contaminants and doesn't leave any unpleasant aftertaste.

If this hasn't convinced you to carry all the water you need, one final admonishment: Be prepared for surprises. Water sources described in the text and shown on maps can change course or dry up completely, especially in late summer. Never run your water bottle dry in expectation of the next source; fill up when water is available, and always keep a little in reserve.

Food While not as critical as water, food is energy and should not be under-emphasized. Avoid foods that are hard to digest, such as sugary candy bars and fatty potato chips. Carry high-energy, fast-digesting foods, such as nutrition bars, dried fruit, jerky, and trail mix. Bring a little extra food—it's good protection against an outing that turns unexpectedly long, perhaps due to foul weather or losing your way.

Optional Items

Map and Compass (and the know-how to use them) Many trails don't require much navigation, so a map and compass aren't always as essential as water or food—but it's a close call. If the trail is remote or infrequently visited, a map and compass are necessities.

A handheld GPS (global positioning system) receiver can also be a useful trail companion, but it's no substitute for a map and compass; knowing your longitude and latitude is not much help without a map.

Cell Phone Most parts of the country, even remote destinations, have some level of cellular coverage, but service is sketchy at best in much of Yellowstone and the Tetons. In extreme circumstances, a cell phone can be a lifesaver, but don't depend on it; even where available, coverage is unpredictable, and batteries fail. And be sure that the occasion warrants the phone call—a blister doesn't justify a call to search and rescue. Smartphones can be useful for hiking; you can load maps, route notes, and photos and use the inbuilt GPS to track your route.

Emergency Kit We never hit the trails without carrying the following: sunscreen, hat, sunglasses, blister kit, bear spray, toilet paper, matches or lighter, water bottle and water-purification method, trekking poles, whistle, rain jacket, and emergency snacks.

Gear Depending on the remoteness and rigor of the trail, there are many additional useful items to consider: pocketknife, flashlight, fire source (waterproof matches, lighter, or flint), and first-aid kit.

Every member of your party should carry the appropriate items described above; groups often split up or get separated along the trail. Solo hikers should be even more disciplined about preparation and carry more gear. Traveling solo is inherently more risky. This isn't meant to discourage solo travel but simply to emphasize the need for extra preparation. Solo hikers should make a habit of carrying a little more gear than is absolutely necessary.

Trail Etiquette

The overriding rule on the trail is "Leave No Trace." Interest in visiting natural areas continues to increase in North America, even as the quantity of unspoiled wilderness shrinks. These pressures make it ever more critical that we leave no trace of our visits.

Never Litter If you carried it in, it's just as easy to carry it out. Leave the trail in the same, if not better, condition than you found it. Try picking up any litter you encounter and packing it out—it's a great feeling. Just one piece of garbage and you've made a difference.

Stay on the Trail Paths have been created, sometimes over many years, for several purposes: to protect the surrounding natural areas, to avoid dangers, and to provide the best route. Leaving the trail can cause damage that takes years to undo. Never cut switchbacks. Shortcutting rarely saves time or energy, and it takes a terrible toll on the land, trampling plant life and hastening erosion. Moreover, safety and consideration intersect on the trail. It's hard to get truly lost if you stay on the trail.

Share the Trail The best trails attract many visitors, and you should be prepared to share the trail with others. Do your part to minimize impact. Commonly accepted trail etiquette dictates that bike riders yield to both hikers and equestrians, hikers yield to horseback riders, downhill hikers yield to

Trail Etiquette

- Leave no trace—never litter.
- Stay on the trail—never cut switchbacks.
- Share the trail—use courtesy and common sense.
- Leave it there—don't disturb plants or wildlife.

Top-Rated Trails

Northwest Yellowstone: Mammoth/Gallatin Country

Northeast Yellowstone: Tower/Roosevelt Country

Central Yellowstone: Norris/Canyon Country

Southeast Yellowstone: Lake Country

Southwest Yellowstone: Cascade and Geyser Country

Grand Teton National Park

uphill hikers, and everyone stays to the right. Not everyone knows these rules of the road, so let common sense and good humor be your ultimate guide.

Leave It There Removal or destruction of plants; animals; or historical, prehistoric, or geological items is certainly unethical and almost always illegal.

Getting Lost If you become lost, stay on the trail. Stop and take stock of the situation. In many cases, a few minutes of calm reflection will yield a solution. Consider all the clues available; use the sun to determine direction if you don't have a compass. If you determine that you are indeed lost, stay on the main trail, and stay put. You are more likely to encounter other people by staying in one place.

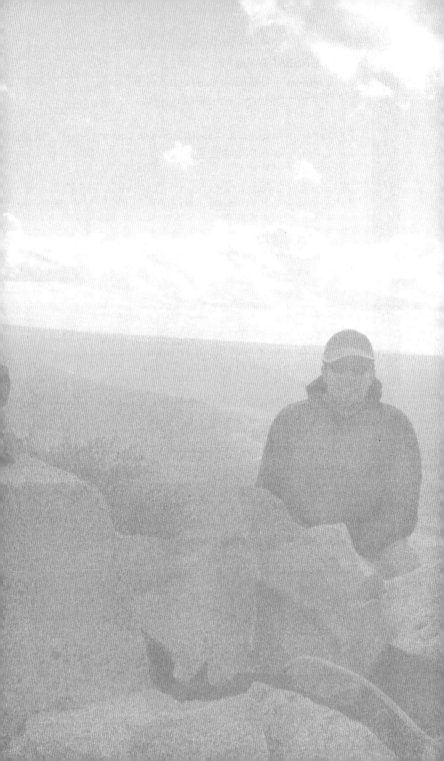

CHAPTER 1

Northwest Yellowstone: Mammoth/Gallatin Country

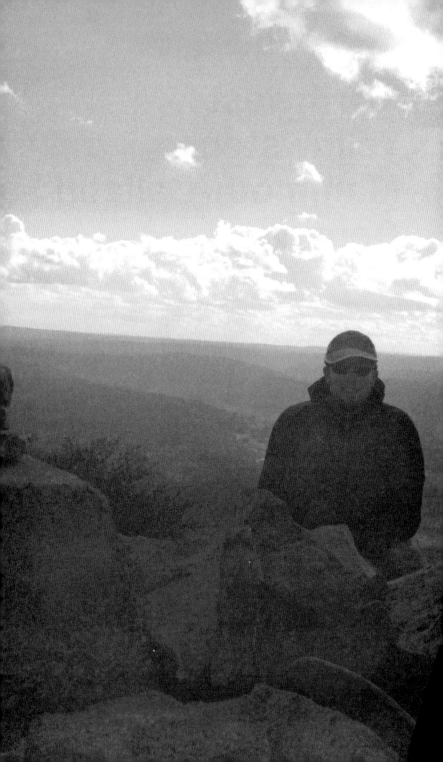

Northwest Yellowstone: Mammoth/Gallatin Country

The northwestern quadrant of Yellowstone National Park includes the developed area around the park's headquarters at **Mammoth Hot Springs** and, to the west, the soaring peaks of the **Gallatin Range.** It is also the park's lowest and driest region, which makes it a great place to visit in spring, fall, and winter.

The **North Entrance,** near the sociable gateway town of Gardiner, Montana, is the only park entrance that remains open year-round; the Grand Loop Road remains open year-round between Gardiner and Cooke City. Just before Mammoth Hot Springs, the first-come, first-served **Mammoth Campground** ($20) is the park's only year-round campground. Eight miles south of Mammoth, the smaller, National Park Service–run **Indian Creek Campground** ($15) is in the thick of moose country and is often closed in the spring season because of bear activity.

The region's diverse terrain includes some of the park's topographic extremes, ranging from desertlike corridors between 5,300 and 6,000 feet near the park's northern boundary to several peaks that top out at more than 10,000 feet. Yellowstone's low-lying **Northern Range,** which straddles the Montana–Wyoming state line, is a vital overwintering area for migrating wildlife such as pronghorn, elk, bighorn sheep, mule deer, bison, and coyotes between November and May. Like the animals, early- and late-season hikers migrate here to seek refuge from the rest of the park's extreme weather. These relatively mild conditions also make Mammoth a popular base camp for winter sports such as snowshoeing and cross-country skiing.

In Mammoth, the main visitor center and backcountry office (where permits are issued) are housed adjacent to the park headquarters in the **Fort Yellowstone–Mammoth Hot Springs Historic District,** in buildings

Overleaf and opposite: *Andrew Dean Nystrom on Bunsen Peak (Trail 3)*

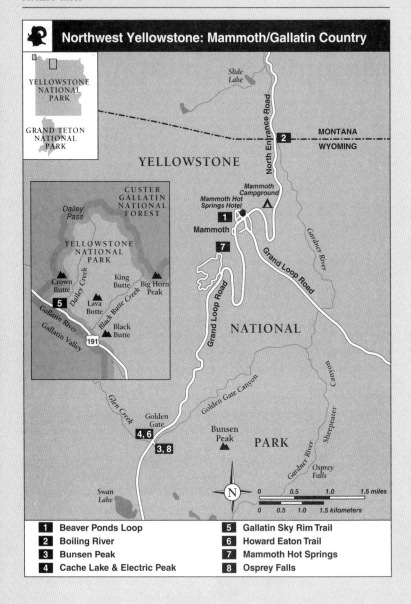

Northwest Yellowstone: Mammoth/Gallatin Country

YELLOWSTONE
NATIONAL
PARK

GRAND TETON
NATIONAL
PARK

Slide Lake

North Entrance Road

2

MONTANA

WYOMING

YELLOWSTONE

Mammoth Campground

Mammoth Hot Springs Hotel

1

Mammoth

7

Gardner River

Grand Loop Road

CUSTER GALLATIN NATIONAL FOREST

Dailey Pass

YELLOWSTONE NATIONAL PARK

Dailey Creek

Crown Butte

King Butte

Big Horn Peak

5

Lava Butte

Black Butte Creek

Black Butte

Gallatin River

Gallatin Valley

191

Grand Loop Road

NATIONAL

Glen Creek

Golden Gate Canyon

Sheepeater Canyon

Golden Gate

4, 6

3, 8

Bunsen Peak

PARK

Gardner River

Osprey Falls

Swan Lake

N

| 0 | 0.5 | 1.0 | 1.5 miles |
| 0 | 0.5 | 1.0 | 1.5 kilometers |

1	Beaver Ponds Loop	**5**	Gallatin Sky Rim Trail
2	Boiling River	**6**	Howard Eaton Trail
3	Bunsen Peak	**7**	Mammoth Hot Springs
4	Cache Lake & Electric Peak	**8**	Osprey Falls

Northwest Yellowstone: Mammoth/Gallatin Country

TRAIL	DIFFICULTY	LENGTH	TYPE	USES & ACCESS	TERRAIN	FLORA & FAUNA	EXPOSURE	OTHER
1	3	5.5						
2	1	1.0						
3	4/5	4.2/7.0						
4	5	11.2–21.5						
5	5	16.3–18.4						
6	3/4	4.0/6.6						
7	1	1.0						
8	5	10.2						

USES & ACCESS
- Day Hiking
- Bicycling
- Horses
- Backpacking
- Child-Friendly
- Wheelchair Access
- Permit

TYPE
- Loop
- Out-and-back
- Point-to-point

DIFFICULTY
- 1 2 3 4 5 +
less   more

TERRAIN
- Canyon
- Mountain
- Summit
- Lake
- Stream
- Waterfall

FLORA & FAUNA
- Autumn Colors
- Wildflowers
- Birds
- Wildlife

EXPOSURE
- Cool & Shady
- Great Views
- Photo Opportunity

OTHER
- Camping
- Swimming
- Historic/Secluded
- Geologic Interest
- Geothermal
- Moonlight
- Steep

constructed by the US Army during its tenure as park custodian (1886–1918). Nearby, portions of the updated **Mammoth Hot Springs Hotel** date back to 1911. Nightly room rates run $150–$262, with cabins available from $98; call 307-344-7311 for information and reservations. The hotel will be closed for renovations during winter 2017.

Just outside the North Entrance, which was the park's first major gateway, the large stone **Roosevelt Arch** was designed by Old Faithful architect Robert Reamer in 1903 to commemorate the completion of the Northern Pacific railway spur line from Livingston to Gardiner, Montana, and the subsequent visit of President Theodore Roosevelt. The top of the arch is inscribed FOR THE BENEFIT AND ENJOYMENT OF THE PEOPLE, a quote from the Organic Act of 1872, the enabling legislation for what was then the world's first national park. Inside the arch is a sealed time capsule that includes period postcards and a photo of Roosevelt. It was here that the park celebrated the centenary of the National Park Service in 2016.

The railroad's plans to lay spur lines through the fragile geyser basins and monopolize public access to the park were countered by the lobbying efforts of President Roosevelt's Boone & Crockett Club, a politically influential pro-hunting group. By 1905 the US Army Corps of Engineers had established the beginnings of today's Grand Loop Road, and in 1915 the first private automobiles were admitted to the park. In 1916 the newly constituted National Park Service banned horse-drawn wagons from all park roads.

Today, you can still drive or cycle the original gravel stagecoach road (one-way only, except for bicycles and hikers) from Mammoth to Gardiner. It starts behind the Mammoth Hot Springs Hotel and winds down 5 miles to the North Entrance gate.

Permits and Maps

The year-round **Albright Visitor Center and Museum** sells a good selection of maps and field guides and is the only place in Yellowstone Park to offer free Wi-Fi. A small museum focuses on history and has a good exhibit on predators and prey upstairs. Rangers also hand out free day-hiking brochures and are a good source of trail updates and general advice. Call 307-344-2263; open daily, 8 a.m.–7 p.m. in summer, 9 a.m.–5 p.m. in winter. For more detailed trail information, head downstairs to the summer-only **backcountry office**, which issues boating, fishing, and backcountry camping permits and is a wealth of hiking and backpacking information. Call 307-344-2160; the office is open 8 a.m.–noon and 1–4:30 p.m. In spring, fall, and winter, call the park's operator at 307-344-7381 for advice about where to obtain permits.

National Geographic's *Trails Illustrated Mammoth Hot Springs* (no. 303, scale 1:63,360) map depicts all of the trails, trailheads, and campsites mentioned in this chapter. The similar *Trails Illustrated Yellowstone National Park* (no. 201, scale 1:126,720) map, with trails and mileage way points, has sufficient detail for trip planning and frontcountry hiking but does not depict trailheads or backcountry campsites. A good compromise is Beartooth Publishing's *Yellowstone North* (1:80,000).

Northwest Yellowstone: Mammoth/Gallatin Country

Beaver Ponds Loop............ 39

The most popular moderately strenuous day hike in the Mammoth area traverses forested gulches, aspen-dotted meadows, and open sagelands, providing the opportunity to see a wide variety of wildlife, including the occasional moose and black bear. Wildlife is at its most active in the late afternoon.

TRAIL 1

Hike
5.5 miles, Loop
Difficulty: 1 2 **3** 4 5

Boiling River 45

Yellowstone's premier legal frontcountry soak is a dynamic series of five-star hot pots formed by the confluence of an impressive thermal stream and an icy river. It's an easily accessible stroll through an attractive river canyon, popular with families, and—for hot-springs aficionados—definitely not to be missed.

TRAIL 2

Hike, Swim
1.0 mile, Out-and-back
Difficulty: **1** 2 3 4 5

Bunsen Peak 51

This quick, scenic ascent above timberline is a popular early-season altitude acclimatization route and will give you a real cardio workout. On a clear day, it's relatively easy way to gain a panoramic overview of the Northern Range. Waterfall lovers will not want to miss the steep but rewarding side trip to Osprey Falls.

TRAIL 3

Hike
4.2 miles, Out-and-back, or 7 miles, Loop
Difficulty: 1 2 3 **4 5**

Cache Lake and Electric Peak...... 57

An ambitious and challenging summit hike that offers some of the park's best views, along with a big sense of achievement and a side trip to a charming lake. It's best done as an overnighter.

TRAIL 4

Hike, Backpack
21.5 miles, Out-and-back
Difficulty: 1 2 3 4 **5**

TRAIL 5

Hike

16.3 or 18.4 miles, Loop

Difficulty: 1 2 3 4 **5**

Gallatin Sky Rim Trail 63

A demanding but scenic ridgeline hike in the north-west corner of the park that promises rugged peaks, volcanic cliffs, and huge views.

TRAIL 6

Hike

4 miles, Point-to-point, or 6.6 miles, Loop

Difficulty: 1 2 **3 4** 5

Howard Eaton Trail 70

This short downhill section of Yellowstone's long-est trail traverses good wildlife habitat and a wide variety of picturesque terrain, including geothermal areas, boulder fields, and the scenic shoulder of Terrace Mountain. It's most enjoyable if you can arrange a shuttle.

TRAIL 7

Hike

1 mile, Loop

Difficulty: **1** 2 3 4 5

Mammoth Hot Springs 74

A network of wooden boardwalks offers a close-up look at the most accessible thermal area in the northern half of the park. While Yellowstone's most famous geysers wow audiences with their predict-able, instantly gratifying performances, Mammoth's mercurial hot-spring terraces are impressive for both their human history and their drawn-out natu-ral development.

TRAIL 8

Hike, Bike

10.0 miles,

Out-and-back,

or 10.2 miles, Loop

Difficulty: 1 2 3 4 **5**

Osprey Falls. 80

A strenuous add-on to the Bunsen Peak Loop, this infrequently visited waterfall awaits at the head of the impressive Sheepeater Canyon. After a long, flat stretch along an abandoned service road through a regenerating burn area, you plunge 800 feet into the deep, narrow canyon.

Beaver Ponds Loop

The most popular moderately difficult loop near Mammoth traverses a range of habitats and provides the opportunity to see a wide variety of wildlife, including the occasional black bear.

Best Time

The trail is hikable May–October. During summer, the exposed portions of the route are hot and dry. Wildflowers bloom early here, and aspen groves color the hillside starting in September. Wildlife is most abundant in spring, fall, and winter. The beavers are at their busiest in the late afternoon.

Finding the Trail

From the Grand Loop Road junction in front of the Albright Visitor Center, the Sepulcher Mountain/ Beaver Ponds trailhead (1K1) parking area is 0.25 mile south toward Norris Junction. The signed trailhead is at the foot of Clematis Gulch, between an old stone park-employee residence and the dormant hot-spring cone known as Liberty Cap. There are parking lots on both sides of the road, but private vehicles are not allowed to park in the tour bus parking area next to the new restroom facilities.

Logistics

This day hike is one of the only short loop hikes in the northern half of the park and is frequently recommended by rangers at the Albright Visitor Center. It's also a favorite with park employees early and late in the season. Given all this, it can get busy at times.

TRAIL USE
Hike
LENGTH
5.5 miles, 2.5–3 hours
VERTICAL FEET
±400
DIFFICULTY
– 1 2 **3** 4 5 +
TRAIL TYPE
Loop
SURFACE TYPE
Dirt

FEATURES
Child Friendly
Stream
Autumn Colors
Wildflowers
Birds
Wildlife
Great Views
Historic Interest
Geologic Interest
Steep

FACILITIES
Visitor Center
Restrooms
Picnic Tables
Phone
Water

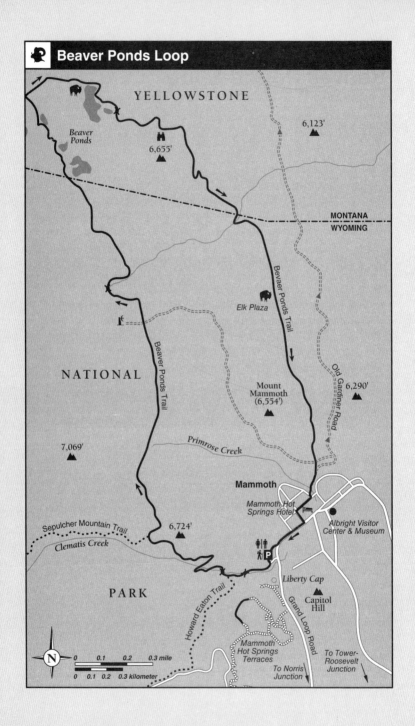

Beaver Ponds Loop

YELLOWSTONE

Beaver Ponds

6,123'

6,655'

MONTANA
WYOMING

Beaver Ponds Trail

Elk Plaza

Beaver Ponds Trail

NATIONAL

Old Gardiner Road

6,290'

Mount
Mammoth
(6,554')

7,069'

Primrose Creek

Mammoth

Mammoth Hot
Springs Hotel

Albright Visitor
Center & Museum

Sepulcher Mountain Trail

6,724'

Clematis Creek

P

Liberty Cap

PARK

Capitol
Hill

Howard Eaton Trail

Grand Loop Road

N

0   0.1   0.2   0.3 mile

0   0.1 0.2 0.3 kilometer

*Mammoth
Hot Springs
Terraces*

*To Norris
Junction*

To Tower-
Roosevelt
Junction

Trail Description

From the trailhead parking areas 1 near the northern base of the Mammoth Hot Springs terraces, look for a trailhead sign on the main road pointing the way up Clematis Gulch, between the dormant Liberty Cap hot-spring cone (to your left) and the old stone house next to the restroom facility and tour bus parking area (to your right).

Beyond the Sepulcher Mountain trailhead, ▶2 the path crosses Clematis Creek a couple of times on wooden footbridges as it climbs into shady mixed spruce–fir forest. Ignore the Howard Eaton Trail, which cuts uphill just before the second bridge, and continue to your right across the creek.

Beyond this bridge, the trail swings away from the north bank of the creek and switchbacks sharply

OPTIONS

Starting from Mammoth Hot Springs Hotel

If you'd rather not start out with the steepest part of the hike, you can do the loop in reverse with no difference in elevation gain.

Map Room, Music, and Espresso at Mammoth Hot Springs Hotel

If you have a few minutes to spare, check out the Map Room off the Mammoth Hot Springs Hotel lobby. Constructed in 1937, it features a unique map of the United States fashioned from 16 types of wood from nine countries. The map was designed by architect Robert Reamer, who also envisioned the Old Faithful Inn. If you're staying in the area, check out the schedule of evening talks, slide shows, and live piano music. In the morning (6:30–10 a.m.), there's an espresso cart in the lobby to get you going.

Old Gardiner Road

If you're headed north out of the park after the hike, consider taking the scenic, 5-mile gravel stagecoach route down to the North Entrance station in Gardiner.

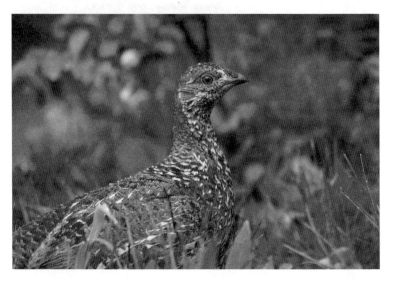

Male grouse *court mates in spring with low-frequency drumming noises they create by rapidly vibrating their wings.*

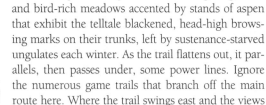

Steep

Viewpoint

Birds

Wildlife

around a juniper- and sagebrush-studded ridge to the Howard Eaton–Golden Gate Trail junction ►3 after 0.3 mile. Keep right to finish the calf-stretching 350-foot climb up to the Beaver Ponds Loop Trail junction, ►4 0.7 mile from the parking areas.

Beyond this junction, views of Mammoth Hot Springs, Bunsen Peak, and the Lava Creek Bridge on the Mammoth–Tower road open up to the east, with Mount Everts (7,842 feet) tilting to your left in the north. Watch and listen here for strutting sage grouse alongside the trail, especially in early spring.

The slope eases up as it rolls through sagelands and bird-rich meadows accented by stands of aspen that exhibit the telltale blackened, head-high browsing marks on their trunks, left by sustenance-starved ungulates each winter. As the trail flattens out, it parallels, then passes under, some power lines. Ignore the numerous game trails that branch off the main route here. Where the trail swings east and the views really open up, watch for elk, mule deer, and pronghorn grazing in the sagelands below to your right.

After passing several mature stands of heavily browsed aspen and crossing a National Park Service service road (which leads up the hill to a radio tower), the trail descends gently through meadows and spruce–fir forest. You cross a seasonal stream via a bridge before reaching the first of several shallow, cattail-fringed beaver ponds ▶5 after 2.5 miles. Look for evidence of the amphibious, hydrological engineers in the form of gnawed-down logs around the shore. The paddle-tailed rodents lie low during the day and are busiest in the late afternoon. Moose are also occasionally spotted browsing nearby in the willow thickets.

Stream

Wildlife

The trail undulates and meanders past a couple of small, marshy ponds and crosses four seasonal streams on footbridges over 0.5 mile before arriving at the last and largest of the unnamed ponds. ▶6 Listen for birds as you approach through the trees. The edges of the mixed forest are also a favored haunt of black bears, so make plenty of noise to avoid unpleasant surprises. The trail loops around along the shore, passing a variety of idyllic spots to stop for a picnic lunch. At the outlet, you can admire some of the beavers' handiwork before carefully crossing over the stream on a simple bridge.

The trail climbs away from the ponds through open grassland and shady forest, back under more power lines, and past the ruins of an old log cabin before entering a wide-open plateau known as Elk Plaza and more rolling sagelands. Here you get an eye-level view of the geologic layers of the ridgelike Mount Everts across the Gardner River Valley to the north (left).

Historic
Interest

Geologic
Interest

Beyond the Mammoth Area Trails notice board, a trailhead sign ▶7 announces your return to civilization. Continue straight ahead at the old service road intersection, ▶8 and drop down 100 yards on a narrow, rocky trail to the beginning of the gravel, one-way Old Gardiner Road, ▶9 an early stagecoach route that drops 1,000 feet in 5 miles to the park's North Entrance station.

To return to the trailhead parking areas, ▶10 walk behind the Mammoth Hot Springs Hotel and left out to the main road. Then turn right and head for Liberty Cap.

🚶	MILESTONES
▶1	0.0 Start at Sepulcher Mountain/Beaver Ponds parking areas
▶2	0.1 Sepulcher Mountain/Beaver Ponds trailhead
▶3	0.3 Right at Howard Eaton–Golden Gate Trail junction
▶4	0.7 Right at Beaver Ponds Loop Trail junction
▶5	2.5 First of several beaver ponds
▶6	3.0 Last and largest beaver pond
▶7	5.0 Beaver Ponds/Clematis Creek trailhead
▶8	5.1 Straight through old service road intersection
▶9	5.25 Start of Old Gardiner Road
▶10	5.5 Return to trailhead parking areas

Boiling River

Yellowstone's premier frontcountry soak is a dynamic series of five-star hot pots formed by the confluence of an icy river and an impressive thermal stream. It's fun for the entire family and, as one of few remaining places to legally soak in the US national parks, it's definitely not to be missed.

Best Time

Soaking in the mix of cool and near-boiling water is most enjoyable in early morning or late afternoon and best avoided in the midday summer sun. Visiting in the winter is a special treat. The area is normally open for soaking July–April, but access is restricted by the National Park Service (NPS) during periods of high spring runoff.

Finding the Trail

The springs do not appear on official NPS park maps and are not named on most other maps, but they are still easy to find. The unsigned turnoff for the parking areas is off the North Entrance Road, almost exactly halfway between the North Entrance gate and the Mammoth Hot Springs Junction, 2.3 miles from either point. Officially, these are the parking areas for the Lava Creek Trail, which leads to the bathing area. The only signs near the parking areas—the main one on the east side of the road and an overflow lot with shady picnic tables on the west side—announce the Wyoming–Montana state line (if headed south from Gardiner) and 45TH PARALLEL OF LATITUDE: HALFWAY BETWEEN EQUATOR AND NORTH POLE (if headed north from

TRAIL USE
Hike

LENGTH
1.0 mile, 1–2 hours,
including soaking

VERTICAL FEET
Negligible (±300)

DIFFICULTY
– **1** 2 3 4 5 +

TRAIL TYPE
Out-and-back

SURFACE TYPE
Dirt

FEATURES
Child Friendly
Handicap Access
Stream
Swimming
Geothermal

FACILITIES
Restrooms
Picnic Tables

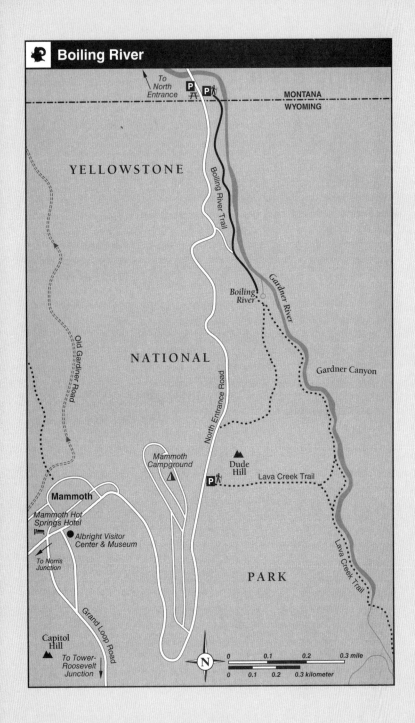

Boiling River

MONTANA
WYOMING

To
North
Entrance

YELLOWSTONE

Boiling River Trail

Gardner River

Boiling
River

Gardner Canyon

NATIONAL

North Entrance Road

Old Gardiner Road

Mammoth
Campground

Dude
Hill

Lava Creek Trail

Mammoth

Mammoth Hot
Springs Hotel

Albright Visitor
Center & Museum

To Norris
Junction

PARK

Lava Creek Trail

Grand Loop Road

Capitol
Hill

To Tower-
Roosevelt
Junction

N

| 0 | 0.1 | 0.2 | 0.3 mile |

| 0 | 0.1 | 0.2 | 0.3 kilometer |

Mammoth). The signed Lava Creek trailhead (1N3) is on the northeast side of the road, behind the restrooms on the far east side of the gravel parking lot.

Logistics

The Boiling River is generally open for soaking sunrise–sunset, or as late as 5 a.m.–9 p.m. in the high season. Check with the visitor center in Mammoth for the current status. Even though there are few signs, the area is one of the park's worst-kept secrets and receives up to 200 visitors per day.

Bring drinking water, hiking sandals (flip-flops will fall off in the river), and a towel, plus a flashlight if visiting around sunset. The only changing area is inside the restroom at the trailhead.

Trail Description

From the far east side of the main parking area ►1 on the east side of the North Entrance Road, a wide, flat gravel path heads upstream alongside the Gardner River (yes, the river and the town of Gardiner are spelled differently, for no good reason except that Montana is quirky) for about half a mile.

The 45th parallel also passes through Minneapolis–Saint Paul, Nova Scotia, Bordeaux, the Black Sea, the Caspian Sea, Mongolia, and the northern tip of the Japanese islands.

 Stream

OPTIONS

Mammoth Campground Trail

If you are staying at Mammoth Campground, it's worth knowing that an alternative path, which is roughly as long as the trail from the parking lot but much steeper, descends 250 feet in elevation from the far northeastern corner of the camping area. The unsigned trailhead is across the North Entrance Road, to the left of the prominent Dude Hill, but there's no parking here. It's not uncommon to confuse this route with the signed Lava Creek Trail that starts at a turnout parking area just to the south. The campground office can point you in the right direction.

Geothermal

Swimming

The steep, unnamed path from the Mammoth Campground ▶2 joins the Lava Creek Trail (also called the Boiling River Trail) just before the main trail winds around the thermal source that emanates from an off-limits cave, thought to be resurfacing runoff from distant Mammoth Hot Springs. The official Boiling River soaking area, ▶3 indicated by split-rail log fencing, is at the far end of the trail, 0.5 mile from the trailhead.

Signs warn of the possible presence of the pathogenic bacteria *Naegleria fowleri,* but no cases of the rare meningitis caused by the microscopic amoeba have ever been reported here. Just to be safe, do not submerge your head or nose below the water—the amoeba enters the brain via the nasal passages. Symptoms include a runny nose, a sore throat, a severe headache, and in the worst cases, possible death within a few days.

Bathing in the near-scalding main thermal channel would be fatal and is prohibited. (See "Bathers Beware" on page 20.) The actual composition of the dynamic bathing area changes daily and with the seasons. Seek out spots where other soakers are congregating, and beware of direct contact with undiluted thermal water. If you have trouble finding a calm spot where the current does not wash you downstream, try placing a big river stone in your lap.

Do not overdo the soaking, especially if you have to make the steep alternative hike back up to Mammoth Campground afterward. When finished, retrace your steps to the campground or parking areas. ▶4

MILESTONES

▶1   0.0 Start at Boiling River/Lava Creek trailhead
▶2   0.4 Junction with trail from Mammoth Campground
▶3   0.5 Boiling River soaking area
▶4   1.0 Return to parking lots

Authors' Favorite Legally Soakable Hot Springs in Greater Yellowstone

A soak in the natural Boiling River (Trail 2, page 45) is a no-brainer if you're crossing the 45th parallel in the right season. It's a brilliant hot pot in winter but is closed by spring runoff, often until midsummer. Soaking is most enjoyable here around sunrise or sunset.

North of Yellowstone, in the Paradise Valley, the family-friendly Chico Hot Springs Resort (chicohotsprings.com) is open year-round for swimming and soaking in open-air mineral spring–fed swimming pools.

South of Jackson and east of Hoback Junction, in the Bridger-Teton National Forest, two appealing year-round soaking options await (with U.S. Forest Service campgrounds nearby): the developed Granite Creek Hot Springs pools and the adjacent, undeveloped Granite Creek Falls Hot Springs. Both require a bit of driving (or snowmobiling or dogsledding in winter) to access, and the undeveloped option requires a sometimes-tricky and icy-cold creek ford, but the consensus is that the juice is well worth the squeeze.

For our money, the Bechler's Dunanda Falls Creek Hot Springs (Trail 27, page 220) and the Ferris Fork natural whirlpool (aka Mr. Bubbles; Trail 25, see page 212 for a photo) are the holy grail of primitive backcountry Wyoming soaking spots. Both require lengthy hikes to access, and there's good camping nearby. Dunanda Falls can be visited in a day, but Ferris Fork requires a backpacking trip. En route to Union Falls (Trail 34, page 263), Ouzel Pool (aka Scout Pool) is a soothing warm-water swimming hole. Nearby, thermally fed Mountain Ash Creek is yet another swell option for refreshing weary bones.

If you're still desperate for a hot soak but can't find one, the hot public showers at Old Faithful Inn (see page 199) are passable surrogates, as I first discovered after bicycling through Yellowstone on a frosty July morning, when my hands were so frozen that I could no longer properly clamp down on the brakes!

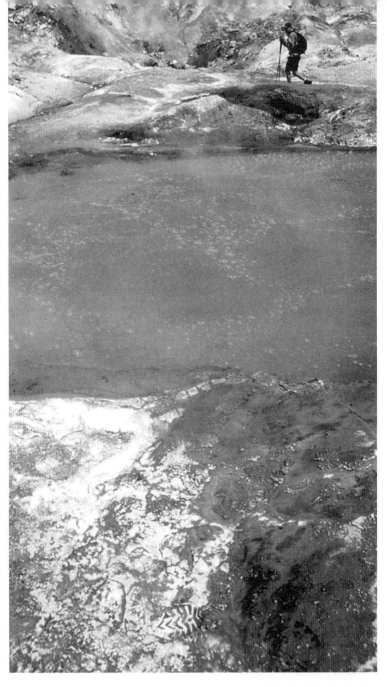

Washburn Hot Springs, *an optional destination for the Mount Washburn hike (Trail 18)*

Bunsen Peak

This scenic, heart-pumping ascent is a popular early-season altitude acclimatization route. Many folks hike in jeans and tennis shoes, but boots and trekking poles come in handy for the scree slopes, especially if you opt for the full loop or the steep side trip to Osprey Falls.

Best Time

The trail is hikable May–October: snow lingers on the trail near the summit as late as June, but the south-facing slope is free of heavy snow earlier than most peaks in the park. Other than snowmelt, there is no water along the entire route. There is precious little shade along the way, so it is best to hike early in the morning or late in the afternoon. Early afternoon thundershowers (locally known as rollers)—and lightning—are common. No matter what the weather is like at the trailhead, pack a jacket for the typically brisk weather up top.

Finding the Trail

From Mammoth, go 4.5 miles south on Grand Loop Road (US 89) and turn left into the gravel Bunsen Peak trailhead (1K4) parking area on the east side of the road (just past the Golden Gate). From Norris Canyon Road, go 16.5 miles north on Grand Loop Road and turn right into the parking area. Get here early to secure a space in this small and popular lot. If the parking area is full, try the smaller pullouts farther along the main road.

TRAIL USE
Hike

LENGTH
4.2 miles, 3 hours, or
7.0 miles, 5.5 hours

VERTICAL FEET
±1300

DIFFICULTY
– 1 2 3 **4 5** +

TRAIL TYPE
Out-and-back or Loop

SURFACE TYPE
Dirt

FEATURES
Mountain
Summit
Wildflowers
Wildlife
Great Views
Photo Opportunity
Geologic Interest
Steep

FACILITIES
None

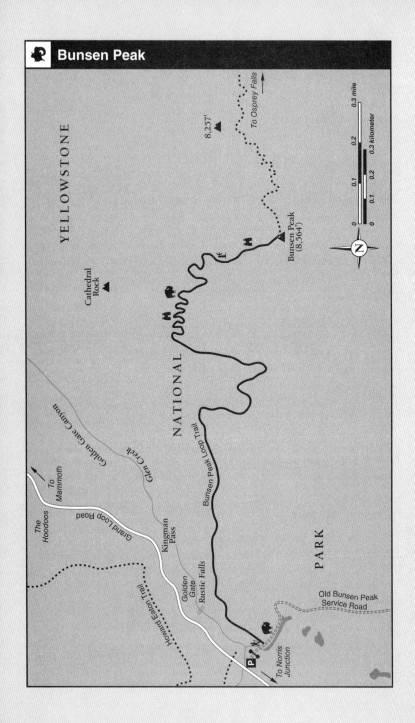

Bunsen Peak

YELLOWSTONE

Cathedral Rock ▲

8,257' ▲

To Osprey Falls

Bunsen Peak (8,564') ▲

NATIONAL

Golden Gate Canyon

Glen Creek

To Mammoth

The Hoodoos

Grand Loop Road

Kingman Pass

Golden Gate

Rustic Falls

Howard Eaton Trail

Bunsen Peak Loop Trail

PARK

Old Bunsen Peak Service Road

P

To Norris Junction

0.3 mile

0.3 kilometer

0   0.1   0.2

0   0.1   0.2

N

Trail Description

From beyond the service road barrier at the Bunsen Peak trailhead ►1 parking area, the singletrack earthen trail splits off from Old Bunsen Peak Road at a signed junction ►2 opposite a few waterfowl-rich ponds. Just up the hill through some sagebrush, a notice board ►3 has a map of trails in the Mammoth region.

The doubletrack gravel trail winds gently up through lodgepole pines in a regenerating burn mosaic created by the 1988 North Fork Fire. Thanks to the burn, in spring and summer this section is often festooned with wildflowers. The trail climbs scenically above Rustic Falls and the Golden Gate, with the Howard Eaton Trail sometimes visible off to the left above the rocky white jumble known as The Hoodoos.

From here, you can also spot your destination atop Bunsen Peak, just to the right of the telecommunications equipment. Behind you are expansive views back over Gardner's Hole, Swan Lake Flat, and beyond to the Gallatin Range. The trail flattens out through an area dotted with snags as it swings away from Grand Loop Road and heads for the summit.

As you climb through remnants of a mature spruce–fir forest on the southwest-facing slope, heading toward the first switchbacks, watch for

The patchwork "burn mosaic" pattern left by the 1988 fires, most evident from Grand Loop Road, demonstrates how supposedly catastrophic fires can actually open up new ecological niches.

 Viewpoint

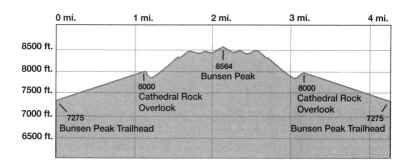

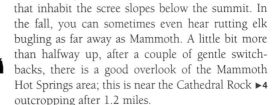

Osprey Falls and Loop Trails

To make this trail into a loop, drop down the east side of Bunsen Peak after summiting, and return to the parking area via the Old Bunsen Peak Road, a wide, relatively flat, paved service road that is now unused. This abandoned road is also a popular cross-country ski route; the northern end is an alternative trailhead that is used by park employees but is largely inaccessible to park visitors. Plan on about five hours for the full loop, plus 2.8 miles and an extra couple of hours if you opt to take the steep detour down to Osprey Falls.

Wildlife

the stoic bighorn sheep (some with radio collars) that inhabit the scree slopes below the summit. In the fall, you can sometimes even hear rutting elk bugling as far away as Mammoth. A little bit more than halfway up, after a couple of gentle switch-backs, there is a good overlook of the Mammoth Hot Springs area; this is near the Cathedral Rock ▶4 outcropping after 1.2 miles.

Viewpoint

Beyond the overlook, the trail traverses several scree slopes. Avoid the temptation to shortcut switchbacks here as they get shorter, steeper, and more frequent. The trail tread remains good, but it is slow going—all the better for spotting ripe raspberries. As the trail wraps around the northwest slope of the summit, it passes under a power line that feeds the antennae on the first of three small summits, ▶5 at 2 miles from the trailhead.

Steep

Viewpoint

Expansive panoramic views of the Absaroka Range and Beartooth Wilderness open up to the north and northeast as you pass several precariously anchored antennae. The true summit, Bunsen Peak (8,564 feet), ▶6 is a few hundred yards farther along, down through a small, rocky saddle. At last check, the summit register consisted of a rusty metal box filled with dog-eared scraps of paper

Summit

and tucked under some rocks in the middle of the remains of a lookout foundation.

Whoa! The unobstructed, 360-degree views here are superb: Electric Peak and the Gallatin Range to the northwest and west; Mount Holmes to the southwest; the Central Plateau to the south; Mount Washburn and the southern Absarokas to the southeast; and Sheep Mountain and the vast Custer Gallatin National Forest to the north. Far below to the northeast is the Yellowstone River drainage, with Swan Lake Flat and the upper Gardner River drainage to the south.

After absorbing the views, it is time to make your first and only real decision of the hike. Your options are to retrace your steps for an hour or so back to the trailhead parking area ▶7 or descend the rocky, marginally steeper northeast slope on an unsigned but well-blazed and well-maintained route through heavily burned elk habitat to join Old Bunsen Peak Road and complete a longer 8.4-mile loop. The latter option includes the detour to seldom-seen Osprey Falls (described in Trail 8, page 80).

Geologists theorize that Bunsen Peak, which dates back some 50 million years, is the eroded remains of a volcano. Evidence of the lava and volcanic rocks that once enclosed the peak is visible far below in the Gardner River Canyon.

HISTORY

Bunsen, Geysers, and Burners

The peak was named after German chemist and physicist Robert Wilhelm Bunsen—as was his invention, the burner (remember high school science lab?). Bunsen also did pioneering theoretical research about the inner workings of Iceland's geysers, which his burner resembles.

Absaroka Range

The Absaroka (pronounced ab-SOR-ka) Range is named after one of the region's numerous American Indian tribes, known today in English as the Crow.

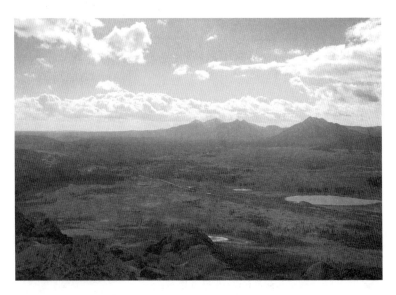

Looking southwest *from Bunsen Peak over Gardner's Hole and Swan Lake Flat*

🚶 MILESTONES

▶1　0.0 Start at Bunsen Peak trailhead parking area

▶2　0.1 Left at Bunsen Peak–Osprey Falls trail junction

▶3　0.2 Straight past Mammoth Area Trails notice board

▶4　1.2 Cathedral Rock overlook

▶5　2.0 Telecommunications equipment; first of three summits

▶6　2.1 Bunsen Peak

▶7　4.2 Return to parking area

Cache Lake and Electric Peak

Superhumans can tackle Electric Peak (without Cache Lake) as a day hike, but even fit hikers will likely want to make this a moderate overnighter, combining some of the park's best summit views with a lovely, forest-lined lake.

Best Time

Mid-July–September is the best time to climb Electric Peak. Before and after these months, you should be prepared to encounter snow on the peak. Check the weather forecast before attempting Electric Peak, and don't consider the ascent if an afternoon storm is brewing. Lightning is a real possibility; there's a reason it's called Electric Peak.

Finding the Trail

From the north, go 4.5 miles south on Grand Loop Road from Mammoth (just past the Golden Gate) and turn left into the gravel Bunsen Peak trailhead parking area on the east side of the road. From the south, go 16.5 miles north from Norris Canyon Road on Grand Loop Road and turn right into the parking area. Get here early to secure a space in this small and popular lot. If the parking area is full, try the smaller turnouts farther south along the main road.

Logistics

The best way to tackle Electric Peak is to get a backcountry permit for one of the two campsites (1G3 and 1G4) at the base of Electric Peak, allowing you

TRAIL USE
Hike, Backpack

LENGTH
11.2 miles, 6 hours, or
21.5 miles, 2 days

VERTICAL FEET
±3,670

DIFFICULTY
– 1 2 3 4 **5** +

TRAIL TYPE
Out-and-back

SURFACE TYPE
Dirt, Rock

FEATURES
Backcountry Permit
Mountain
Summit
Lake
Stream
Great Views
Geologic Interest
Wildlife
Steep
Camping

FACILITIES
None

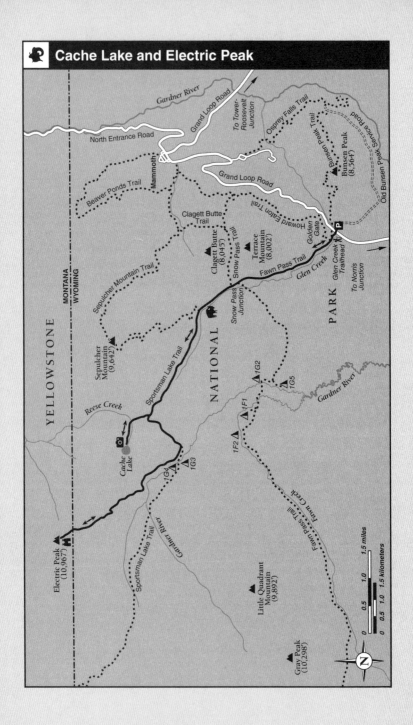

Cache Lake and Electric Peak

to ascend the peak the next morning when skies are normally at their clearest.

Both Electric Peak and Cache Lake are in the Gallatin Bear Management Area, which means that from May 1 to November 10 hiking is allowed only on designated trails (this includes the trail up to Electric Peak). Groups of four or more are recommended. Bring bear spray and take all the normal precautions, including hanging your food on the provided food poles and sleeping 100 yards from where you cook.

Trail Description

The hike starts at the Glen Creek trailhead (1K3) ▶1, across the road from the busy Bunsen Peak parking area. The trail starts off as a doubletrack through the sagebrush valley of Swan Lake Flat, following the meandering Glen Creek. After about 100 yards you continue straight at the junction with the Howard Eaton Trail ▶2, beside the trailhead information board (see Trail 6, page 70). As the trail swings to the right you'll follow the power lines and metal posts used to mark the winter cross-country skiing route. Pass underneath the power lines, and ignore the path to the right to meet the Snow Pass junction. ▶3 Trails branch left here to Fawn Pass and right to Mammoth, but our trail continues straight. Continue straight again a minute later as a second shortcut trail leads off to join the Mammoth Trail and then head into the forested gully ahead.

 Stream

The next section of trail climbs gently above a lush, green, meandering valley, where you might spot moose in the morning and afternoon. Cross a small stream to the junction with the Sepulcher Mountain Trail, ▶4 and take the left branch, continuing up the Glen Creek valley through patches of meadow and forest as Electric Peak looms on the horizon. After a short climb through forest,

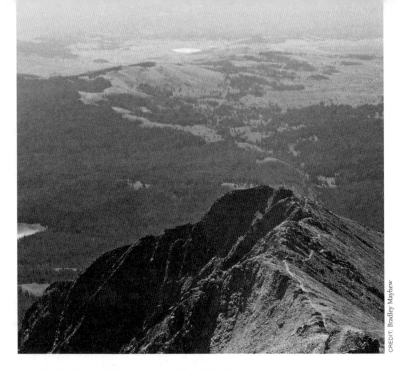

CREDIT: Bradley Mayhew

Looking back *toward Swan Lake from Electric Peak*

you meet the signed junction with Cache Lake. ►5 Depending on the time, you could visit the lake now or detour to it on the way back from Electric Peak. The trail is signposted as 1.2 miles to Cache Lake, ►6 but it's more like 0.7 mile. Electric Peak towers above the calm waters, allowing you to reflect on tomorrow's climb and maybe spot moose browsing the lake's shores. If you decide not to tackle Electric Peak, the out-and-back walk to Cache Lake is a moderate, largely flat day hike of 11.2 miles.

Lake 〰

Back at the junction ►7 with Cache Lake, follow the signed trail toward Sportsman Lake, climbing a forested gully lined with fallen trees. You soon reach the top of a spur ridge where the signed junction to Electric Peak ►8 leads off to the right. If camping, continue straight at this junction, and descend to the Gardner River. The river ford here isn't difficult, but it helps to have hiking poles if you don't want to get your feet wet. Look for an easier crossing just before the ford, at a small clearing with a sign that

says NO CAMPING BUILD NO FIRES. Campsite
1G3 is signed just after the stream crossing, and site
1G4 is a couple of minutes farther to the right. ▶9
Both campsites are secluded and about a 15-minute
walk from the turnoff to Electric Peak, a total of
about three hours from the trailhead.

 Camping

The next morning, return the 15 minutes up
to the junction ▶10 with Electric Peak to start the
ridge climb. Fill up with water at the Gardner River
first because there's no water once you start climbing the ridge. Figure on a three-hour climb, gaining
some 2,800 feet, followed by a two-hour descent.
The trail climbs above last night's campsite, dipping
briefly into a side valley and then curving around a
cliff area; be sure to take the main trail to the right,
not the game trails that stay lower on the hillside.
As the views open up, you'll see Gray Peak to the
southwest, Electric Pass and the trail leading to
Sportsman Lake to the west, and views of Swan Lake
Flat to the southeast. As you pass the final clump of
trees, the trail steepens and heads straight up a gully
along the spine of the ridge, sometimes crossing
the ridgeline to the left. Essentially you are headed
straight up the ridgeline. To the right you can see
Cache Lake below and Sepulcher Mountain beyond.

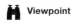 Steep

 Viewpoint

Finally you reach a saddle just before the peak
proper, which is a good place to take a breather.
From here on, you need to be comfortable with
basic route-finding skills and a bit of scrambling.
The faint trail follows the west side of the final
ridge, and you need to keep your eyes open to follow it; if you find yourself doing anything more
than a scramble, then you are on the wrong path.
Just before the rust-colored summit, you climb one
last section on unstable talus, which requires some
nerves but no technical skills. At the 10,969-foot
summit ▶11 you'll find a couple of memorials and
some antlers, along with fabulous views down to
Gardiner, the Absaroka Mountains, the Paradise

 Summit

Wildlife Valley, and beyond—essentially the whole north-west quarter of the park. Keep your eyes peeled for bighorn sheep and pikas. Savor your achievement, for this is truly a mighty view.

From the summit you simply return to Glen Creek trailhead ►12 the way you came, with the option of the 1.4-mile detour to Cache Lake if you didn't visit it on the way up. Figure on a 4.5-hour walk from the summit back to the trailhead, longer if you detour to Cache Lake.

MILESTONES

►1	0.0 Start at Glen Creek trailhead
►2	0.1 Junction with Howard Eaton Trail
►3	2.1 Snow Pass/Fawn Pass junction
►4	2.9 Junction with Sepulcher Mountain Trail
►5	4.9 Junction with Cache Lake
►6	5.6 Cache Lake (0.7-mile detour)
►7	6.3 Junction with Cache Lake
►8	7.2 Turnoff to SE Electric Peak Trail
►9	7.3 Campsites
►10	7.4 Turnoff to SE Electric Peak Trail
►11	11.6 Electric Peak summit
►12	21.5 Glen Creek trailhead

Gallatin Sky Rim Trail

This spectacular trail on the edge of the park is a long day's hike, but don't be put off—the rewards are some of Yellowstone's most rugged and impressive scenery, with mountain views spilling deep into Montana.

Best Time

The ridgeline is free from snow mid-July–September. It's a good idea to get an early start as this is a long hike and afternoon clouds can obscure views. Check the weather forecast before setting off. Much of the hike is on an exposed ridgeline and is not a place to be caught in a thunderstorm.

Finding the Trail

To get to this far northwestern section of the park, you actually have to leave it, exiting the park at West Yellowstone and then driving 30 miles north on US 191 toward Big Sky and Bozeman. From the north, head south 18 miles from the Big Sky turnoff and park in the Dailey Creek Trailhead (WK1). It's a great hike to slot in between the park and Bozeman.

Logistics

It's a good idea to bring Beartooth Publishing's Bozeman, Big Sky, West Yellowstone map, not to navigate this trail but to help identify the surrounding ranges and peaks. Note that the park's mile markers are a bit suspect here—the total trail distance is anywhere from 16 to 19 miles, depending

TRAIL USE
Hike

LENGTH
16.3 or 18.4 miles,
9–11 hours

VERTICAL FEET
±3,835

DIFFICULTY
– 1 2 3 4 **5** +

TRAIL TYPE
Loop

SURFACE TYPE
Dirt

FEATURES
Mountain
Summit
Great Views
Photo Opportunity
Steep
Geologic Interest
Camping

FACILITIES
None

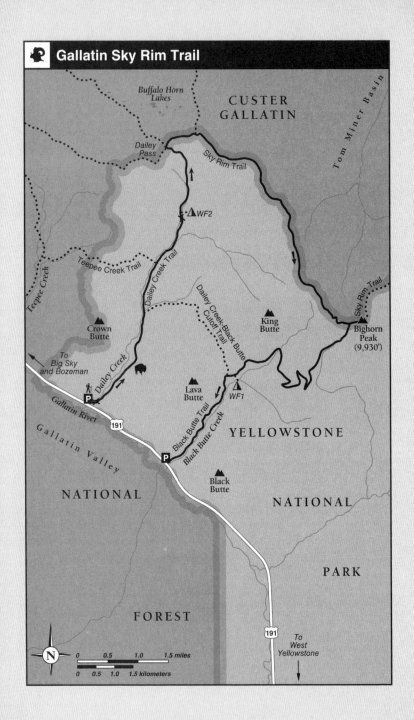

Gallatin Sky Rim Trail

CUSTER GALLATIN

Buffalo Horn Lakes

Dailey Pass

Sky Rim Trail

Tom Miner Basin

WF2

Teepee Creek Trail

Teepee Creek

Dailey Creek Trail

Crown Butte

Dailey Creek–Black Butte Cutoff Trail

King Butte

Sky Rim Trail

Bighorn Peak (9,930')

To Big Sky and Bozeman

Dailey Creek

Lava Butte

WF1

P

Gallatin River

191

Black Butte Trail

Black Butte Creek

YELLOWSTONE

Gallatin Valley

P

Black Butte

NATIONAL

NATIONAL

PARK

FOREST

191

To West Yellowstone

N

| 0 | 0.5 | 1.0 | 1.5 miles |
| 0 | 0.5 | 1.0 | 1.5 kilometers |

on which of the signs you believe. There is no water on the ridgeline, so pack an extra bottle. There is no entry fee for this section of the park.

Trail Description

From the parking lot ▶1 the trail heads up Dailey Creek, crossing the stream on a log bridge after a few minutes as Crown Butte rises to the left. After 40 minutes or so, you pass the junction with the Dailey Creek–Black Butte Cutoff Trail, ▶2 where you will rejoin the main trail at the end of the loop if you don't want to arrange a shuttle or walk along the road. After another 20 minutes, a side trail branches left to Teepee Creek ▶3 and the Yellowstone National Park boundary. As you continue straight up the valley, the terrain starts to close in and you can see the ridgeline wall at the end of the valley. As you cross Dailey Creek on a log bridge, be sure to fill your spare water bottle as this is the last reliable water source, especially in late summer. Just 15 minutes farther is backcountry campsite WF2, ▶4 next to a trickle of a stream.

The trail arcs left through patches of forest and meadow before swinging left to make the gradual ascent to Dailey Pass. ▶5 At the top of the pass you'll be faced with a red-and-white park boundary post and a four-way junction. Straight on takes you down to dispersed camping sites in the Buffalo Horn Lakes region, if you want to make this an overnighter. Our hike follows the right-hand trail climbing along the ridgeline.

Fine views start to open up on the dirt ridge toward the Taylor Peaks and Monument Mountain of the Madison range in the Lee Metcalf Wilderness, plus Sphinx Mountain, Lone Peak, and Ramshorn Peak to the north.

A 30-minute uphill section with a couple of switchbacks takes you up past volcanic breccia

This northwestern section of Yellowstone Park was added in 1927, making it the most recent section of the park.

 Camping

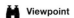 **Viewpoint**

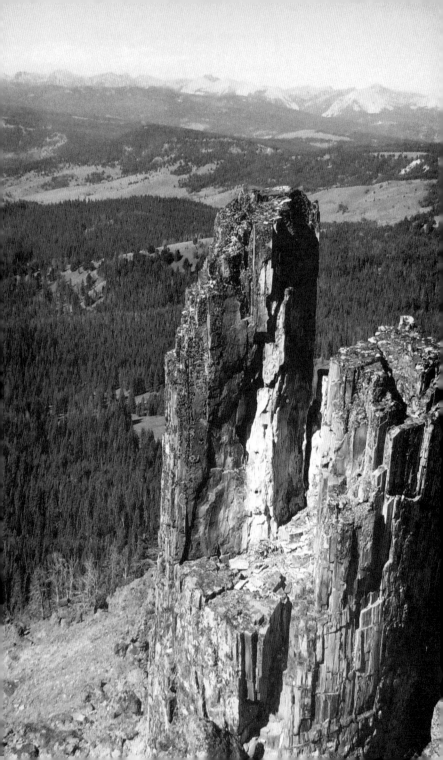

bluffs to join the ridgetop Sky Rim Trail. ▶6 To the east is the Tom Miner Basin, with Ramshorn and the Twin Peaks to the left, and Paradise Valley and the Absaroka Mountains beyond. A park sign says you have walked 7 miles, one of several examples along this trail where the signed distances are unreliable.

You might assume that the uphill sections are behind you at this point, but the next 5 miles of ridgeline walk are almost all up and down. As you climb again through patchy forest, look for a faint trail to the right that opens up to views of a fabulous petrified tree, buried 50 million years ago by a volcanic lahar (mudflow) and part of the wide-ranging Gallatin Petrified Forest.

The trail passes the first of many General Land Office metal survey posts, climbs to a crest, and then descends, only to climb again as it traverses several minor peaks and dips. The top of one peak offers 360-degree views and a pleasant ridgetop stroll before descending and climbing steeply again. As you descend again, look to the right to see two arches eroded in a breccia curtain, part of a wider bowl of volcanic rock outcrops.

As you climb onto a grassy plateau, the path becomes increasingly faint; if in doubt keep heading for the park boundary markers. It feels like you are on top of the world here, but the bad news is that from here you descend to a col, only to then make a very steep 600-foot climb—so steep in fact that there's not even a trail; you just have to follow the orange markers straight up the hillside. Atop the plateau you'll meet an important junction, ▶7 where the Sky Rim Trail and Black Butte Trail converge. Figure on six hours of hiking to this point.

From the junction it's well worth making the 10-minute detour on the daunting-looking trail

Dailey Creek (sometimes misspelled Daly Creek) was named for Andrew Dailey, an early homesteader who wintered in the Paradise Valley in 1866 and later returned to settle there.

Photo Opportunity

Geologic Interest

Steep

Opposite: *Petrified tree, as seen from the ridgeline of the Sky Rim Trail*
CREDIT: Bradley Mayhew

Summit that winds around dramatic, crumbling cliffs to the summit of Bighorn Peak (9,889 feet). ►8 From here you can see the Sky Rim Trail continuing along the ridgeline to Shelf Lake, 3 miles away, with Sheep Mountain (and its telecom tower) just beyond and Electric Peak visible to the right.

Viewpoint

Return to the junction and get ready to say good-bye to the high ground. The faint trail descends the grassy hill, dropping as it curves to the right to follow the ridge, but never dropping too steeply, traversing sagebrush hills interspersed with patches of forest. Keep your eyes open for bears on this section.

To the right King Butte towers like a giant melted candle. Around 1.25 hours from the plateau, you reach two streams, your first water source for six hours or more. The trail descends through pockets of aspen to backcountry campsite WF1 and then crosses a meadow to the junction ►9 with the Dailey Creek–Black Butte Cutoff Trail. From here it's 2 miles down the valley to Black Butte trailhead ►10 and US 191, where you can meet your vehicle or hike along the highway 1.7 miles to reach the Dailey Creek Trailhead. Alternatively, hike 2.2 miles uphill via the Dailey Creek–Black Butte Cutoff Trail

Camping

Overnight Options

It's possible to turn this hike into an overnighter by booking park backcountry campsites WF1 or WF2, in Black Butte Creek and Dailey Creek respectively, but both are only 2 miles from the highway, so it's hard to justify carrying all the extra weight. A better option for an overnight backpacking trip is to detour to the Buffalo Horn Lakes region and its free, dispersed camping, just outside the park boundary in the Custer Gallatin National Forest. One other option is to continue from Bighorn Peak along the Sky Rim Trail 3 miles to Shelf Lake and its two backcountry campsites, WE7 and WE5. This adds 6 miles to this hike.

OPTIONS

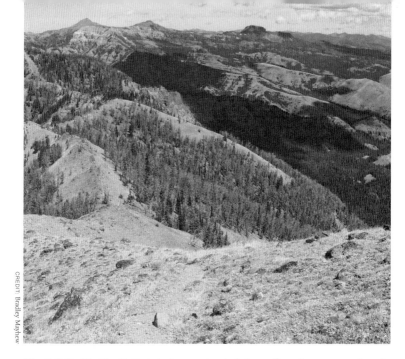

The Gallatin Sky Rim Trail *winds along a series of ridgelines, offering fine views on either side.*

and its patrol cabin to rejoin the Dailey Creek Trail, and descend 1.8 miles down the valley to the Dailey Creek trailhead. Figure on a total of 2.5 hours of walking from the plateau to the trailheads.

🚶	MILESTONES
▶1	0.0 Trailhead parking lot
▶2	1.8 Junction with Dailey Creek–Black Butte Cutoff Trail
▶3	2.6 Junction with Teepee Creek Trail
▶4	3.5 Campsite WF2
▶5	4.9 Dailey Pass
▶6	5.7 Sky Rim Trail
▶7	10.0 Junction with Black Butte Trail
▶8	10.2 Bighorn Peak
▶9	14.4 Dailey Creek–Black Butte Cutoff
▶10	16.3 Black Butte trailhead, or 18.4 Dailey Creek trailhead

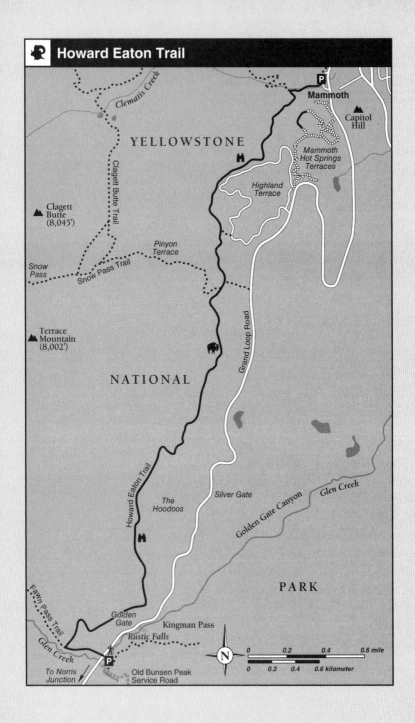

Howard Eaton Trail

Clematis Creek

YELLOWSTONE

P
Mammoth

▲ Capitol Hill

Mammoth Hot Springs Terraces

Highland Terrace

▲ Clagett Butte (8,045')

Clagett Butte Trail

Pinyon Terrace

Snow Pass

Snow Pass Trail

▲ Terrace Mountain (8,002')

NATIONAL

Grand Loop Road

Howard Eaton Trail

The Hoodoos

Silver Gate

Golden Gate Canyon

Glen Creek

PARK

Fawn Pass Trail

Glen Creek

Golden Gate

Kingman Pass

Rustic Falls

P

To Norris Junction

Old Bunsen Peak Service Road

N

| 0 | 0.2 | 0.4 | 0.6 mile |
| 0 | 0.2 | 0.4 | 0.6 kilometer |

Howard Eaton Trail

Named after a pioneering Yellowstone outfitter and guide, this short downhill section of Yellowstone's longest trail (much of which is no longer maintained because it parallels Grand Loop Road) traverses a wide variety of scenic terrain from the Golden Gate to Mammoth Hot Springs.

Best Time

The trail is hikable May–October; some exposed stretches make early morning and late afternoon the most pleasant times to hike here.

Finding the Trail

From the north, go 4.6 miles south on Grand Loop Road from Mammoth and turn right into the busy Glen Creek trailhead (1K3) parking turnout (just past the Golden Gate). From the south, go 16.4 miles north from Norris Canyon Road on Grand Loop Road and turn left into the parking turnout.

Logistics

Arranging a car shuttle is the first order of business to make this an easy hike; leave a car in one of the parking turnouts near the bottom of the Mammoth Hot Springs Terraces. Otherwise, you can try to arrange a ride from Mammoth uphill to the Glen Creek trailhead before you start hiking.

TRAIL USE
Hike

LENGTH
4 miles, 2 hours, or
6.6 miles, 4 hours

VERTICAL FEET
+250/–850

DIFFICULTY
– 1 2 **3 4** 5 +

TRAIL TYPE
Point-to-point or Loop

SURFACE TYPE
Dirt

FEATURES
Autumn Colors
Wildflowers
Wildlife
Great Views
Photo Opportunity
Geologic Interest
Geothermal

FACILITIES
None

Snow Pass and Terrace Mountain Loop

If you are unable to arrange a car shuttle, you can loop around between Clagett Butte and Terrace Mountain on the Snow Pass Trail instead of finishing the hike in Mammoth. This option adds 2.6 miles and up to two hours because of the added elevation gain of more than 1,000 feet, which nearly doubles the difficulty of the hike.

The Hoodoos were named for their ghostly appearance but bear little resemblance to the park's other natural rock pinnacles, which are more classical examples of the form.

Geologic
Interest

Wildlife

Trail Description

From the Glen Creek trailhead, ▶1 head west through the sagelands of Swan Lake Flat toward Quadrant Mountain (10,216 feet) and the Gallatin Range.

After a few hundred yards, you reach a notice board and the Howard Eaton–Fawn Pass Trail junction. ▶2 Turn right and climb sharply several hundred feet into the forest. Bunsen Peak juts up to your right, with the lichen-encrusted Golden Gate and Rustic Falls gorge far below.

Stop to admire the expansive views of the Gallatins to the west, where the trail reaches its high point (7,500 feet) along the shoulder of Terrace Mountain (8,006 feet). After 1.3 miles, the trail drops down into the eerie rockscape known as The Hoodoos, ▶3 a massive jumble of ancient limestone hot-spring deposits that sheared off of Terrace Mountain during landslides. The travertine boulder field provides prime habitat for yellow-bellied marmots (also known as rock chucks) and is a favorite playground of rock climbers.

Beyond The Hoodoos, the trail jogs left, away from Grand Loop Road, and starts to descend gradually through a burn area and aspen groves to another notice board and the Snow Pass Trail junction, ▶4 2.8 miles from the trailhead. Watch for moose and, in late summer, black bears (and less frequently grizzlies) prowling this scenic stretch for buffalo berries. To be safe, make plenty of noise where sight lines are restricted.

If you are not completing the loop option, keep straight downhill 0.5 mile past the junction, through pine and juniper forest, to reach a short spur trail for the Mammoth Hot Springs Terraces. ▶5 You can take a detour here along Upper Terrace Drive, but the most interesting thermal features are more accessible at the end of the hike, near Liberty Cap. As the trail wraps around the Upper Terraces, you will enjoy views to the north of the historic Fort Yellowstone area.

Drop another 0.5 mile past the travertine Narrow Gauge Terrace through sagebrush and shady Douglas-fir forest to the Beaver Ponds Trail junction. ▶6 Turn right and continue 0.2 mile down Clematis Gulch to end up at the Sepulcher Mountain trailhead. ▶7

Terrace Mountain was an active thermal area 65,000 years ago. Notice how the bright grayish-white travertine of The Hoodoos is similar to the dormant areas around the Mammoth Hot Springs Terraces.

🚶 MILESTONES

▶1   0.0 Start at Glen Creek trailhead parking turnout

▶2   0.3 Right at Howard Eaton–Fawn Pass Trail junction

▶3   1.3 The Hoodoos

▶4   2.8 Straight at Snow Pass Trail junction

▶5   3.3 Straight past Mammoth Hot Springs Terraces

▶6   3.8 Right at Beaver Ponds Trail junction

▶7   4.0 Arrive at Sepulcher Mountain trailhead

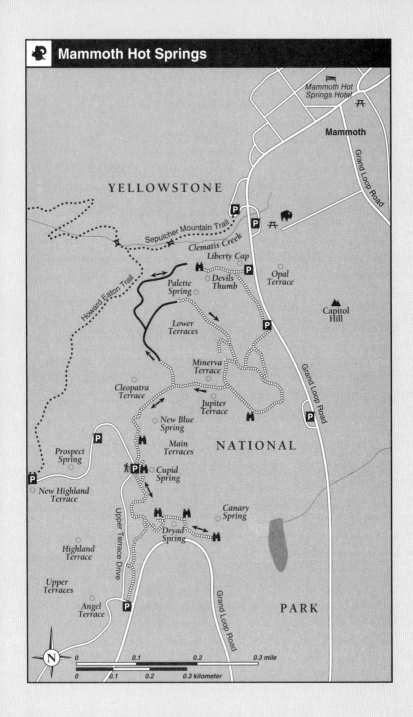

Mammoth Hot Springs

YELLOWSTONE

Mammoth Hot Springs Hotel

Mammoth

Grand Loop Road

Sepulcher Mountain Trail

Clematis Creek

Liberty Cap

Opal Terrace

Palette Spring

Devils Thumb

Howard Eaton Trail

Capitol Hill

Lower Terraces

Minerva Terrace

Cleopatra Terrace

Jupiter Terrace

New Blue Spring

Grand Loop Road

Prospect Spring

Main Terraces

NATIONAL

New Highland Terrace

Cupid Spring

Canary Spring

Upper Terrace Drive

Dryad Spring

Highland Terrace

Upper Terraces

Angel Terrace

Grand Loop Road

PARK

N

0	0.1	0.2	0.3 mile

0	0.1	0.2	0.3 kilometer

Mammoth Hot Springs

While many of Yellowstone's most famous hydro-thermal areas wow audiences with their dramatic antics and predictable, instantly gratifying performances, Mammoth's mercurial hot-spring terraces are impressive more for their important place in the history of the park and their long-term natural development. A network of boardwalks provides numerous options for exploring the most accessible thermal area in the northern half of the park.

Best Time

You can explore at least some portion of the terraces year-round. When boardwalks are iced over in winter, the fringes of the thermal area are fascinating to explore on skis or snowshoes. There is no shade on the boardwalks, so bring plenty of water and sun protection.

Finding the Trail

From Mammoth Junction, either walk 0.25 mile south to the Lower Terraces boardwalk or drive 2 miles south on Grand Loop Road toward Norris. Go past a paved overlook turnout, and turn right at the well-signed entrance gate to reach the main Upper Terrace Drive parking lot, where the route begins.

Logistics

All visitor facilities are located near the parking lots at the Upper and Lower Terraces. Rangers lead free, 90-minute walks (no reservations necessary) that

TRAIL USE
Hike

LENGTH
1.0 mile, 1–1.5 hours

VERTICAL FEET
±300

DIFFICULTY
– **1** 2 3 4 5 +

TRAIL TYPE
Loop

SURFACE TYPE
Boardwalk

FEATURES
Child Friendly
Handicap Accessible
Great Views
Photo Opportunity
Historic Interest
Geologic Interest
Geothermal
Moonlight Hiking

FACILITIES
Visitor Center
Restrooms
Picnic Tables
Phone
Water

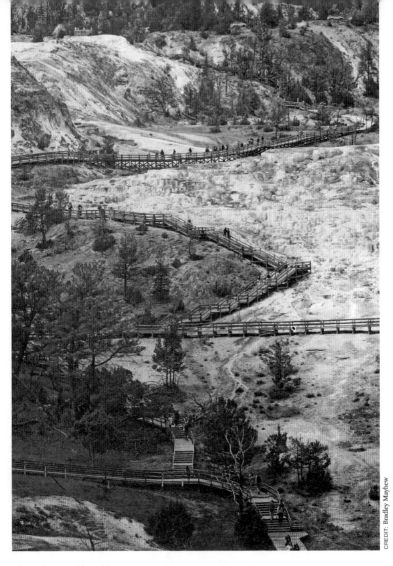

Boardwalks crisscross *the travertine terraces of Mammoth Hot Springs.*

depart from the Upper Terraces parking lot at 9 a.m. daily between Memorial Day and Labor Day.

Before heading out, pick up a helpful Mammoth Hot Springs Trail Guide ($1 donation requested) from the visitor center or the metal box below the map on the east side of the main parking area.

Trail Description

After surveying the views of Fort Yellowstone and the Main Terrace from the overlook (6,590 feet) near the main parking area, ▶1 follow the boardwalk to the right, past the short boardwalk leading to the white and orange Cupid Spring, down to the first of three platforms overlooking the travertine terraces below the source of Canary Spring. ▶2 Note: there is a less steep, wheelchair-accessible boardwalk by the parking area at the junction with the main road.

Named for its bright yellow color, the huge mound of Canary Spring owes its brilliance to filamentous bacteria living around its vent. The rest of the impressive geothermally heated runoff channel exhibits more oranges, browns, and greens, indicating the presence of thermophiles that prefer cooler temperatures. Grey sinter remains in areas where water has stopped flowing. The lower overlook platform provides the best up-close look at how calcium carbonate, which dissolves from the sedimentary limestone layers, crystallizes on the plant matter that falls onto the terraces.

 Geothermal

 Geologic Interest

It's estimated that as many as 65 species of algae and bacteria live in Mammoth's hot springs, and that up to 2 tons of travertine are deposited here daily.

Retrace your steps along the boardwalk back up to the parking area and main overlook, ▶3 where a different boardwalk ▶4 leads straight ahead to another overlook of the mostly dormant New Blue Spring. Follow the stairs down to the Lower Terraces and another junction, ▶5 where there is yet another trail map signboard. To your left is the multilayered Cleopatra Terrace; to your right is Minerva Terrace, definitely a highlight of the tour.

Named for the Roman goddess of artists and sculptors, many of Minerva's ornately layered terraces took shape in the early 1990s. At last look, the spring was inactive, but a photo on the interpretive sign shows what the area looked like during

Geologists speculate that the hot water surfacing here in the small fissures may flow as far as 21 miles underground along a fault line from the Norris Geyser Basin. Some of the same water is thought to resurface farther downhill at the Boiling River.

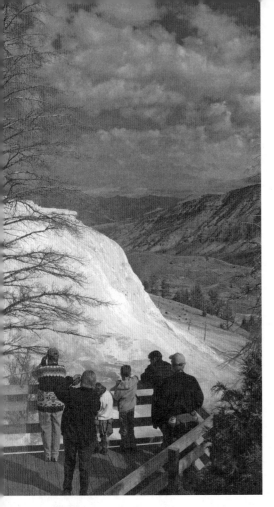

Canary Spring: *Family at the lower Canary Spring Overlook*

a period of activity in 1977. Believe it or not, during one particularly active cycle, minerals deposited by Minerva buried the boardwalk you are now standing on. In the dry areas, look for elk tracks in the gravel and evidence of how fragile the crust is where bison hoofs have caused cave-ins.

From the junction, follow the paved path down to your right about 100 yards to Palette Spring, ▶6 a good example of how thermophiles (heat-tolerant bacteria) lend different colors to runoff channels.

Back at the trail map sign, detour to your right down the steep gravel path for a close-up look at the dormant, 37-foot-tall hot-spring

OPTIONS

Lower Terraces from Mammoth

You can walk five minutes from the visitor center in Mammoth and join this hike halfway, at Liberty Cap. If you want to explore more, you can bicycle or drive around the 1.5-mile, one-way Upper Terrace Drive past several more active hot-spring terraces.

cone that was named Liberty Cap ▶7 in 1871 for its resemblance to the peaked caps worn during the French Revolution. There are picnic tables across the road near the dormant Opal Terrace (a favorite springtime hangout of elk), and restrooms to the left past the bus parking area. The easiest way to do this hike is to get picked up here or get dropped at the beginning of the hike and walk all the way back to the Mammoth Hot Springs Hotel.

Retrace your steps back past Palette Spring, and turn left on the boardwalk at the junction ▶8 to loop around the lower side of Minerva Terrace. Even where all appears dry and dormant, watch closely for steam puffing out of small cracks in the hillside, hinting at future hydrothermal activity. At Jupiter Terrace, ▶9 interpretive signs display historical photos and explain the terrace's varied cycles of activity.

Head right (uphill) on the boardwalk, and climb the stairs starting at the foot of the Main Terrace to return to the Upper Terrace overlook and parking area. ▶10

The bubbling visible at the surface of the hot springs is due to carbon dioxide gas expanding, not water boiling. Groundwater temperatures have been measured at around 170°F.

🚶	**MILESTONES**
▶1	0.0 Start at Upper Terrace Drive parking area
▶2	0.1 Right on boardwalk to Canary Spring
▶3	0.2 Back at parking area and overlook
▶4	0.25 Straight on boardwalk to New Blue Spring overlook
▶5	0.4 Left on paved path at Cleopatra–Minerva Terrace junction
▶6	0.5 Right down gravel path at Palette Spring junction
▶7	0.6 North (right) on gravel path to Liberty Cap; return by retracing your steps
▶8	0.7 Left on boardwalk at Palette Spring junction
▶9	0.85 Right on boardwalk at Mound–Jupiter Terraces junction
▶10	1.0 Return to Upper Terrace Drive parking area

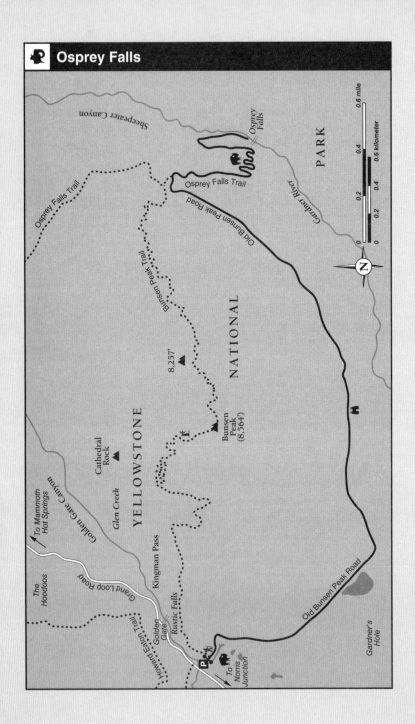

Osprey Falls

Sheepeater Canyon

Osprey Falls

PARK

Osprey Falls Trail

Osprey Falls Trail

Old Bunsen Peak Road

Gardiner River

Bunsen Peak Trail

8,257'

NATIONAL

Bunsen Peak
(8,564')

Cathedral Rock

YELLOWSTONE

Glen Creek

Golden Gate Canyon

To Mammoth Hot Springs

Kingman Pass

The Hoodoos

Grand Loop Road

Old Bunsen Peak Road

Howard Eaton Trail

Golden Gate

Rustic Falls

Gardner's Hole

To Norris Junction

0   0.2   0.4   0.6 mile
0   0.2   0.4   0.6 kilometer

Osprey Falls

This hike on an old service road ends with a steep out-and-back drop to the secluded base of a scenic falls at the head of an impressive canyon. The route can be extended to a slightly longer and more strenuous loop by combining it with Trail 3 (page 51) to see both sides of Bunsen Peak.

Best Time

Old Bunsen Peak Road is open for travel whenever the park is open to visitors. The hiking and biking season runs roughly May–October. On hot days and for spotting wildlife, it's best to hike in the early morning or late afternoon.

Finding the Trail

From the north, go 4.5 miles south on Grand Loop Road from Mammoth and turn left into the Bunsen Peak trailhead parking area on the east side of the road (just past the Golden Gate). From the south, go 16.5 miles north from Norris Canyon Road on Grand Loop Road and turn right into the parking area. If the parking area is full, try the smaller Glen Creek trailhead turnout on the opposite side of the road.

Logistics

There's no water at the trailhead, and the only water along the trail is at the falls. If doing this hike as part of the full Bunsen Peak Loop (starting as described in Trail 3), watch carefully for orange blazes (metallic flags tacked to tree trunks) marking the way to the cutoff for Osprey Falls as you finish the descent

TRAIL USE
Hike, Bike

LENGTH
10.0 or 10.2 miles,
5–7 hours

VERTICAL FEET
±850

DIFFICULTY
– 1 2 3 4 **5** +

TRAIL TYPE
Out-and-back or Loop

SURFACE TYPE
Dirt, Road

FEATURES
Canyon
Waterfall
Wildflowers
Birds
Wildlife
Steep

FACILITIES
None

off the back side of Bunsen Peak. Bicyclists are allowed on the gravel service road but must park their bikes before descending to Osprey Falls. The northeast end of Old Bunsen Peak Road is an alternative trailhead, used primarily by park employees.

Trail Description

Beyond the service road barrier at the Bunsen Peak trailhead parking area, ▶1 continue straight on Old Bunsen Peak Road at the signed Bunsen Peak Trail junction ▶2 across from some waterfowl-rich ponds.

Wildlife The relatively level gravel service road heads east out across the rolling sagebrush meadows of Gardner's Hole and passes through prime bison and elk habitat. Watch for scats and tracks along the road. This stretch of abandoned road is also a popular mountain bike and cross-country ski track, so you could easily combine hiking and biking on this trip.

After skirting a couple of ponds, the road swings around the foothills and southern base of Bunsen Peak (8,564 feet). The regenerating forest is more than head-high here, obscuring the views in places. **Canyon** Eventually the road approaches an overlook that affords a glimpse of the Gardner River at the bottom of Sheepeater Canyon.

The canyon is named after the park's only original year-round residents, a subgroup of the Shoshone Nation who referred to themselves as the Tukuarika but were called the Sheepeater by Western settlers. In 1871, the year before Yellowstone was declared a park, they were forcibly relocated to the Wind River Reservation.

Although osprey rarely nest near their namesake falls, if you're lucky you might spot them circling over the river looking for prey, as well as bald eagles.

At the signed Osprey Falls–Bunsen Peak Trail junction, ▶3 3.4 miles from the trailhead, turn right where the old road continues straight ahead and drops down into a National Park Service (NPS) maintenance area. The road dead-ends at an alternative trailhead that is used by NPS employees but that visitors are discouraged from using. The rim of Sheepeater Canyon ▶4 is several hundred yards beyond the bike parking rail. Bikes are not allowed past this point due to the extreme steepness of the trail to Osprey Falls.

Do not let the posted signs warning about treacherous conditions on the Osprey Falls Trail scare you. Yes, the steep trail's tread is in poorer condition than most of the superbly maintained trails in the park, but with a reasonable dose of caution it is safely manageable under normal circumstances. It plunges nearly 800 feet in a little over 0.5 mile to the base of the impressive 150-foot Osprey Falls, ▶5 a total of 5 miles from the trailhead.

The misty area near the base of the falls makes a fine spot for a picnic as you ponder the stiff climb back out to the trailhead parking area. ▶6

Besides bighorn sheep, the Tukuarika hunted bison, elk, and deer with bows fashioned from ram's horns and ornamented with porcupine quills, using arrows tipped with obsidian. Evidence of chutes used to herd bighorn off cliffs has been uncovered near Rustic Falls.

 Waterfall

🚶 MILESTONES

▶1   0.0 Start at Bunsen Peak trailhead parking area

▶2   0.1 Straight on road at Bunsen Peak–Osprey Falls Trail junction

▶3   3.4 Right at Osprey Falls–Bunsen Peak Trail junction

▶4   3.8 Sheepeater Canyon rim

▶5   5.0 Osprey Falls

▶6   10.0 Return to trailhead parking area

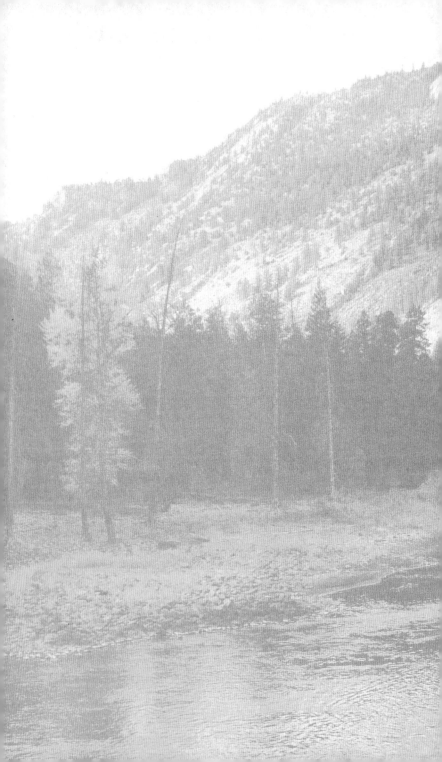

CHAPTER 2

Northeast Yellowstone: Tower/Roosevelt Country

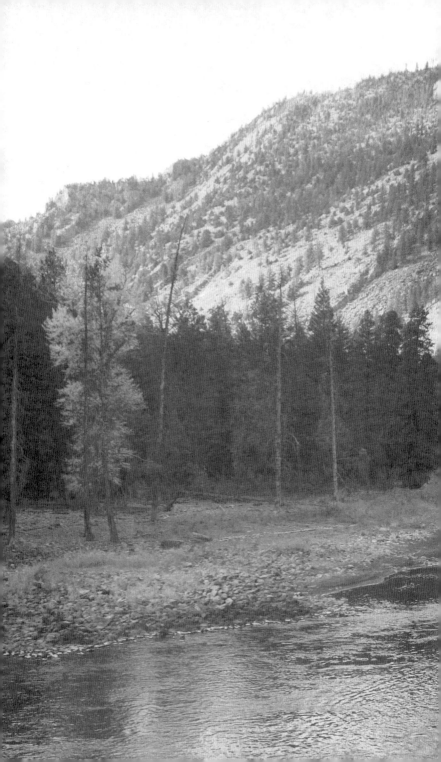

Northeast Yellowstone: Tower/Roosevelt Country

Yellowstone's northeastern quadrant encompasses the core of the park's wildlife-rich Northern Range. It includes the developed areas around Tower Fall and Tower Junction (6,270 feet), the lower Yellowstone River drainage, and the Lamar River Valley. These unique areas include distinct ecological niches but when grouped together offer some of the most diverse and rewarding hikes in the park.

Grand Loop Road—the region's only paved route—remains open to wheeled vehicles year-round between the North Entrance and Cooke City, just east of the Northeast Entrance (7,365 feet) in the park's top-right corner. In winter, chains or snow tires may be required. The region is very popular with anglers and wildlife-watchers, who frequently fill the small and less-developed, National Park Service–run Slough Creek ($15) and Pebble Creek ($15) campgrounds to capacity, even outside of the high season. Another agreeable option is the 32-site Tower Fall Campground ($15), tucked away above Tower Creek in a pleasant forest.

Beyond the Northeast Entrance, the spectacular Beartooth Highway (US 212) was dubbed "the most beautiful drive in America" by roving TV journalist Charles Kuralt. The National Scenic Byway traverses the Beartooth Pass (10,947 feet; typically open Memorial Day weekend–mid-October; call 888-285-4636 for recorded travel conditions, construction, and alternate-route updates, or visit beartoothhighway.com) and a total of 65 stunning miles en route to the appealing outdoor base camp of Red Lodge, Montana. The route also provides easy access to many U.S. Forest Service campgrounds, trailheads, and scenic alpine hikes and backpacking routes in the Absaroka–Beartooth Wilderness.

Overleaf and opposite: *Looking downriver, deep inside the lower Black Canyon of the Yellowstone (Trail 9)*

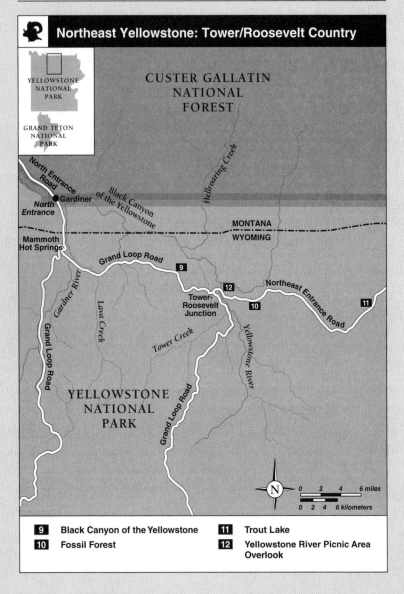

Northeast Yellowstone: Tower/Roosevelt Country

CUSTER GALLATIN
NATIONAL
FOREST

YELLOWSTONE
NATIONAL
PARK

GRAND TETON
NATIONAL
PARK

North Entrance Road

Gardiner

North
Entrance

Black Canyon
of the Yellowstone

Hellroaring Creek

MONTANA
WYOMING

Mammoth
Hot Springs

Grand Loop Road

9

12

Northeast Entrance Road

11

Gardner River

Lava Creek

Tower Creek

Tower-
Roosevelt
Junction

10

Yellowstone River

Grand Loop Road

YELLOWSTONE
NATIONAL
PARK

Grand Loop Road

N

0   2   4   6 miles

0   2   4   6 kilometers

| **9** | Black Canyon of the Yellowstone | **11** | Trout Lake |
| **10** | Fossil Forest | **12** | Yellowstone River Picnic Area Overlook |

Wildlife flocks to Yellowstone's northeast corner for its lush riparian zones, wide-open expanses of grazing meadows, and attractive denning habitat. The Lamar Valley, often referred to as the Serengeti of America, is

Northeast Yellowstone: Tower/Roosevelt Country

TRAIL	DIFFICULTY	LENGTH	TYPE	USES & ACCESS	TERRAIN	FLORA & FAUNA	EXPOSURE	OTHER
9	5	18.5	↘	🚶🚴🐎🎒🛡	🏞📶🏔	🍂🌼🦅🐃	🌳📷	⛺🏊🏛🗺🔺
10	4	3.0	↗	🚶	🏔🔺	🍂🌼🦅🐃	🌳📷	🏛🗺🔺
11	1	1.8	↗	🚶👫	🏔🌊	🐃🔭		
12	2	4.0	↗	🚶👫	🏞	🌼🦅🐃	🌳📷	🗺🔥

USES & ACCESS	TYPE	TERRAIN	FLORA & FAUNA	OTHER
🚶 Day Hiking	↻ Loop	🏞 Canyon	🍂 Autumn Colors	▲ Camping
🚴 Bicycling	↗ Out-and-back	🏔 Mountain	🌼 Wildflowers	⟰ Swimming
🐎 Horses	↘ Point-to-point	△ Summit	🦅 Birds	🏛 Historic/Secluded
🎒 Backpacking		≋ Lake	🐃 Wildlife	🗺 Geologic Interest
👫 Child-Friendly	DIFFICULTY	📶 Stream		🔺 Geothermal
♿ Wheelchair Access	- 1 2 3 4 5 +	🌊 Waterfall	EXPOSURE	☽ Moonlight
	less more		🌳 Cool & Shady	🔻 Steep
🛡 Permit			🔭 Great Views	
			📷 Photo Opportunity	

one of the most popular places in Greater Yellowstone for spotting wolves, elk, bison, and coyotes. Both black and grizzly bears frequently cause roadside "bear jams" around Tower Junction.

The hiking terrain here runs the gamut, from low-lying overnight routes that trace the depths of the Black Canyon of the Yellowstone to high-altitude ascents that top out above timberline for never-ending views of the surrounding wildlands.

The rustic cabins at the summer-only Roosevelt Lodge (circa 1916; rates $89–$142), near President Theodore Roosevelt's favorite campsite, are a popular base camp for families and anglers. The Yellowstone Association Institute (yellowstoneassociation.org) bases many of its field-study seminars nearby at the historic Lamar Valley Buffalo Ranch complex, where the United States' last known mountain bison once survived in captivity. After the Yellowstone herd was counted at 23 in 1902, Great Plains bison were reintroduced, and ultimately the two species were allowed to interbreed in 1915. The ranch is generally not open to the public.

The last of Yellowstone's once-extensive gray wolf population was exterminated in the Lamar Valley in the 1920s. In 1995 an unprecedented wolf reintroduction effort began with the release of 14 wild-captured Canadian gray wolves near Soda Butte and Druid Peak. The Montana state legislature unceremoniously responded to the federally sponsored reintroduction efforts by proposing that wolves be reintroduced smack-dab in the middle of pro-wolf territory: Central Park in New York City, the Presidio in San Francisco, and on the National Mall in Washington, D.C.

The last two of Yellowstone's 31 reintroduced wolves died in early 2004. In 2015 there were 99 wolves running in 10 packs inside Yellowstone National Park, down from 170 wolves in 2007. Up to 500 wolves live in Greater Yellowstone.

After extensive, multiyear construction that widened Grand Loop Road over Dunraven Pass (8,859 feet) to accommodate modern RVs and improve safety, the route once again provides seasonal access to the Chittenden Road parking area (which provides access to the north slope of Mount Washburn) and Canyon Junction. Call 307-344-2117 for Dunraven opening dates and Yellowstone road-construction updates.

Permits and Maps

The only permits required here are for fishing and backcountry campsites along the Blacktail Deer Creek and Yellowstone River trails.

There's no visitor center in the region, but the Tower Ranger Station (open 8 a.m.–4:30 p.m. daily in summer), housed in a reconstructed historic soldier station near Roosevelt Lodge, issues backcountry and fishing permits and can advise about current hiking conditions. The rustic, log cabin–style Northeast Entrance Ranger Station, a National Historic Landmark and a fine example of National Park Service "parkitecture" built between 1934 and 1935, may issue permits as well, depending on seasonal staffing levels.

The Trails Illustrated Tower/Canyon (no. 304, scale 1:63,360) map covers all of the hikes, trailheads, and campgrounds described in this chapter, except the Blacktail Deer Creek Trail and the western half of the Yellowstone River Trail, which appear on the Mammoth Hot Springs (no. 303, scale 1:63,360) and Yellowstone National Park (no. 201, scale 1:126,720) sheets in the same series. Beartooth Publishing's Yellowstone North (1:80,000) covers the whole area.

Northeast Yellowstone: Tower/Roosevelt Country

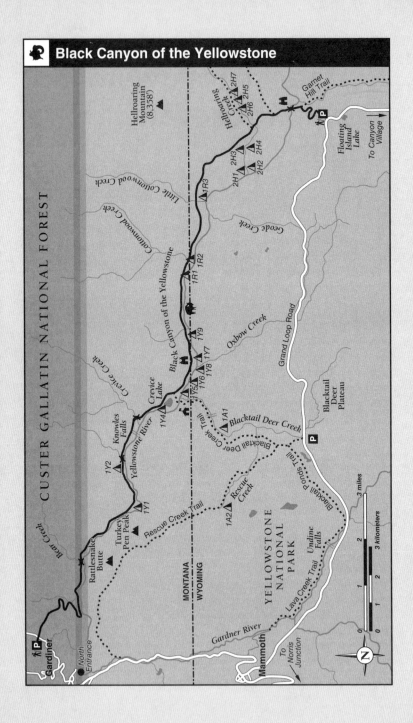

Black Canyon of the Yellowstone

Black Canyon of the Yellowstone

This classic downhill hike is an early- and late-season favorite of park employees because the campsites are snow-free as soon as early May and as late as October. It's just far enough away from the road for you to start feeling like you're in the wilderness and is a prime route for fishing and wildlife-watching.

Best Time

The trail is typically dry enough for hiking by mid-May. The ford of Hellroaring Creek, however, can be waist-deep and tricky as late as August during years of high runoff. Ticks are a nuisance in spring and early summer. The route is hot at midday in summer and can be frosty in the early morning but is bug- and snow-free early and late in the season, when many of the park's higher-elevation trails are in worse shape.

Finding the Trail

From the west, go 14.1 miles east from Mammoth (toward the Tower–Roosevelt junction) on Grand Loop Road and turn left into the signed Hellroaring trailhead (2K8) parking area (labeled a "gravel pit" on some older maps), which is 0.3 mile down a good gravel road on the north side of the road. From the east, go 3.4 miles west (toward Mammoth) from Tower–Roosevelt junction on Grand Loop Road and turn right into the parking area.

The exit (western) trailhead used to be in the town of Gardiner, Montana, but a private landowner withdrew permission for hikers to cross a section of

TRAIL USE
Hike, Backpack, Horse

LENGTH
18.5 miles, 1–4 days

VERTICAL FEET
+1,800/–1,250

DIFFICULTY
– 1 2 3 4 **5** +

TRAIL TYPE
Point-to-point

SURFACE TYPE
Dirt

FEATURES
Backcountry Permit
Canyon
Stream
Waterfall
Autumn Colors
Wildflowers
Birds
Wildlife
Great Views
Photo Opportunity
Camping
Swimming
Secluded
Geologic Interest
Steep

FACILITIES
Horse Staging

land, so the trail has been rerouted in the last couple of years. The trailhead is now beside the horse corrals at the National Forestry Service–run Eagle Creek Campground, just northeast of Gardiner. From the park's North Entrance, pass through the Roosevelt Arch and turn right on Park Street. After a couple of blocks, turn left on Second Street and cross the Yellowstone River Bridge. Turn right on Jardine Road and head uphill 2.2 miles to Eagle Creek Campground. The corral parking is at the end of one of the campground's loop roads. Eagle Creek has 15 exposed campsites ($7) but no water. For details, contact the Custer Gallatin National Forest office at 805 Scott St. W. in Gardiner; call 406-848-7375.

Logistics

Most people prefer to do this hike one-way in the downhill direction (east to west), which requires a car shuttle. If in doubt about fording Hellroaring Creek, use the stock bridge crossing upstream. It's an extremely long, strenuous day hike, so consider spreading it over two to four days to allow ample time for fishing, easygoing hiking, and plenty of relaxing. You really can't go wrong with any of the campsites along the route, though all prohibit wood fires. Your selection will likely be determined by availability and how many nights you will be camping.

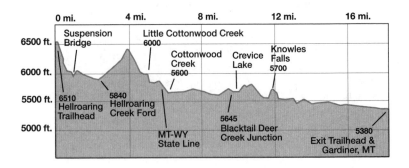

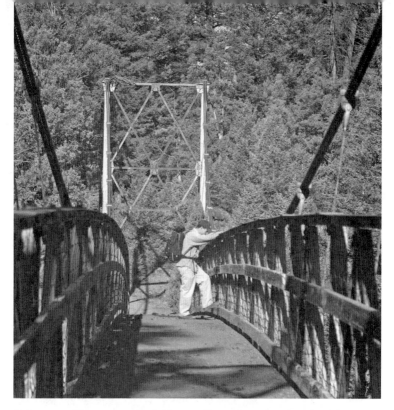

Yellowstone River suspension bridge: *Bradley Mayhew contemplates the whitewater raging through the narrows far below.*

Trail Description

From the Hellroaring trailhead ►1 (2K8) parking lot, a singletrack, earthen trail that receives heavy horse use winds down through damp Douglas-fir forest to an overlook of the Yellowstone River, with Garnet Hill looming to the right across Elk Creek.

 Viewpoint

Starting at a small burn area, the trail switchbacks down steeply for a total of 600 feet over the first mile, past the Garnet Hill Trail junction ►2 after 0.7 mile, through open grasslands dotted with wildflowers to the brawny steel Yellowstone River suspension bridge, ►3 which is bookended by juniper trees and just wide enough for two skinny horses.

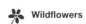 Wildflowers

Blacktail Deer Creek Shortcut

By starting at the Blacktail Deer Creek (1N5) trailhead, you can shorten the route by about 5 miles, joining the main canyon trail near the Lower Blacktail Patrol Cabin. Another short alternative is to make an out-and-back jaunt to the Yellowstone River bridge—a short but steep day hike, with a 1,600-foot total elevation change and a length of 2 miles round-trip.

Gardiner's Best Burger

After a grueling hike, the only thing better than a soak in the Boiling River (see Trail 2, page 45) is a half-pound buffalo cheeseburger and thick huckleberry shake at the Wild West Corral Drive-In (406-848-7627, 711 W. Scott St.), on the western end of the main drag in Gardiner.

After checking out the whitewater roaring far below, you climb away from the river through a rocky canyon and over a sagebrush plateau, past the Buffalo Plateau–Coyote Creek Trail junction ►4 to Hellroaring junction, ►5 at 2 miles from the trailhead, where Hellroaring Mountain (8,358 feet), the park's biggest exposed granite outcropping, looms in the background.

Geologic Interest ✎

Your next move depends on the season and your destination. Before August, you'll want to scout the condition of the potentially tricky Hellroaring Creek ford, ►6 a few hundred yards beyond the junction and around the left side of the glacial lake basin (which is dry by late summer), to decide whether you would rather use the stock bridge, 1.5 miles upstream from the junction. All even-numbered campsites along Hellroaring Creek are on the south bank, and odd-numbered sites are on the north bank. These sites are the obvious first-night choice if you're planning a three-night trip.

Camping ▲

Hellroaring Creek was named by an early explorer who reported that it was a "real hell roarer."

From the junction on the north side of Hellroaring Creek, ►7 east-to-west-trending trails lead off to more campsites. If you've crossed via the stock bridge, turn right at this intersection. Fronting the confluence of Hellroaring Creek and the Yellowstone

River, the ideal campsite, 2H1, ▶8 is accessed either along the north bank of the creek via the spur trail for campsite 2H3 or a few hundred yards later via a cutoff from the main trail. Both of these watercourses are blue-ribbon fishing spots for cutthroat trout after high waters recede, starting around mid-July.

The trail climbs away from the river, crossing a varied landscape of minor marshes, small glacial lakes, and open sagelands. As you switchback more than 300 feet up a ridge, the impressive outline of Electric Peak (10,992 feet) comes into view near the crest. The trail descends to the roomy campsite 1R3, ▶9 perched high above the river 4.3 miles from the trailhead, before crossing Little Cottonwood Creek. ▶10 The views here down into the beginnings of the Black Canyon of the Yellowstone are stunning.

Appropriately, there's no signage announcing the Wyoming–Montana state line, ▶11 as this abstract political delineation 5.7 miles from the trailhead has no effect on your experience. A few hundred yards farther along, campsites 1R2 ▶12 (hiker-only) and mixed-use 1R1 ▶13 are equally attractive, situated well off the trail on benches high above the river, with easy access to water around the mouth of Cottonwood Creek.

Watch for elk antlers protruding from trees and ankle-busting badger burrows in the trail as it descends for a long, flat, forested stretch alongside the river. A couple of miles farther, past trailside bison wallows, hiker-only campsites 1Y9 ▶14 and 1Y7 ▶15 are 8.3 and 9 miles from the trailhead, respectively. Both sites are superb first-night riverfront options if you're making a two-day trip. Late in the season, sandy swimming beaches are exposed below the towering outcroppings of columnar basalt.

Just before the Blacktail Bridge and 9.8 miles from the trailhead, hiker-only campsite 1Y5 ▶16 enjoys a secluded riverfront setting. If you've opted

The Black Canyon of the Yellowstone has one of the densest collections of predators in the Lower 48, with one wolf, mountain lion, or grizzly bear for every 2 square miles.

 Canyon

 Camping

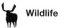 Wildlife

 Swimming

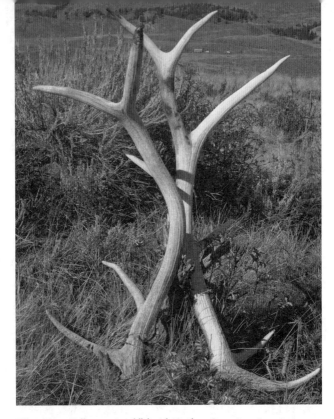

Elk antlers: *Yellowstone's wildlife-rich Northern Range is an important over-wintering refuge for elk and other large mammals.*

Camping ⚠

for the Blacktail Deer Creek Trail shortcut, you'll join the Yellowstone River Trail at the junction, ▶17 several hundred yards ahead on the north side of the bridge. The hiker-only campsites 1Y6 and 1Y8 are across the bridge, east of the Lower Blacktail Patrol Cabin, 0.4 and 0.8 mile, respectively, down a spur trail along the south bank of the river.

The trail skirts the northern shore of the fishless, aquamarine Crevice Lake, ▶18 which has no inlet or outlet but is a nice spot for a cool dip on a hot day. Because of the steep banks and lack of shade around the lake, the best spots for breaking your daylong hike in half with a picnic lunch are just before the lake or a few hundred yards beyond it, near the riverfront, hiker-only campsite 1Y4, ▶**19** 10.6 miles from the trailhead.

The trail leaves the river again to cross Crevice Creek ▶**20** on a sturdy bridge 11.4 miles from the trailhead. This is a good place to tank up on water before the final bone-dry homestretch. Note: Most maps incorrectly depict an abandoned trail here heading right up the creek to a patrol cabin and the park's northern boundary.

Beyond, the trail begins an alternating pattern of climbing up above the river and winding through massive fields of scree and lichen-encrusted glacial boulders before switchbacking down steeply to the river. Beyond the first such climb and descent, a short spur trail leads down to the viewpoint for the 15-foot Knowles Falls, ▶**21** 11.8 miles from the trailhead, where the cascade's volume is more impressive than its height.

 Waterfall

Next you reach flats leading to the hiker-only campsites 1Y2 ▶**22** (12.4 miles from the trailhead) and 1Y1, ▶**23** which is beyond an impressive narrows, 13.5 miles from the trailhead. Both of these sites front the river but are not entirely secluded from the trail. Beyond the campsites, keep an eye out for snakes on the trail and bald eagles perched in the cottonwoods. As the river calms below the falls and changes color from jade green to ashy gray, you'll see more willows along the shore and cacti near the trail. This change in flora ushers in the final hot and dry 5-mile stretch, which some hikers opt to skip by exiting via the Blacktail Deer Creek trailhead (1N5).

A Camping

The head-high browse lines visible on tree trunks indicate just how desperate some animals become during the depths of the six-month winter.

The trail slaloms through park boundary markers en route to a sturdy old wooden bridge over the appealing Bear Creek. Just past the bridge, the newly rerouted trail branches to the right, near a large, dormant thermal terrace, and starts the hot, tiring final climb up to Eagle Creek Campground, climbing 800 feet over the next 2 miles or so. After dipping into the drainage of Bear Creek, the trail switchbacks up a ridge to cross the main Gardiner–Jardine road and finally arrives at the horse corrals of Eagle Creek Campground ►24.

🚶 MILESTONES

►1   0.0 Start at Hellroaring trailhead parking lot

►2   0.7 Left at Garnet Hill Trail junction

►3   1.0 Yellowstone River suspension bridge

►4   1.6 Left at Buffalo Plateau–Coyote Creek Trail junction

►5   2.0 Left at Hellroaring junction for low-water Hellroaring Creek ford and campsites 2H2 and 2H4; right for high-water stock bridge crossing and campsites 2H6, 2H8, and 2H9

►6   2.2 Hellroaring Creek ford

►7   2.3 Straight at junction; left for campsites 2H3 and 2H1; right for campsites 2H5 and 2H7

►8   2.6 Campsite 2H1 cutoff/spur trail

►9   4.3 Campsite 1R3 spur trail

►10   4.5 Little Cottonwood Creek

►11   5.7 Wyoming–Montana state line (no sign)

►12   5.9 Campsite 1R2 spur trail

►13   6.0 Campsite 1R1; Cottonwood Creek

►14   8.3 Campsite 1Y9 spur trail

►15   9.0 Campsite 1Y7 spur trail

►16   9.8 Campsite 1Y5 spur trail

►17   10.0 Right at Blacktail Deer Creek Trail junction; left for bridge, patrol cabin, and campsites 1Y6 and 1Y8

►18   10.3 Crevice Lake

►19   10.6 Campsite 1Y4 spur trail

►20   11.4 Crevice Creek bridge

►21   11.8 Knowles Falls

►22   12.4 Campsite 1Y2 spur trail

►23   13.5 Campsite 1Y1 spur trail

►24   18.5 Arrive at Eagle Creek Campground

Fossil Forest

This short but steep and challenging ascent is the most direct of several unmarked routes that end up at Yellowstone's most fascinating and significant petrified forest, located high up a ridge, with amazing, endless views.

Best Time

There is neither shade nor water at the trailhead or along the route, so early morning or later in the afternoon is best, and be sure to carry enough water. The primary hiking season is June–October. Wildflowers are abundant after the snowmelt in July and August.

Finding the Trail

Finding the unsigned trailhead takes a bit of extra attention. From the west, head 4.1 miles east on the Northeast Entrance Road from the Tower–Roosevelt junction—1.2 miles past the signed Specimen Ridge trailhead parking area—and watch for a small, unsigned, paved turnout on the south (right) side of the road. From the east, go past the turnoff for Slough Creek Campground on Northeast Entrance Road, then 0.5 mile past the bridge over the Lamar River. Don't confuse the parking turnout you want with another signed trailhead and parking area that has a designated handicapped parking spot and is just 0.2 mile past the bridge, where an old service road heads south up the Crystal Creek drainage.

TRAIL USE
Hike

LENGTH
3.0 miles, 2–3 hours

VERTICAL FEET
±1,350

DIFFICULTY
– 1 2 3 **4** 5 +

TRAIL TYPE
Out-and-back

SURFACE TYPE
Dirt, Paved

FEATURES
Mountain
Summit
Autumn Colors
Wildflowers
Birds
Wildlife
Great Views
Photo Opportunity
Secluded
Geologic Interest
Steep

FACILITIES
None

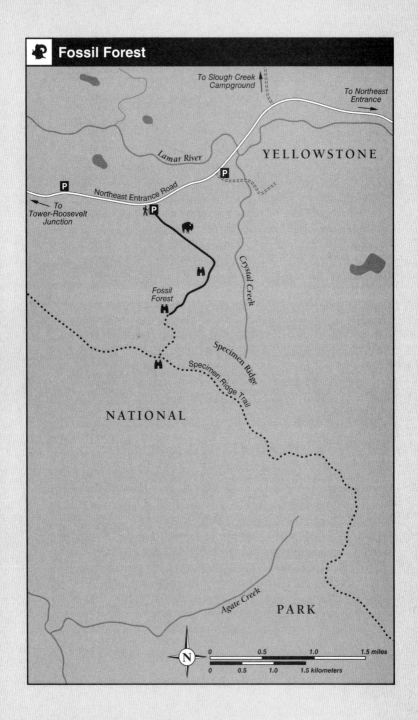

Fossil Forest

To Slough Creek
Campground

To Northeast
Entrance

YELLOWSTONE

Lamar River

P

Northeast Entrance Road

P

To
Tower-Roosevelt
Junction

P

Crystal Creek

Fossil
Forest

Specimen Ridge

Specimen Ridge Trail

NATIONAL

Agate Creek

PARK

N

0   0.5   1.0   1.5 miles

0   0.5   1.0   1.5 kilometers

Logistics

If you have binoculars, before you head out, scan the ridge from the roadside turnouts to identify your destination: a pair of large, rocky outcroppings next to a forested patch below the crest of Specimen Ridge. Once you've found the correct parking area, you should be able to identify the trail heading up the ridge with the naked eye. Be aware that the temperature changes as fast as the elevation gain. Bring a jacket, as afternoon thundershowers are common and it can get a bit brisk up top.

Trail Description

From the parking turnout, ▶1 an unsigned but well-beaten path heads south across the sagebrush foothills, through several bison wallows toward a group of lichen-encrusted, granitic glacial erratic boulders ▶2 situated atop a small rise about 0.3 mile from the road. The ensuing steep beeline up the hillside will really get your calves and heart pumping. When tired, stop and smell the blossoms: the meadows here are usually bursting with wildflowers by July.

 Wildflowers

    Watch closely as you climb, and you may begin to notice small fossilized shards. Trust me, you will be looking down at your feet a lot during this

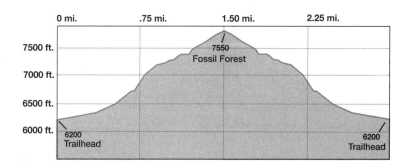

Steep athletic climb. At times it feels like you are on a StairMaster set at 10-plus.

You will begin to notice small, upright fossilized stumps off to the left as spur trails branch off near the top of the ridge. Fall colors peak here around the end of September, a bit later than elsewhere in the park. Behind you, views of the Northern Range are unsurpassed.

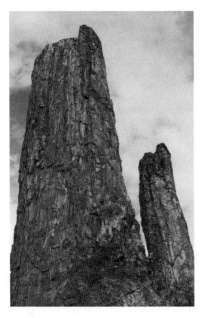

Twin petrified pine trees, *some 50 million years old, stand upright in the Fossil Forest below Specimen Ridge.*

Literally acres are littered with small shards of petrified material; you can hardly pitch a horseshoe here off the various informal trails without hitting an ossified stump: dogwoods, magnolias, oaks, walnuts, maples, and even avocado and breadfruit. As you crest the ridge, the trail joins another path trending northwest–southeast along the ridgeline. Look back north toward the trailhead to see the footprint of glacial lakes and the Absaroka Range.

Follow the ridgeline, keeping a burn area to your left and a Douglas-fir forest to your right, exploring the various unofficial "social" paths if you have the energy. Upon emerging from **Geologic Interest** a small patch of forest, a gigantic upright fossilized redwood stump ▶3 and two smaller standing pine trunks appear about 1.5 miles from the parking area. Take care on the rocky slope if you descend to inspect the redwood's exposed root structures. The silica-induced petrification occurred during volcanic phases over a 15-million-year period, starting perhaps as far back as 55 million years ago.

The National Park Service strictly prohibits the collection of any fossilized materials; please leave this mind-boggling place as you found it. (For a sad example of what can result from illegal souvenir hunting, visit the greatly diminished Petrified Tree near the Tower–Roosevelt junction. If you must take a piece of geologic history home with you, the Custer Gallatin National Forest issues permits for small-scale collection in the Tom Miner Basin).

**Geologic
Interest**

From here, you have three options: climb straight up, go straight down, or retrace your steps back to the trailhead. If you have a reserve of energy, the brisk 400-foot climb up to the top of Specimen Ridge is highly recommended. You'll be rewarded by a scenic picnic spot with breathtaking views southwest across the Grand Canyon of the Yellowstone to Mount Washburn (the lookout tower is barely visible). From the summit it's about one hour back to the trailhead. Less advisable are the steep, unstable social paths that plunge higgledy-piggledy down along the western edge of the forest.

Steep

The adjacent Crystal Creek drainage was used as an elk-trapping site in the early 1950s and was home to one of three acclimatization pens during the 1995 wolf reintroduction.

If you are feeling less spry, poke around a bit for more stumps, and then retrace your steps for the gentlest way back down to the trailhead parking area. ▶4

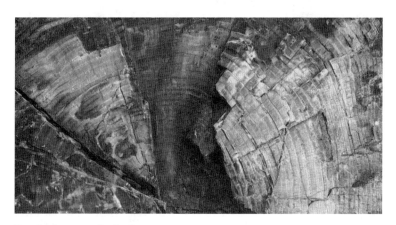

Details *of rings on a fossilized tree stump*

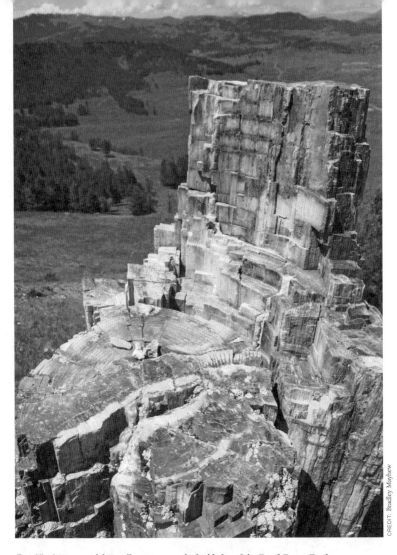

Petrified trees *and fine valley views are the highlights of the Fossil Forest Trail.*

🚶	MILESTONES
▶1	0.0 Start at unsigned parking turnout
▶2	0.3 Glacial boulders
▶3	1.5 Fossil Forest
▶4	3.0 Return to trailhead

Trout Lake

This easy, family-friendly stroll to a charming pond is especially lovely in the early-morning light, and there's some scope for simple off-trail exploring. It's a popular trail with anglers.

Best Time

The trail is accessible year-round, as the Northeast Entrance Road from Mammoth to Cooke City is open year-round, but you'll need snowshoes in winter. The trail gets warm on summer afternoons.

Finding the Trail

From the west, drive 18 miles east on the Northeast Entrance Road from Tower Junction, passing the Lamar Valley and Soda Butte before turning into the small signed parking lot on the left.

From the Northeast Entrance it's an 11-mile drive on the Northeast Entrance Road; the parking lot is 1.5 miles past the Pebble Creek Campground. The small parking lot holds only a half-dozen vehicles, so get here early. There is no toilet or water at the trailhead, but there are nearby picnic spots at the Soda Butte picnic area.

Logistics

Trout Lake is popular with anglers who come for cutthroat and rainbow trout; the cutthroat are catch-and-release only, the rainbow must be killed.

TRAIL USE
Hike

LENGTH
1.8 miles, 1.5 hours

VERTICAL FEET
Negligible (±230)

DIFFICULTY
− **1** 2 3 4 5 +

TRAIL TYPE
Out-and-back

SURFACE TYPE
Dirt

FEATURES
Child Friendly
Mountain
Lake
Cool & Shady
Great Views

FACILITIES
None

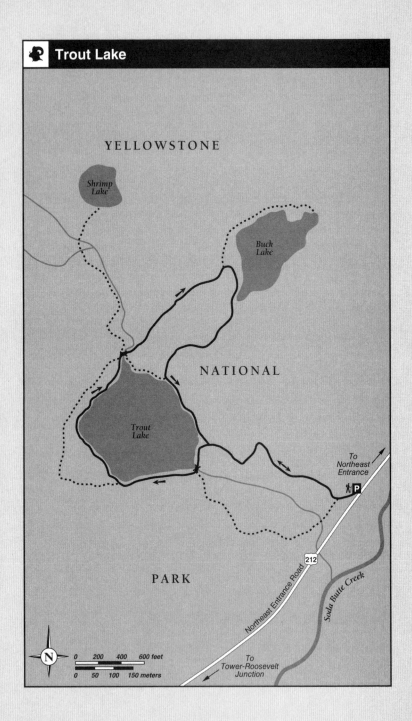

Trout Lake

YELLOWSTONE

Shrimp Lake

Buck Lake

NATIONAL

Trout Lake

To Northeast Entrance

212

Northeast Entrance Road

Soda Butte Creek

PARK

N

0   200   400   600 feet

0   50   100   150 meters

To Tower-Roosevelt Junction

Fishing starts on the Saturday of Memorial Day weekend. The inlet stream is closed to fishing at any time. You will need a Yellowstone National Park fishing permit, not a Wyoming permit.

Trail Description

As you leave the parking lot ►**1** the immediate climb might put off young families, but don't worry—the uphill section lasts less than 10 minutes. The trail climbs within earshot of the lake's outlet stream past a meadow offering views of The Thunderer peak before curving around to reach the natural bowl of Trout Lake. ►**2** Follow the trail clockwise around the lake, crossing a sturdy log bridge over the outlet stream. The craggy ridge of Mount Hornaday (10,036 feet) looms behind the lovely lake. A small clearing on the southeast side of the lake marks a minor junction where an unofficial path heads southeast for five minutes to a forested knoll boasting views of Soda Butte and the Lamar Valley beyond. Head back to the junction and continue left on the upper of two trails that offer views above the lake.

On the north side of the lake, you'll cross the inlet stream. ►**3** For the shortest version of this hike, continue around the lake and back to the parking area for a 1.2-mile hike. If you are willing to explore a bit, add on 30 minutes of walking by taking the middle path just after the inlet bridge on an unofficial but clear trail, and briefly climb a miniature ridge for an overview of Trout Lake. The clear trail then continues for five minutes to Buck Lake, ►**4** with its views of Amphitheater (10,662 feet) and Abiathar (10,928 feet) peaks near the park's northeastern border near Silver Gate.

Continue a short way around the left shore, and you'll see the main trail leading back to Trout Lake. ►**5**

Bad-weather day, or need to keep the kids occupied? Pick up the *Yellowstone: Color It Wild* coloring book, published by the Yellowstone Association, or the national park's version of Monopoly. Both are available in bookstores at the park's major visitor centers.

 Viewpoint

 Viewpoint

 Lake

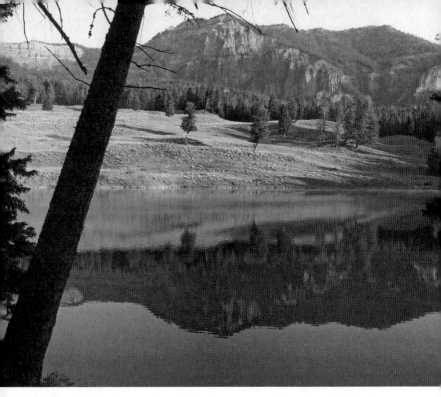

Peaceful Trout Lake *in morning light*

From Trout Lake it's a 10-minute walk downhill back to the parking lot. ►6 Back at the inlet bridge, explorers can follow paths that climb the left side of the Trout Lake inlet stream, eventually crossing the stream to climb to overgrown Shrimp Lake.

🚶	MILESTONES	
►1	0.0	Start at parking lot
►2	0.3	Trout Lake
►3	0.7	North Inlet
►4	1.0	Buck Lake
►5	1.25	Trout Lake
►6	1.8	Parking lot

Yellowstone River Picnic Area Overlook

Bring your binoculars: this easy, family-friendly hike provides opportunities to spot wildlife and offers quick access to unobstructed views of both the Grand Canyon of the Yellowstone and the Absaroka Range. Turn around wherever you like, or complete the loop by following the start of the Specimen Ridge Trail.

Best Time

The exposed trail can get hot in the summer, but it's enjoyable whenever the weather is decent. The hiking season runs May–October, making it a good early- and late-season choice. Wildflower-watchers are happiest here in spring.

Finding the Trail

From the west, go 17.5 miles east from Mammoth Hot Springs on Grand Loop Road to the Tower–Roosevelt junction. Turn left (northeast) on the Northeast Entrance Road and go 1.2 miles (0.5 mile past the Yellowstone River bridge) before turning right into a parking area just west of the signed picnic area and trailhead on the south side of the road. Leave the parking spots at the trailhead for cars using the picnic area.

From the Northeast Entrance, go 27.8 miles southwest on the Northeast Entrance Road, and turn left into the parking lot.

From Canyon Village to the south, go 19 miles north over Dunraven Pass (8,859 feet) on Grand Loop Road, and turn right (northeast) at Tower Junction; then continue 1.2 miles, and turn right into the picnic area.

TRAIL USE
Hike

LENGTH
4.0 miles, 1.5–2 hours

VERTICAL FEET
+200

DIFFICULTY
– 1 **2** 3 4 5 +

TRAIL TYPE
Out-and-back or Loop

SURFACE TYPE
Dirt

FEATURES
Child Friendly
Canyon
Wildflowers
Birds
Wildlife
Great Views
Photo Opportunity
Geologic Interest
Geothermal

FACILITIES
Restrooms
Picnic Tables

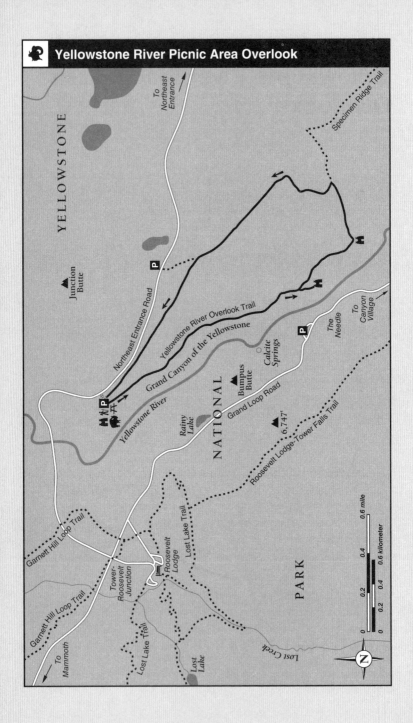

YELLOWSTONE

To Northeast Entrance

Specimen Ridge Trail

Junction Butte

P

Northeast Entrance Road

Yellowstone River Overlook Trail

Grand Canyon of the Yellowstone

To Canyon Village

The Needle

P

Calcite Springs

Bumpus Butte

Yellowstone River

Grand Loop Road

NATIONAL

Rainy Lake

6,747'

Roosevelt Lodge–Tower Falls Trail

Garnett Hill Loop Trail

Lost Lake Trail

Tower Roosevelt Junction

Roosevelt Lodge

Garnett Hill Loop Trail

To Mammoth

Lost Lake Trail

Lost Lake

Lost Creek

PARK

0.6 mile

0.4

0.6 kilometer

0.2

0.4

0.2

0

0

N

In the parking area, ignore several unofficial social trails; the official (signed) trailhead is by the picnic table just to the left (east) of the restroom. All the trails end up in the same place.

Trail Description

In the picnic area, ▶1 look for the trailhead on the east side of the parking lot. The earthen trail climbs 200 feet in the first few hundred yards for a breathtaking start to a breathtaking hike.

Once atop the hill, stop for a peek down into The Narrows of the Grand Canyon of the Yellowstone ▶2 some 800 feet below. Can you hear the river roar? Take extra care with the kids near the precipitous canyon rim—there are no safety railings here in the backcountry. The Tower–Canyon road and its overhanging cliffs of columnar basalt, remnants of former lava flows, are visible across the canyon. Keep your eyes out for bighorn sheep scampering along the canyon's sheer walls.

 Canyon

 Wildlife

About halfway along the trail, at 1.2 miles, you don't need an acute sense of smell to pick up on the sulfur odor wafting out of the active Calcite Springs ▶3 thermal area on the opposite side of the canyon. Look for ospreys in the canyon, as fabulous views open up of the breccia towers that loom above the Yellowstone River.

 Geothermal

After 2 miles, the route reaches a viewpoint and potential picnic spot at a three-way junction with the Specimen Ridge Trail. ▶4 Below you lies the Bannock Ford, a wide and shallow crossing of the Yellowstone River that was a favorite of Bannock hunters as they traversed the park. From here, you can either retrace your steps to the trailhead or continue along the trail, taking the left fork at the junction with the Specimen Ridge Trail toward the Specimen Ridge trailhead (2K4) to finally loop left back to the picnic area and parking lot. ▶5

Bannock Trail

The Bannock Trail was probably used off and on for centuries by American Indian tribes. Its current name comes from its frequent use in the 1800s by the Bannock, who crossed the Yellowstone Plateau when heading for the plains east of the park to hunt bison, after the totem animal was exterminated from the Snake River Plains, the tribe's homeland. They crossed the Yellowstone River upstream from its confluence with Tower Creek, in the canyon far below the junction with the Specimen Ridge Trail. Many people have assumed this ford was an ancient crossing. However, archaeological investigations have found no evidence of repeated, long-term use.

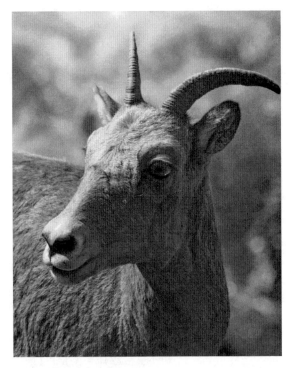

Female bighorn sheep *are frequently seen scampering down-canyon to the Yellowstone River.*

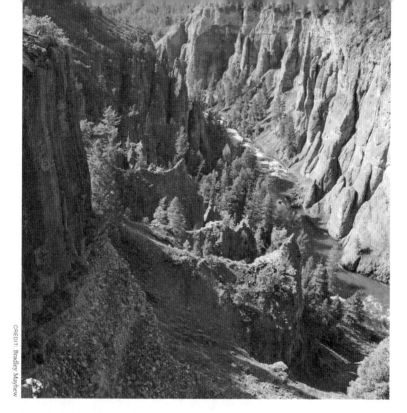

Basalt cliffs *line the Narrows section of the Yellowstone River.*

Both return routes require approximately the same amount of time and effort. If opting for the loop, watch closely for an unsigned and easily missed path heading off to the left just before you reach the road to avoid having to finish up this otherwise scenic final stretch on the pavement.

MILESTONES

▶1   0.0 Start at Yellowstone River Picnic Area trailhead
▶2   0.2 Grand Canyon of the Yellowstone overlook
▶3   1.2 Calcite Springs Overlook
▶4   2.0 Specimen Ridge Trail junction
▶5   4.0 Return to parking lot

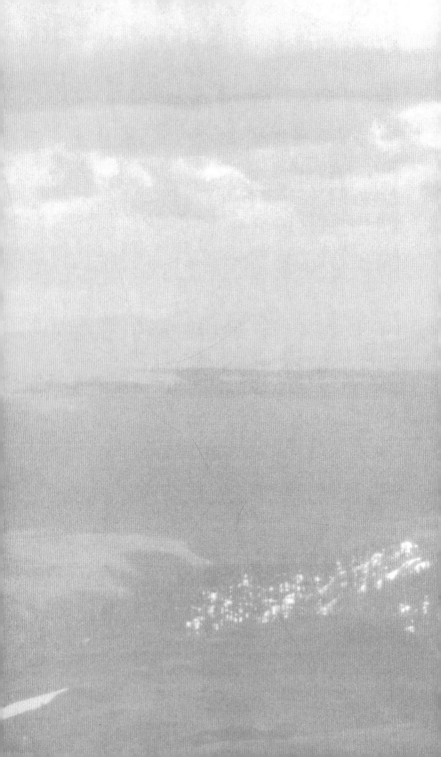

Central Yellowstone: Norris/Canyon Country

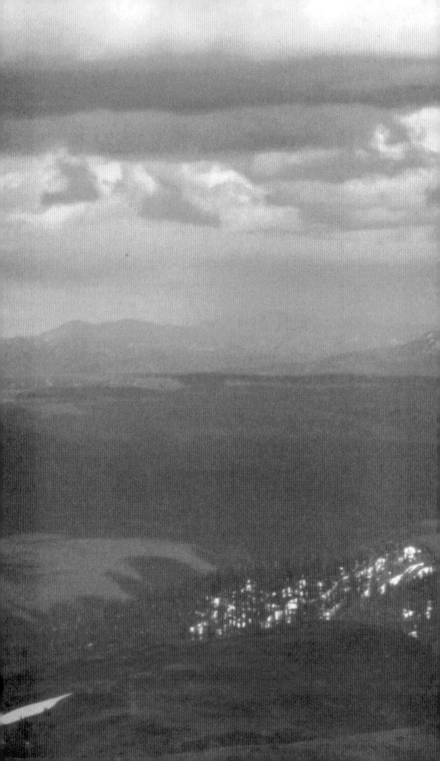

Central Yellowstone: Norris/Canyon Country

After the area around Old Faithful, Yellowstone's varied central core is the most heavily visited region of the park. The biggest crowds congregate around Canyon Village, as it is home to a concentration of visitor services, as well as the sprawling Canyon Lodge complex ($140–$265) and the forested, Xanterra-run Canyon campground ($28, including two hot showers), both open from around Memorial Day to early to mid-September.

The region's singular must-see attraction? It's the dramatic Grand Canyon of the Yellowstone. The canyon's scenic upper stretch is flush with huge waterfalls and is easily accessed from North and South Rim drives via several easy paths, scenic overlooks, and short spur trails.

The best place in the region—many say in North America—to spot wildlife is the broad Hayden Valley, a former arm of Yellowstone Lake between Canyon and Lake Junctions that attracts flocks of birds with its rich aquatic vegetation, and hordes of charismatic megafauna with its vast grasslands. Some researchers have attributed the treeless valley's lack of typical aspens and cottonwoods to the long-term absence of wolves, which allowed elk to heavily browse all the saplings. Others have suggested that flooding may have played an important role.

In the fall, legions of bison migrate across the infrequently visited Central Plateau via the Nez Perce Creek–Mary Mountain corridor to the warmth of the Firehole River Basin, as they make their way to the low-lying areas outside the park's western boundary, around West Yellowstone.

After the explosive Norris Geyser Basin, adjacent to the well-situated, National Park Service–run Norris Campground ($20, open mid-May–late September), the region's second-most dynamic thermal area is the fault-riddled Mud Volcano complex, where there's a short but worthwhile self-guided interpretive loop. The boardwalks afford a close-up whiff of several

Overleaf and opposite: *Looking north from Mount Washburn toward the Gallatin National Forest and Absaroka Range (Trail 18)*

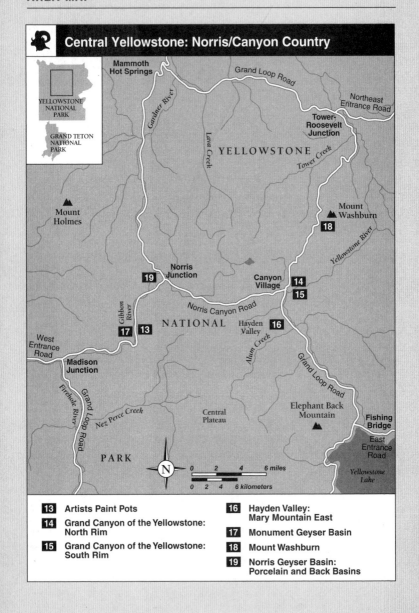

Central Yellowstone: Norris/Canyon Country

YELLOWSTONE NATIONAL PARK

GRAND TETON NATIONAL PARK

Mammoth Hot Springs

Grand Loop Road

Northeast Entrance Road

Gardner River

Lava Creek

Tower-Roosevelt Junction

Tower Creek

YELLOWSTONE

Mount Holmes

Mount Washburn

18

Yellowstone River

Norris Junction

19

Canyon Village

14

15

Norris Canyon Road

Gibbon River

17 **13**

NATIONAL

Hayden Valley

16

Alum Creek

West Entrance Road

Madison Junction

Grand Loop Road

Firehole River

Nez Perce Creek

Central Plateau

Elephant Back Mountain

Grand Loop Road

Fishing Bridge

East Entrance Road

PARK

N

| 0 | 2 | 4 | 6 miles |
| 0 | 2 | 4 | 6 kilometers |

Yellowstone Lake

13 Artists Paint Pots

14 Grand Canyon of the Yellowstone: North Rim

15 Grand Canyon of the Yellowstone: South Rim

16 Hayden Valley: Mary Mountain East

17 Monument Geyser Basin

18 Mount Washburn

19 Norris Geyser Basin: Porcelain and Back Basins

Central Yellowstone: Norris/Canyon Country

TRAIL	DIFFICULTY	LENGTH	TYPE	USES & ACCESS	TERRAIN	FLORA & FAUNA	EXPOSURE	OTHER
13	1	1.2	Loop	Day Hiking, Child-Friendly			Photo Opportunity	Geothermal, Moonlight
14	2	3.8	Point-to-point	Day Hiking, Child-Friendly, Wheelchair Access	Canyon, Stream, Waterfall	Birds	Great Views, Photo Opportunity	Geothermal, Moonlight
15	2	3.0	Point-to-point	Day Hiking, Child-Friendly, Wheelchair Access	Canyon, Stream, Waterfall	Birds	Great Views, Photo Opportunity	Historic/Secluded, Geologic Interest, Geothermal, Steep
16	4	10.0	Out-and-back	Day Hiking	Stream	Autumn Colors, Wildflowers, Birds, Wildlife	Great Views, Photo Opportunity	Geologic Interest, Geothermal
17	3	3.0	Out-and-back	Day Hiking			Great Views, Photo Opportunity	Geothermal, Geothermal, Steep
18	4	6.0	Out-and-back	Day Hiking, Bicycling, Backpacking	Mountain, Summit	Autumn Colors, Wildflowers, Birds, Wildlife	Great Views, Photo Opportunity	Camping, Historic/Secluded, Geologic Interest, Steep
19	2	2.0	Loop	Day Hiking, Child-Friendly, Wheelchair Access			Photo Opportunity	Geologic Interest, Geothermal, Moonlight

USES & ACCESS
- Day Hiking
- Bicycling
- Horses
- Backpacking
- Child-Friendly
- Wheelchair Access
- Permit

TYPE
- Loop
- Out-and-back
- Point-to-point

DIFFICULTY
- 1 2 3 4 5 +
less   more

TERRAIN
- Canyon
- Mountain
- Summit
- Lake
- Stream
- Waterfall

FLORA & FAUNA
- Autumn Colors
- Wildflowers
- Birds
- Wildlife

EXPOSURE
- Cool & Shady
- Great Views
- Photo Opportunity

OTHER
- Camping
- Swimming
- Historic/Secluded
- Geologic Interest
- Geothermal
- Moonlight
- Steep

pungent, sulfur-stinking mudpots and some of the park's most acidic hydrothermal features, which have a pH of 1–2, similar to stomach fluids or battery acid.

Adjacent to Madison Junction, the RV-friendly, Xanterra-run Madison Campground (open early May–mid-October; $23.50) is the closest camping option to Old Faithful (16 miles south) and a favorite with anglers thanks to its easy access to the world-famous Madison River. The closest showers are also in Old Faithful, but there are some nice tent-only campsites near the river, evening ranger programs, and lots of good wildlife-watching and summertime swimming nearby in the Firehole River Canyon.

During summer, rangers lead several outings around Norris and Canyon, including a 90-minute canyon rim walk from Uncle Tom's parking lot and ranger talks at Artist Point, as well as a daily 45-minute evening talk at the outdoor Canyon Campground Amphitheater. Check the current program schedule in the park newspaper, or download it from the park website.

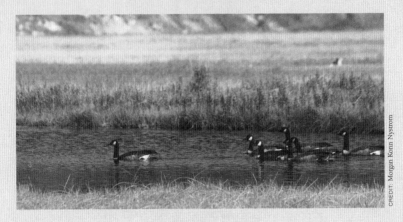

Canada geese

The 12-mile-long Norris–Canyon Road traverses the divide between the Central and Solfatara Plateaus to connect Canyon (7,734 feet) and Norris (7,484 feet) junctions via one of the park's least scenic stretches of road, known locally as "lodgepole alley."

Call 307-344-2117 before heading north from Canyon toward Tower Junction on Grand Loop Road to confirm the status of Dunraven Pass (8,859 feet) and for general Yellowstone road-construction updates.

Permits and Maps

Except for the optional overnight add-on trip to Seven Mile Hole (see Trail 18 Options, page 156), none of the hikes in this chapter requires backcountry permits.

The Canyon Visitor Education Center, which focuses on Yellowstone's volcanic landscape, features a 3-D relief map of Greater Yellowstone and interactive displays about the region's bison, the Yellowstone Volcano Observatory, and the park's geothermal features.

There's also well-stocked Yellowstone Association bookstore and a backcountry office (307-242-2550; open daily 8 a.m.–7 p.m. during the summer). You can also rent bear spray canisters for around $10 per day or $28 per week at the Bear Aware kiosk outside the Canyon visitor center; call 406-224-536 or visit bearaware.com for details.

At the entrance to the geyser basin, the Norris Geyser Basin Museum & Information Station also has helpful staff and a good bookstore (307-344-2812; open late May–October 10, daily, 9 a.m.–5 p.m.).

Fourteen miles east of the park's West Entrance (open mid-April–mid-November), the Madison Information Station has a smaller bookstore and rangers on duty until October 10 (307-344-2821; open daily, 9 a.m.–5 p.m., during the summer). The Junior Ranger Station here is a great place to bring the kids, who can get started on the park's Junior Ranger program.

National Park Service rangers and U.S. Forest Service staff are also on duty year-round, just outside the park's West Entrance at the recently expanded West Yellowstone Chamber of Commerce Visitor Center, which also houses a park backcountry office (406-646-4403; open daily, 8 a.m.–8 p.m., during the summer; winter hours are shorter). Free Wi-Fi is available here.

National Geographic's *Trails Illustrated* Yellowstone National Park map (no. 201, scale 1:126,720) depicts all the trails described in this chapter. In the same series, the individual 1:63,360 maps Tower/Canyon (no. 304), Mammoth Hot Springs (no. 303), and Old Faithful (no. 302) show the trails in greater detail and include trailheads and backcountry campsites. All of the trails are covered by single maps, with the exception of the Mary Mountain trail, which appears on portions of all three.

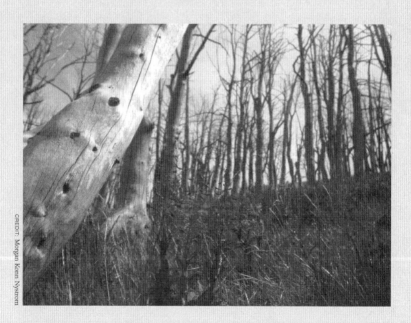

CREDIT: Morgan Konn Nystrom

Dead trees in *Mount Washburn burn area. Vegetation has regenerated since the 1988 fire, including legendary displays of summer wildflowers.*

Central Yellowstone: Norris/Canyon Country

Monument Geyser Basin 146

Aficionados of unique thermal areas will enjoy this stiff but scenic and straightforward ascent through a regenerating burn area to a seldom-visited geyser basin. Others may suspect that the lack of switchbacks on the trail is aimed at discouraging visitors.

Mount Washburn............... 151

One of the park's most popular and rewarding day hikes features great views, a gradual climb, wildflowers and loads of wildlife, plus panoramic views from a working fire lookout atop the northern end of the gigantic caldera created by the last eruption of Yellowstone's supervolcano.

Norris Geyser Basin: Porcelain and Back Basins.................... 157

Boardwalks offer an up-close look at Yellowstone's hottest and most volatile hydrothermal area. The basin is home to Steamboat Geyser, the world's largest active geyser, as well as rare acidic geysers and a fascinating assortment of other dynamic thermal features.

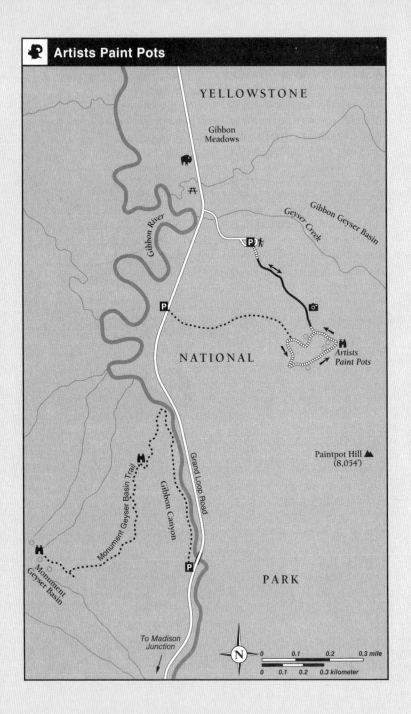

Artists Paint Pots

YELLOWSTONE

Gibbon Meadows

Gibbon River

Gibbon Geyser Basin

Geyser Creek

NATIONAL

Artists Paint Pots

Paintpot Hill ▲
(8,054')

Monument Geyser Basin Trail

Grand Loop Road

Gibbon Canyon

Monument Geyser Basin

PARK

To Madison Junction

N

| 0 | 0.1 | 0.2 | 0.3 mile |

| 0 | 0.1 | 0.2 | 0.3 kilometer |

Artists Paint Pots

Interpretive signs are lacking, but this easy loop provides an intimate overview of several types of hydrothermal features. If thermal areas pique your interest, the hike combines nicely with the steep ramble up to the nearby Monument Geyser Basin.

Best Time

The shadeless route is usually passable as soon as the park opens in late April through October. Visit early in the morning to beat the tour bus crowds. Many of the paint pots' vibrant colors get washed out after heavy precipitation.

Finding the Trail

From the north, go 3.5 miles south from Norris Canyon Road on Grand Loop Road and turn left into the well-signed parking area on the east side of the road. From the south, go 9.5 miles northwest on Grand Loop Road from Madison Junction and turn right into the parking area (which is 1 mile past the Gibbon River bridge).

Trail Description

From the east side of the large parking area, ▶1 look for the wooden footbridge, ▶2 which leads to a wide, flat gravel trail that passes through a regenerating patch of burned lodgepole pines. You can see steam plumes emanating from vents in the paint pot basin against the hillside in the background.

TRAIL USE
Hike

LENGTH
1.2 miles, up to 1 hour

VERTICAL FEET
±100

DIFFICULTY
– **1** 2 3 4 5 +

TRAIL TYPE
Loop

SURFACE TYPE
Mixed

FEATURES
Child Friendly
Photo Opportunity
Geothermal
Moonlight Hiking

FACILITIES
Picnic Tables

Paint pots (also known as mud pots when less colorful) form where sulfuric acid in the groundwater and heat-loving microorganisms conspire to break down rocks. Dissolved minerals then lend a range of red, green, and blue colors to the gloppy sort of clay.

Photo Opportunity

Geothermal

As the trail opens up and cuts right under some power lines, you can see steam from the stark-white Monument Geyser Basin high atop the ridge across Grand Loop Road.

The trail returns to a boardwalk just before reaching a junction ▶3 for the loop portion of the trail, 0.4 mile from the trailhead at the edge of the thermal basin. Many folks walk in the clockwise direction and never make it up this far to see the highlight of the trail.

Heading counterclockwise, the trail winds around past an abandoned trail, up some stairs to the biggest and best of the mud pots for an ono-matopoetic "bloop, blap, plop, ploop" symphony paired with a sulfurous beef-jerky smell—a real feast of mixed messages for the senses.

Complete the full loop for a good overview of the entire basin. Gibbon Meadows and the thermal areas around Sylvan and Evening Primrose Springs stretch out to the west, with Purple Mountain (8,391 feet) in the background to the left and Mount Holmes (10,336 feet) to the far right. The geyser and other hydrothermal features down below are actually best viewed from above.

Loop down past some fumaroles, a steamy perpetual spouter, and a connected roiling pool to a bridge spanning the thermal outlet channel. Back at the first junction, ▶4 retrace your steps to the parking area. ▶5

🚶 MILESTONES

▶1 0.0 Start at Artists Paint Pots parking area
▶2 0.1 Bridge on northeast side of parking area
▶3 0.4 Right at loop trail junction
▶4 0.8 Right at same loop trail junction
▶5 1.2 Return to parking area

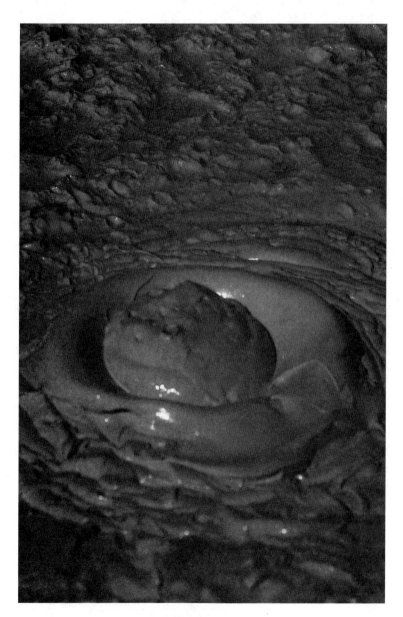

A mud pot *(also known as a paint pot) about to burp*

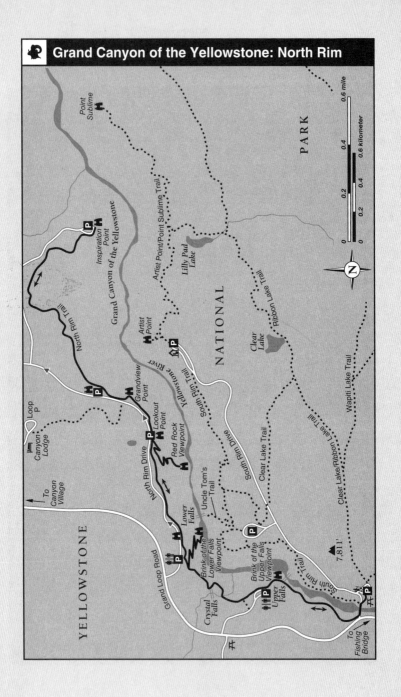

Grand Canyon of the Yellowstone: North Rim

Grand Canyon of the Yellowstone: North Rim

Although it often parallels a busy road, this popular route leads past a series of overlooks and scenic viewpoints, with a couple of opportunities to take steep detours below the canyon rim for close encounters with the impressive falls.

Best Time

The trails are most enjoyable in the early morning before the crowds descend, or around sunset. Most of the detours down to the falls can be icy in cold weather and are closed in winter. Check for seasonal closures at any visitor center.

Finding the Trail

From Canyon Village, go 2.2 miles south on Grand Loop Road and turn left (east) on South Rim Drive. Cross over the Yellowstone River on Chittenden Bridge and park in the large lot on your right, signed for the Wapiti Lake trailhead and picnic area. From the south, go 13.8 miles north on Grand Loop Road from the Fishing Bridge junction and turn right (east) at South Rim Drive.

Logistics

Set up a shuttle by leaving a vehicle in the parking loop at Inspiration Point, 1.6 miles southeast of Canyon Village at the end of a well-signed dead-end road, just past the smaller turnout for the Glacial Boulder trailhead. Otherwise, it's a 3-mile walk back along the road or trail to Chittenden Bridge.

TRAIL USE
Hike

LENGTH
3.8 miles, 2–3 hours

VERTICAL FEET
±1,200 including detours

DIFFICULTY
– 1 **2** 3 4 5 +

TRAIL TYPE
Point-to-point

SURFACE TYPE
Dirt, Paved

FEATURES
Child Friendly
Handicap Access
Canyon
Stream
Waterfall
Birds
Great Views
Photo Opportunity
Geothermal
Moonlight Hiking

FACILITIES
Visitor Center
Restrooms
Picnic Tables
Phone

Construction projects are scheduled in the Canyon region until 2020. Inspiration Point and the section of trail around Crystal Falls were closed to visitors in 2016 but should have reopened by the time you read this. Other viewpoints on the north rim are due for renovation in the coming years and could be inaccessible. Check with the visitor center to see if this hike has been affected.

You can make a leisurely full day of it by combining this hike with the canyon's equally impressive South Rim route (see Trail 15, page 136).

Trail Description

Ignore the Howard Eaton and Wapiti Lake Trails that head out from the far (east) side of the parking area. ▶1 Instead, walk back across Chittenden Bridge, and watch for traffic as you cross the road to the start of the North Rim Trail. ▶2

Follow the old road as it traces the western bank of the Yellowstone River 0.5 mile to the signed turnoff on your right for the overlook of the gushing Brink of the Upper Falls. ▶3 A short set of steps leads down and around to the actual brink, ▶4 where the Yellowstone River plummets 109 feet—stop before you get to the bottom to look for rainbows and to listen to the roar. Afterward, retrace your steps to the large parking lot at the top of the staircase. ▶5

Continue to your right through the parking lot and past the restrooms a few hundred yards; then turn right on the signed continuation of the North Rim Trail. ▶6 After the trail approaches the canyon rim, detour to your right on a short path to an overlook of the much smaller, three-stage Crystal Falls, ▶7 the graceful tail end of Cascade Creek.

Glacial meltwater carved out the canyon some 14,000 years ago. The colorful patches of orange, green, and brown rocks in the canyon walls near the river indicate active thermal areas.

Waterfall ▐▌

Waterfall ▐▌

Opposite: *Visitors enjoy dramatic views over the Lower Falls of the Yellowstone River from the Brink of the Lower Falls viewpoint.*

CREDIT: Bradley Mayhew

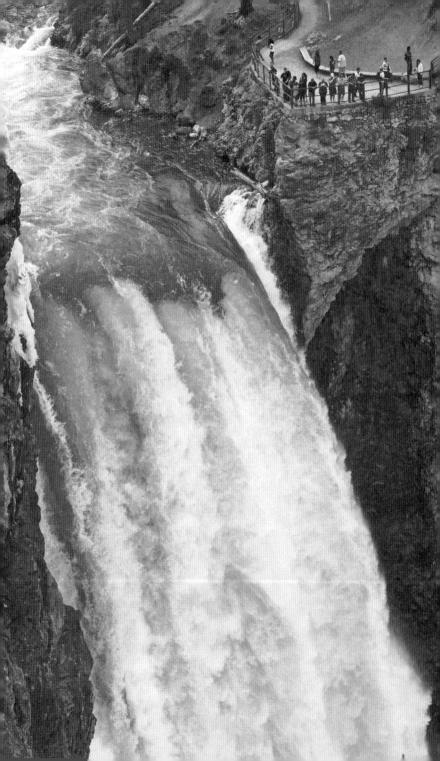

The Grand Canyon of the Yellowstone is 20 miles long, 800–1,200 feet deep, and 1,500–4,000 feet wide.

It's best viewed from across the canyon at Uncle Tom's Point.

Follow the trail away from the canyon rim and turn right at the signed path to the viewpoint for the Brink of the Lower Falls, ▶8 where a series of switchbacks drops down 600 feet toward the base of the stupendous, 308-foot cataract. Not far down the 0.5-mile side trail ▶9 (closed in winter), you'll see the brink and can catch a glimpse of the Upper Falls upstream. Even if you aren't inclined to hike all the way down to the bottom to look for rainbows and feel the spray, ▶10 it's worth at least a short detour.

If you haven't set up a shuttle, the Lower Falls overlook is a logical point to retrace your steps to the trailhead parking lot.

Back up top, turn right and walk alongside the one-way road paralleling the canyon rim for a few hundred yards past some restrooms. Turn right on the paved trail at the parking turnout for Lookout Point ▶11 for the best views of the Lower Falls. Visible below to your right is the steep paved Red Rock Trail, ▶12 which drops 500 feet in 0.25 mile for yet another scenic and misty look up-canyon.

Back at the Lookout Point parking area, ▶13 turn right and follow the path alongside the road up to the parking area for Grandview Point, ▶14 where benches hewn from glacial boulders provide a nice picnic spot with views down the colorful canyon.

Viewpoint

Photo Opportunity

Here, the unpaved trail forks to the right, away from the road, to end up at the Inspiration Point ▶15 parking loop. Steps (which were renovated in 2016) lead down past inviting benches with views of birds and thermal features in the multicolored canyon to yet another dramatic overlook.

🚶	**MILESTONES**
▶1	0.0 Start at Wapiti Lake parking area
▶2	0.1 Right at North Rim Trail
▶3	0.5 Right at Brink of the Upper Falls overlook
▶4	0.7 Brink of the Upper Falls
▶5	0.9 Right at Upper Falls parking lot
▶6	1.0 Right on North Rim Trail
▶7	1.1 Right to Crystal Falls overlook
▶8	1.3 Right at Brink of the Lower Falls overlook
▶9	1.8 Brink of the Lower Falls
▶10	2.3 Right on North Rim Trail
▶11	2.5 Right at Lookout Point
▶12	2.75 Viewpoint at end of Red Rock Trail
▶13	3.0 Right on road
▶14	3.2 Grandview Point
▶15	3.8 Arrive at Inspiration Point parking area

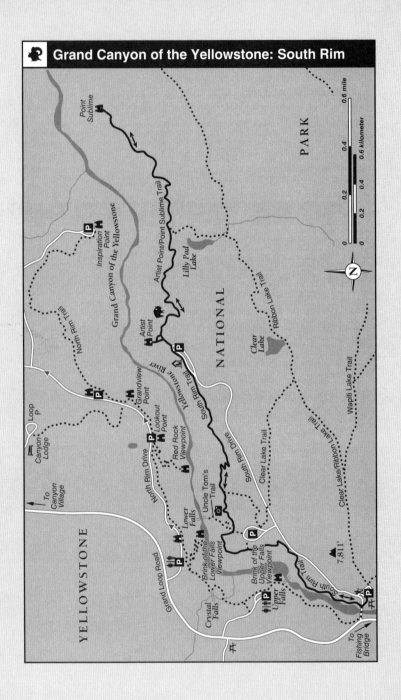

Point Sublime

Artist Point/Point Sublime Trail

Inspiration Point

Grand Canyon of the Yellowstone

Lilly Pad Lake

PARK

Artist Point

Yellowstone River

North Rim Trail

Grandview Point

Lookout Point

Red Rock Viewpoint

North Rim Drive

Canyon Lodge

Loop P

To Canyon Village

South Rim Trail

NATIONAL

Clear Lake

Ribbon Lake Trail

Wapiti Lake Trail

South Rim Drive

Clear Lake Trail

Lake Trail

Clear Lake/Ribbon Lake Trail

Uncle Tom's Trail

Lower Falls

Brink of the Lower Falls Viewpoint

Brink of the Upper Falls Viewpoint

Grand Loop Road

Crystal Falls

Upper Falls

7,811'

South Rim Trail

To Fishing Bridge

YELLOWSTONE

Grand Canyon of the Yellowstone: South Rim

Although parts of this popular route parallel the busy South Rim Drive, the partially paved trail winds in and out of enough forests to provide some serenity. It's a great place to get out of the car to stretch your legs and lungs during a long drive around the Grand Loop.

Best Time

The colors in the canyon are most vibrant at sunrise and especially sunset, when crowds are thinnest. Uncle Tom's Trail is closed all winter, and in spring and fall if icy. Check for seasonal closures at any visitor center.

Finding the Trail

From Canyon Village, go 2.2 miles south on Grand Loop Road and turn left (east) on South Rim Drive. Cross over the Yellowstone River on Chittenden Bridge and park in the large lot on your right, signed for the Wapiti Lake trailhead and picnic area. From the south, go 13.8 miles north on Grand Loop Road from the Fishing Bridge junction and turn right (east) at South Rim Drive.

Logistics

Arrange a shuttle by leaving a car at the busy Artist Point parking lot. Doing this hike in the opposite direction and combining it with the canyon's equally impressive North Rim Trail makes for a leisurely, full-day excursion of around 8 miles (see Trail 14, page 130).

TRAIL USE
Hike

LENGTH
4.0 miles, 1.5–2.5 hours

VERTICAL FEET
±500 including Uncle Tom's Trail

DIFFICULTY
– 1 **2** 3 4 5 +

TRAIL TYPE
Point-to-point

SURFACE TYPE
Dirt, Paved

FEATURES
Child Friendly
Handicap Access
Canyon
Steep
Stream
Waterfall
Birds
Great Views
Photo Opportunity
Historic Interest
Geologic Interest
Geothermal
Moonlight Hiking

FACILITIES
Restrooms
Picnic Tables

137

Construction projects in the canyon region are scheduled until 2020, so check with the visitor center to see which viewpoints are off-limits and if this hike has been affected.

Trail Description

Ignore the Howard Eaton and Wapiti Lake Trails that head out from the far (east) side of the parking area. ►1 Instead, walk back toward Chittenden Bridge, and watch for traffic as you cross the road just before the bridge to the start of the South Rim Trail. ►2

Waterfall

Viewpoint

The trail rises slightly, then drops down alongside the river after 0.6 mile for stellar views from the Upper Falls overlook, ►3 just before the restrooms and parking loop for Uncle Tom's Trail. ►4 When not closed in winter or due to icy conditions, the steep paved paths and hundreds of steel stairs, which descend 500 feet along a historic route, provide an unparalleled, close-up view of the Lower Falls. From the platform at the bottom, ►5 you not only see but also hear and feel the 308-foot falls'

OPTIONS

Ribbon Lake Overnight

Ribbon Lake is a great first-time overnight option, just over 2 miles (about an hour) from the Artist Point/Ribbon Lake trailhead. Take care with wandering kids along this trail—there's a refreshing lack of railings here.

Loop Options

To avoid the hassle of arranging a shuttle, it's possible to do a longer 5.6-mile loop by taking the trail to the south at Lilly Pad Lake Cutoff, halfway between Artist Point and Point Sublime. Then return west along Ribbon Lake Trail, past a minor thermal area around Clear Lake, all the way to the Wapiti Lake Trailhead.

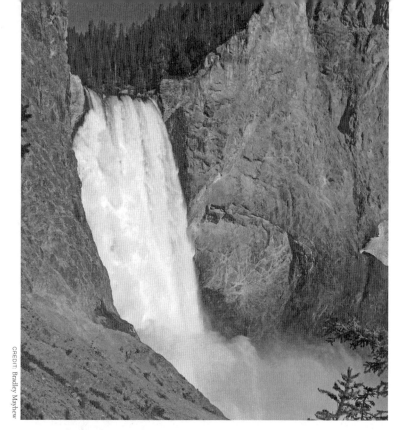

Lower Falls of the Yellowstone River, *seen from Uncle Tom's Trail on the South Rim of the Yellowstone canyon*

might. Not everyone can make this steep, vertigo-inspiring descent, but if you're able, it's worth every huff and puff on the return ascent.

Back up top, steer clear of the parking lot and continue left on the South Rim Trail, ▶6 which traces the canyon rim out of sight of the road for 0.8 mile. You rejoin the road just before the parking loop for Artist Point, ▶7 where a set of stunning overlooks attracts photographers by the busload.

Landscape painter Thomas Moran observed that "the canyon's beautiful tints were beyond the reach of human art," but that doesn't seem to stop folks from trying to capture them. If you have binoculars, it's also a fine point to scan the canyon walls for the nests of raptors, ravens, and swallows.

 Steep

 Viewpoint

 Photo Opportunity

Uncle Tom–Foolery

Uncle Tom Richardson was a pioneering entrepreneurial guide who rigged a Rube Goldberg–esque series of ropes, ladders, and stairs and then charged tourists to scramble 500 feet down into the canyon to the base of the Lower Falls.

Most people turn back here, but even more superlative views await 0.5 mile beyond the Lilly Pad Lake junction ▶8 and a total of 1 mile beyond the Artist Point/Ribbon Lake trailhead (4K8) at Point Sublime, ▶9 a relatively flat, one-hour round-trip from Artist Point. After enjoying the views, return to your car at Artist Point. ▶10

MILESTONES

▶1   0.0 Start at Wapiti Lake parking area
▶2   0.1 Right at South Rim Trail
▶3   0.7 Upper Falls overlook
▶4   0.8 Left at Uncle Tom's Trail
▶5   1.0 Lower Falls viewing platform
▶6   1.2 Left on South Rim Trail
▶7   2.0 Artist Point
▶8   2.5 Straight at Lilly Pad Lake cutoff
▶9   3.0 Arrive at Point Sublime
▶10 4.0 Return to Artist Point

Hayden Valley: Mary Mountain East

The first few miles of the eastern end of this often-overlooked trail meander along the forested northern edge of the wide-open Hayden Valley through open sagelands and prime habitat for bison, coyotes, and grizzlies. Expect to see lots of birds and animals—and to get your feet wet—in one of the best places in the park to see a variety of wildlife. This is a good option for experienced hikers.

Best Time

The low-lying portions of the trail are usually boggy: Check with a ranger station or visitor center for current conditions, especially early or late in the season. The western half of the trail is closed March 10–June 15 from Mary Lake to the western Nez Perce trailhead because of bear-management restrictions.

Finding the Trail

From the north, go 4.5 miles south on Grand Loop Road from Canyon Village and turn left into the small Mary Mountain trailhead parking turnout. The turnout is just north of the Alum Creek pullout on the east side of the road and is sometimes referred to as the Alum Creek trailhead. From the south, go 11.5 miles north on Grand Loop Road from Fishing Bridge and turn right into the turnout.

Logistics

Aside from a possible dip in fishless Mary Lake, this route's most interesting sections are within the first 5 miles of its eastern trailhead. Because overnight

TRAIL USE
Hike

LENGTH
10.0 miles, 5 hours

VERTICAL FEET
Negligible

DIFFICULTY
– 1 2 3 **4** 5 +

TRAIL TYPE
Out-and-back

SURFACE TYPE
Dirt

FEATURES
Stream
Autumn Colors
Wildflowers
Birds
Wildlife
Great Views
Photo Opportunity
Geologic Interest
Geothermal

FACILITIES
None

141

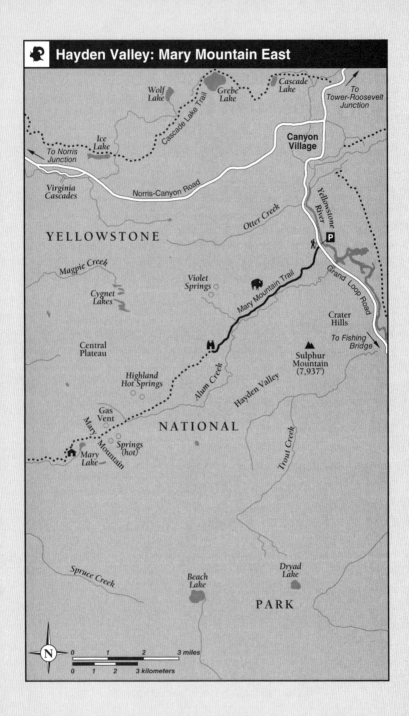

Hayden Valley: Mary Mountain East

Wolf Lake

Grebe Lake

Cascade Lake

Cascade Lake Trail

To Tower-Roosevelt Junction

Ice Lake

Canyon Village

To Norris Junction

Virginia Cascades

Norris-Canyon Road

Otter Creek

Yellowstone River

YELLOWSTONE

Magpie Creek

Cygnet Lakes

Violet Springs

Mary Mountain Trail

Grand Loop Road

Crater Hills

To Fishing Bridge

Central Plateau

Alum Creek

Sulphur Mountain (7,937')

Highland Hot Springs

Hayden Valley

Gas Vent

NATIONAL

Mary Mountain

Springs (hot)

Trout Creek

Mary Lake

Spruce Creek

Beach Lake

Dryad Lake

PARK

N

0   1   2   3 miles
0   1   2   3 kilometers

camping is banned en route due to heavy bear and bison activity, most everyone hikes this trail as an out-and-back route. When open, the Mary Mountain traverse can be done one-way in one long day in either direction with a car shuttle; hiking from west to east adds 400 feet of elevation gain.

Check with the Canyon Ranger Station for updates on current wildlife activity, closures, and restrictions. The trail was closed for much of summer 2016 due to fires and carcasses on the trail. A good topo map, compass, and route-finding skills are often necessary in much of the Hayden Valley, as bison like to use trail markers as scratching posts and knock them down faster than intrepid National Park Service trail crews can resurrect them. Whatever you do, do not attempt to walk through the middle of a bison herd. When in doubt, detour widely or turn around.

If at all possible, hike in a group, avoid hiking at dusk, and bring bear spray. Seasonal park-concessionaire employees have been attacked by grizzlies in the Hayden Valley, and in August 2011 a hiker was killed by a grizzly while hiking alone on the Mary Mountain Trail.

Trail Description

Take care when crossing the busy Grand Loop Road to the Mary Mountain trailhead. ►1 Take a deep breath of fresh air and turn your bison and grizzly sensors on high alert as you start out by skirting the forested northern edge of the wide-open Hayden Valley.

 Wildlife

The perennially boggy trail wanders through rolling sagebrush and traces the treeline above the appealing, thermally fed Alum Creek. Keep your binoculars at the ready not only to spot potentially hazardous wildlife encounters but also to scan the creek's mud flats for abundant raptors and water birds, including herons, American dippers, ducks,

 Birds

Mary Lake and Mary Mountain Traverse

Although camping is prohibited along the route, it's possible to traverse the vast, undeveloped Central Plateau by climbing a total of 500 feet in 21 miles in an epic day hike; you'll end up in the Firehole River basin and so will need to arrange a shuttle. Check with backcountry rangers before planning this hike, however, since it's often off-limits due to wildlife activity.

Seven miles beyond the eastern trailhead, the route enters an unburned alley of lodgepole pines—a veritable bison highway—atop the wild Central Plateau. The trail climbs gradually for 2 miles past dusty bison wallows and sulfurous gas vents to the barren Highland Hot Springs thermal area, beyond an easy ford of an unnamed creek.

Following the historic Mary Mountain stagecoach route, the trail tops out near the western shore of the tranquil 20-acre Mary Lake. The fishless lake attracts lots of birds and is a nice spot for a shady picnic or a refreshing quick dip in the middle of a long, hot day.

geese, pelicans, bald eagles, northern harriers, and nesting sandhill cranes.

Fortunately, the lack of trees in the valley, caused by deposits of fine-grained glacial sediments some 13,000 or 14,000 years ago, means the vistas are mostly open. Meadows outcompete trees in the resulting impermeable clay soils here, so the few lodgepole islands appear in outcroppings of volcanic rock. Grizzlies like to lurk around the valley's forested edges, however, especially in the spring and early summer, when they prey on newborn bison and elk calves. Mature bison are often hidden while they sleep behind large sagebrush bushes and are most unpredictable during the fall mating season, which starts in late July or early August.

Most day hikers take their time and make it only 4 miles from the trailhead, to the easy ford of Violet Creek, ►2 where there are several interesting off-trail thermal areas. Over the next mile, you'll climb a few hundred feet to reach a nice viewpoint

Viewpoint 🔭

▶3 above the western end of the Hayden Valley; it's a great place to watch wildlife. Take care to stick to the main trail: the orange-blazed posts are often toppled by itchy bison.

If you are not continuing on the optional extension to Mary Lake (see left), retrace your steps to return to the eastern Mary Mountain trailhead. ▶4

🚶 MILESTONES

▶1   0.0 Start at Mary Mountain trailhead
▶2   4.0 Cross Violet Creek
▶3   5.0 Hayden Valley viewpoint
▶4   10.0 Return to Mary Mountain trailhead

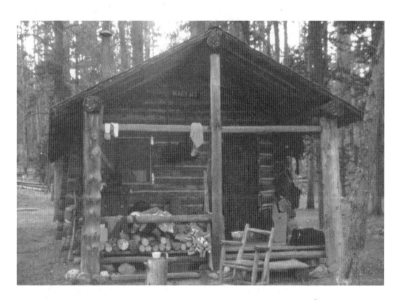

Mary Mountain Patrol Cabin: *Sorry—for National Park Service use only!*

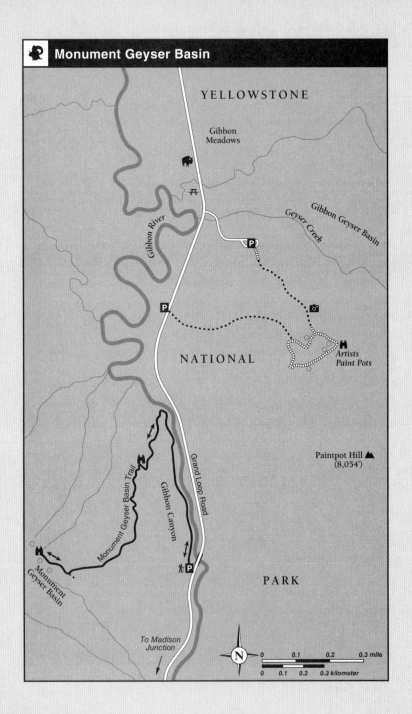

Monument Geyser Basin

YELLOWSTONE

Gibbon Meadows

Gibbon River

Geyser Creek

Gibbon Geyser Basin

P

NATIONAL

Artists Paint Pots

P

Monument Geyser Basin Trail

Gibbon Canyon

Grand Loop Road

Paintpot Hill (8,054')

PARK

Monument Geyser Basin

To Madison Junction

N

| 0 | 0.1 | 0.2 | 0.3 mile |

| 0 | 0.1 | 0.2 | 0.3 kilometer |

Monument Geyser Basin

Since there are few switchbacks, you may get the feeling that this route to a seldom-visited geyser basin was designed to discourage visitors. If you are an aficionado of geothermal activity, however, the unique juice at the end of the stiff, shadeless climb is worth the squeeze.

Best Time

Because the remote basin tops out around 8,000 feet, it's best to wait until snow has melted off the steep trail, usually by late June or early July. Check conditions with rangers before heading out in October. There is little shade and no water along the trail, so plan accordingly.

Finding the Trail

From the north, go 4.6 miles south from Norris Canyon Road (a mile south of the Artists Paint Pots, just past the Gibbon River bridge) on Grand Loop Road and turn right into the small gravel parking pullout on the west (right) side of the road (if this is full, there is another just to the south). From the south, go 8.4 miles north of Madison Junction on Grand Loop Road and carefully turn left across oncoming traffic into the turnout just before the bridge. Look for a trailhead signboard just off the road to confirm that you are on the right track.

TRAIL USE
Hike

LENGTH
3.0 miles, 1.5–2 hours

VERTICAL FEET
±650

DIFFICULTY
– 1 2 **3** 4 5 +

TRAIL TYPE
Out-and-back

SURFACE TYPE
Dirt

FEATURES
Steep
Birds
Great Views
Photo Opportunity
Secluded
Geothermal

FACILITIES
None

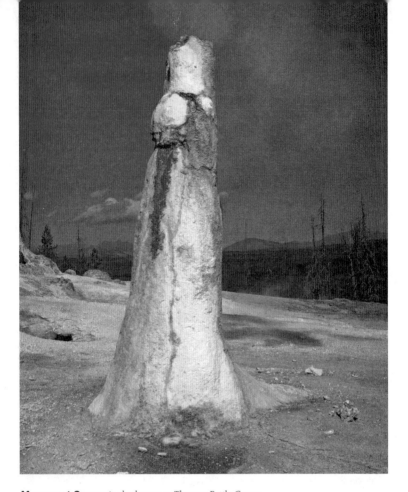

Monument Geyser is also known as Thermos Bottle Geyser.

Trail Description

From the small parking turnout, ▶1 sign in at the trailhead register ▶2 and follow the single-track earthen trail upstream along the crystal-clear Gibbon River. The narrow trail is hemmed in by dense stands of lodgepole saplings that have enthusiastically sprouted since the 1988 North Fork fire.

Steep

Birds

After 0.3 mile ▶3 the trail swings around the ridge and away from the river and begins its short but stiff and unrelenting ascent. For a break, look for honking Canada geese and browsing elk below, around the oxbows in the vast Gibbon Meadows. The small thermal areas visible along both banks of the Gibbon only hint at what awaits up top.

The straight-ahead climb lacks switchbacks and shade. Catch your breath in the shadow of one of the few remaining lodgepole pine snags, and enjoy the ever-expanding views north and south.

Whew! The trail finally tops out at an unsigned junction ▶4 near an overlook of Gibbon Canyon. Head right along the flat ridgetop and follow your nose to the sulfur smell and the most active part of the thought-provoking Monument Geyser Basin. ▶5

 Viewpoint

The highlight of the basin is the eponymous Monument Geyser (also known as Thermos Bottle Geyser), a steaming, 8-foot-tall spire on the far side of the basin that was created when silica precipitated out of water. Other visible thermal features include a variety of active and inactive geyser spires, steaming fumaroles (scalding steam vents), bubbling frying pans, turbid milky pools, and highly acidic

 Geothermal

Stick to the Edges

The thin crust in the basin is extremely fragile, and the subsurface is superheated. Stay behind the downed limbs marking the solid edge of the basin and check things out from near the treeline. The shady areas here make a nice picnic spot.

Submerged Geyser Basin Spires

Geoscientists recently discovered that the profile of Monument Geyser Basin's spires closely resembles that of submerged spire fields beneath Yellowstone Lake. Researchers continue to study the complex of coalesced spires near Mary Bay with remotely operated underwater vehicles. Diatom fossils and lake sediments collected from Monument Geyser Basin suggest that the area was likely covered by a glacial lake more than 10,000 years ago.

mud pots. For a clue as to why you should not venture out into the basin, listen for hollow thumping sounds coming from beneath your feet.

When you've finished exploring, retrace your steps downhill to the trailhead—don't forget to sign out at the trail register—and parking area. ▶6

🚶	MILESTONES

▶1 0.0 Start at Monument Geyser Basin parking turnout
▶2 0.1 Trailhead sign and trail register
▶3 0.3 Trail swings left above Gibbon Meadows; begin climb
▶4 1.4 Right at unsigned junction and Gibbon Canyon overlook
▶5 1.5 Monument Geyser Basin
▶6 3.0 Return to trailhead parking turnout

Mount Washburn

The park's most popular day hike starts out high and continues climbing gradually along old roads and passes wildlife-rich wildflower meadows en route to a spectacular summit with panoramic views from a working fire lookout.

Best Time

The trail is hikable May–October, with a good chance of encountering passable snowdrifts at higher elevations early and late in the season. Frequent afternoon lightning and thundershowers, and a trailhead that's often full after 10 a.m., mean it's best to head out as early as possible. Wildflower displays are legendary from around late July to early August, while elk, grizzlies, and bighorn sheep (don't feed them, and keep your distance) can be spotted throughout the summer.

Bear-management areas adjacent to Dunraven Pass and the Chittenden Road trail are off-limits for much of the year, so obey posted signs and don't stray from the trail.

Finding the Trail

From the south, go 4.5 miles north from Canyon Village on Grand Loop Road—a couple of miles past the Dunraven Picnic Area—and turn right into the frequently full Dunraven Pass trailhead parking area on the east side of the road. From the north, go 32 miles south from Mammoth on Grand Loop Road and turn left into the Dunraven Pass trailhead parking area.

TRAIL USE
Hike, Bike
LENGTH
6.0 miles, 3–4 hours
VERTICAL FEET
±1,400
DIFFICULTY
– 1 2 3 **4** 5 +
TRAIL TYPE
Out-and-back
SURFACE TYPE
Dirt, Paved

FEATURES
Mountain
Summit
Autumn Colors
Birds
Wildlife
Wildflowers
Great Views
Photo Opportunity
Camping
Historic Interest
Geologic Interest
Steep

FACILITIES
Restrooms
Picnic Tables
Phone
Water

151

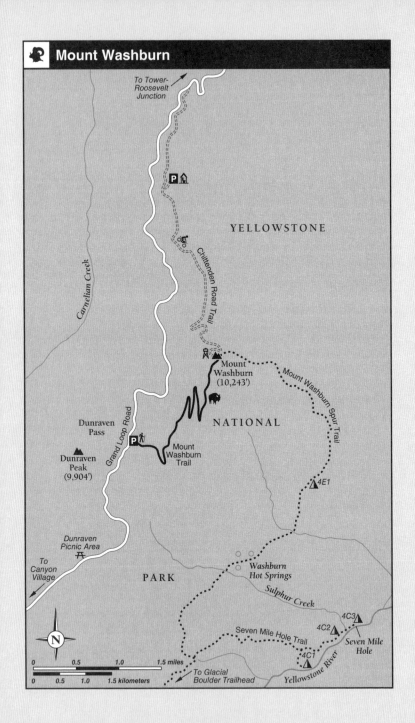

Mount Washburn

To Tower-Roosevelt Junction

YELLOWSTONE

Carnelian Creek

Chittenden Road Trail

Mount Washburn (10,243')

Mount Washburn Spur Trail

NATIONAL

Dunraven Pass

Mount Washburn Trail

Dunraven Peak (9,904')

Grand Loop Road

4E1

Dunraven Picnic Area

To Canyon Village

PARK

Washburn Hot Springs

Sulphur Creek

4C3

4C2

Seven Mile Hole Trail

Seven Mile Hole

4C1

N

Yellowstone River

| 0 | 0.5 | 1.0 | 1.5 miles |
| 0 | 0.5 | 1.0 | 1.5 kilometers |

To Glacial Boulder Trailhead

Logistics

At the time of research, rangers were leading hikes up Mount Washburn once a week. Group size is limited to 20, so reserve a spot by calling 307-344-2550. Check the park newspaper for current schedules as these change often. Pack wind and raingear in case of foul weather up top.

Trail Description

From Dunraven Pass ▶1 (8,859 feet), a wide, abandoned road—originally engineered in 1905 for wagons and stagecoaches—climbs steadily and scenically through subalpine fir forest to a small gap, a nice stop for a short rest.

About halfway up, as glimpses of the lookout atop the summit appear, broad switchbacks swing northeast up the ridge, and views of the Grand Canyon of the Yellowstone and the Yellowstone River drainage open up to the east (right). The higher up you go, the more likely you are to see stunted whitebark pines (a favorite grub source for grizzlies) as well as pikas, marmots, and Rocky Mountain bighorn sheep.

Half a mile beyond the switchbacks, the road reaches a three-way junction ▶2 with the Chittenden

Automobiles were first allowed into the park in 1915. Horse-drawn wagons were banned the next year. Because early Model T Fords lacked fuel pumps, they had to back up the mountain in reverse.

 Wildlife

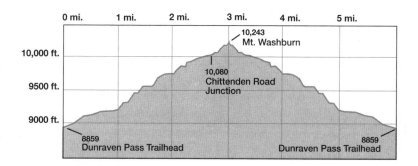

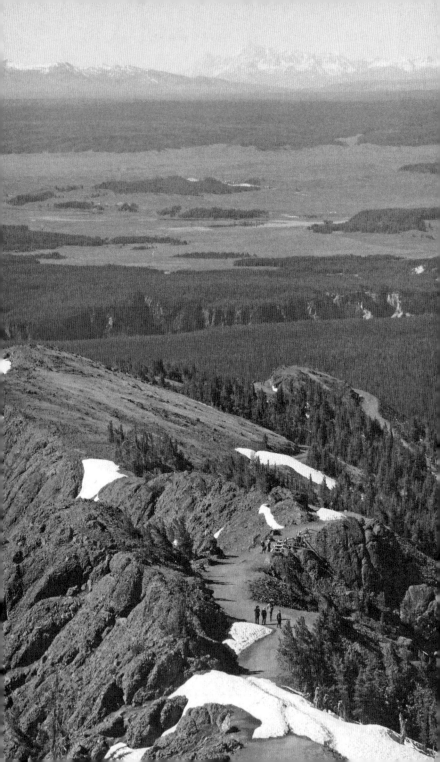

Road Trail and Mount Washburn Spur Trail. Follow the road uphill as it curves around to the left to arrive at the three-story Mount Washburn Lookout Tower (10,243 feet). ▶3

Despite the working fire lookout (the park's only lookout that is staffed all summer), Mount Washburn's slopes burned heavily during the 1988 fires. In addition to an outhouse, a guest logbook, interpretive geology displays, and a powerful telescope in the sheltered ground-level observation room, the lookout offers incredible panoramas of most of the park from upstairs on the outdoor viewing platform. (The Mount Washburn Web cam streams live at tinyurl.com/yellowstonewebcams.) There is no water at the lookout.

On a clear day, the expansive views can stretch anywhere from 20 to 50 miles in all directions. The Absaroka Range extends beyond the park boundaries to the north and east. To the south is the Hayden Valley, Yellowstone Lake, and Mount Sheridan—the southern end of the caldera that extends north to Mount Washburn. To the west is the Gallatin Range. To the southwest you can often see vapor rising from the Norris, Upper, and Lower Geyser Basins, and sometimes you can even see all the way to the Tetons.

The descent from the summit back to the trailhead is easy, taking only 45 minutes to an hour. Retracing your steps, take a hard right at the Chittenden Road–Mount Washburn Trail junction ▶4 to return to the Dunraven Pass parking area. ▶5

> Some 10,000 people hike Mount Washburn each year, making it the park's most popular trail.

 Summit

 Viewpoint

Opposite: *Hikers ascending the Mount Washburn Trail, as viewed from the summit*
CREDIT: Bradley Mayhew

The Chittenden Road Approach

An alternative approach to Mount Washburn starts 5 miles north of the Dunraven Pass trailhead at the Chittenden Road trailhead. This approach is roughly the same length, but bicycles are allowed on the unpaved road, making it a better bike ride than hike. National Park Service vehicles use the road to supply the fire lookout in summer.

Mount Washburn Spur and Seven Mile Hole

You can make a full day of it by setting up a car shuttle at the Glacial Boulder trailhead near Canyon Village and descending from the summit down Mount Washburn's steep, unburned eastern flank. (Alternatively you could hitchhike up to Dunraven Pass to start the hike). The Mount Washburn Spur Trail sees much less traffic than the other two routes to the summit. It passes the Washburn Hot Springs and Inkpot Springs mud pots, the Seven Mile Hole cutoff, and an unsigned overlook of the 1,000-foot Silver Cord Cascade en route to the Glacial Boulder trailhead on Inspiration Point Road (11.5 miles and 6–8 hours total, one-way from Dunraven Pass).

The only overnight camping option along this challenging route is the decent, hiker-only Washburn Meadow campsite 4E1, in prime grizzly habitat 2.5 miles below the summit, with easy access to water.

If you fancy an overnighter, the three riverfront, hiker-only 4C campsites (no wood fires allowed) in Seven Mile Hole are a worthy overnight detour, even though anglers often quip that the descent to the Yellowstone River "feels like 5 miles in, 7 miles out." All told, it's a stiff 4.4-mile add-on trip, requiring a climb of more than 1,000 feet of elevation to get to the Glacial Boulder Trailhead.

MILESTONES

► 1   0.0 Start at Dunraven Pass parking area
► 2   2.6 Sharp left at Chittenden Road–Mount Washburn Trail junction
► 3   3.0 Mount Washburn lookout tower
► 4   3.4 Hard right at Chittenden Road–Mount Washburn Trail junction
► 5   6.0 Return to Dunraven Pass parking area

Norris Geyser Basin: Porcelain and Back Basins

Yellowstone's most hyperactive and acidic hydrothermal area is home to many extremes. It's the park's hottest and most volatile basin, hosting the world's largest active geyser and rare acidic geysers. A leisurely stroll around the boardwalks provides an up-close look at the Earth at play, featuring a complete assortment of geothermal exuberance.

Trying to describe the basin's ever-changing features is futile: wander around to see what you discover, knowing that mysterious noises, new hot spots, and acrid smells await around every bend.

Best Time

There's little shade and no water in the basin. Boardwalks are subject to temporary closure due to thermal activity, but the basin is open whenever access roads are open. Overcast days are best for seeing the features at their steamiest.

Finding the Trail

From the north, go 21 miles south from Mammoth on Grand Loop Road to Norris Canyon Road. You can expect some minor delays on this road due to road construction, at least until 2018. Turn right (west) and continue 0.5 mile to the large Norris Geyser Basin parking loop. From the east, go 11.2 miles west on Norris Canyon Road from Canyon Village and continue straight across Grand Loop Road to enter the parking area. From the south, go 14 miles northeast from Madison Junction on Grand Loop Road and turn (west) left at Norris

TRAIL USE
Hike

LENGTH
2.0 miles, 1–2 hours

VERTICAL FEET
Negligible

DIFFICULTY
– 1 **2** 3 4 5 +

TRAIL TYPE
Loop

SURFACE TYPE
Boardwalk, Gravel

FEATURES
Child Friendly
Handicap Access
Photo Opportunity
Geologic Interest
Geothermal
Moonlight Hiking

FACILITIES
Bookstore
Information Station
Museum
Restrooms
Picnic Tables
Phone

157

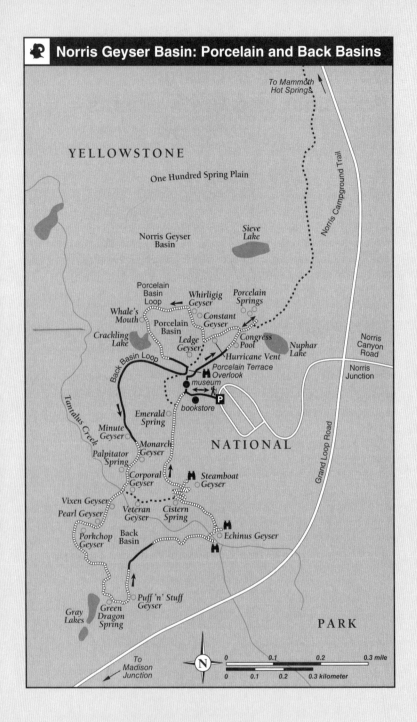

Norris Geyser Basin: Porcelain and Back Basins

YELLOWSTONE

One Hundred Spring Plain

Norris Geyser
Basin

Sieve
Lake

To Mammoth
Hot Springs

Norris Campground Trail

Porcelain
Basin
Loop

Whirligig
Geyser

Porcelain
Springs

Whale's
Mouth

Constant
Geyser

Porcelain
Basin

Crackling
Lake

Ledge
Geyser

Congress
Pool

Nuphar
Lake

Norris
Canyon
Road

Hurricane Vent

Back Basin Loop

Porcelain Terrace
Overlook

Norris
Junction

museum

Tantalus Creek

bookstore

P

Emerald
Spring

NATIONAL

Minute
Geyser

Monarch
Geyser

Palpitator
Spring

Corporal
Geyser

Steamboat
Geyser

Grand Loop Road

Vixen Geyser

Pearl Geyser

Veteran
Geyser

Cistern
Spring

Porkchop
Geyser

Back
Basin

Echinus Geyser

Gray
Lakes

Green
Dragon
Spring

Puff 'n' Stuff
Geyser

PARK

To
Madison
Junction

N

| 0 | 0.1 | 0.2 | 0.3 mile |

| 0 | 0.1 | 0.2 | 0.3 kilometer |

Canyon Road. The boardwalk trails begin near the bookstore and museum, near the northwest corner of the parking area.

Logistics

To hit the basin's highlights in an hour or less, walk clockwise around the Back Basin beginning from the bookstore (take the first left) and turn back when you've seen enough; for most folks, that's at the Echinus Geyser. Or you can cut the Back Basin loop in half by following the boardwalk that parallels Tantalus Creek and returning clockwise to the parking area.

Trail Description

From the parking loop, ▶1 stop by the metal box between the Yellowstone Association bookstore and Norris Museum ▶2 to pick up a self-guided trail map ($1 donation requested). Check here with rangers for updates on recent thermal activity.

After checking out the exhibits about the origins of the world's geothermal features (half of which are in Yellowstone), begin the 0.5-mile Porcelain Basin Loop by turning right on the upper boardwalk. Pause at the Porcelain Terrace ▶3 overlook for a bird's-eye preview of the hundreds of geothermal features packed into the wide-open, blindingly white basin.

After a short gravel stretch, the boardwalk resumes near a solfatara, an unstable volcanic vent area yielding hot vapors and sulfur-rich gases such as sulfuric acid. Nearby, roiling Congress Pool ▶4 is often pale blue but sometimes brown and muddy. Straight ahead on the boardwalk, beyond a trail map sign at the junction, is the overlook of the milky Porcelain Springs, ▶5 which is one of the most dynamic areas and was madly hissing steam at last

Geologists are still trying to determine why sudden, intermittent disturbances (lasting up to a week) cause simultaneous dramatic behavioral changes in the basin's thermal features. It's believed that an underlying plumbing system connects most of the basin.

 Geothermal

look. The 1-mile trail to Norris Campground heads off to the northeast near the overlook.

Back at the boardwalk junction, follow the right fork down past an inviting bench and picnic overlook, and then fork right at the junction near Hurricane Vent. ▶6 Past another bench on your right is Whirligig Geyser, ▶7 which has been dormant since 2000 but makes a rhythmic woosh-woosh sound similar to helicopter blades when it erupts. Nearby Constant Geyser erupts to 30 feet for only a few seconds at surprise intervals. The yellow-orange features and runoff channels here are some of the basin's most colorful.

Continue looping around the back side of the basin on a gravel trail. Near the Whale's Mouth spring, the boardwalk crosses a thermal runoff channel, and the steamy, snap-pop Crackling Lake ▶8 is to your right. Head up the stairs to the seriously stinky Black Growler Steam Vent, ▶9 which

OPTIONS

Norris Ranger-Led Programs

During the summer, ranger-led, 90-minute walks around Norris Geyser Basin depart daily at 9:30 a.m., starting at the museum. Rangers also give 20-minute talks at Steamboat Springs daily at 2 and 3 p.m. At the campground, there are 45-minute campfire talks nightly at 7:30 p.m.; check the park newspaper or visit tinyurl.com/yellowstone-ranger-programs for details.

Norris Campground Trail and Museum

If you are staying at the Norris Campground, a 1-mile trail to the geyser basin starts from near the Museum of the National Park Ranger (open daily, 9 a.m.–5 p.m., in summer), housed in the historic Norris Soldier Station log cabin. There's a video about the history of the National Park Service, and docents and retired rangers share stories about park history and lore.

has been measured at up to 280°F and sounds like a factory when it's going off at full tilt.

Up the short, steep hill at the four-way junction, turn right on the lower gravel path to begin the forested, 1.5-mile Back Basin Loop, ▶10 which was touched by the 1988 fires.

The main park road used to run very close to the once-mighty Minute Geyser, ▶11 which contributed to its getting clogged up in the early stagecoach days. Debris is still visible in the west vent, which used to spout up to 50 feet every 60 seconds. Today, the east vent sputters infrequently.

Continue straight ahead on the boardwalk past the trail sign at the next junction, ▶12 beyond Monarch Geyser Crater and Palpitator Spring. Ahead on your right is the colorful Pearl Geyser, ▶13 where the hissing and steaming sound vaguely like a subway tunnel and sporadic spouts reach up to 8 feet.

Here the boardwalk was rerouted in 2004 after a surprise steam explosion destroyed the route beyond Porkchop Geyser, now a calm spring within a huge blasted rocky hole; interpretive signs near the viewpoint explain the sequence of events. Remember never to venture off-trail in a geyser basin; in 2016 a visitor died after falling into a hot spring after wandering off-trail, joining the at least 21 other people who have died in Yellowstone from hot spring–related injuries.

The new boardwalk loops 0.2 mile around the back side of Porkchop, past the huge Gray Lakes to the noxious Green Dragon Spring, ▶14 where there's a bench that few people use to meditate on the sulfur-lined cavern's murkiness. Nearby, Puff 'n' Stuff Geyser pulsates with steam but rarely erupts.

A combination of boardwalks and sand and gravel paths winds around for 0.3 mile, past several big, steaming pools; runoff channels; and an overlook of Cistern Spring—which is connected to Steamboat Geyser—to end up at a series of benches

Three major faults intersect beneath Norris Geyser Basin, making it Yellowstone's hottest and most seismically active geyser basin. Many of the fumaroles and hot springs exceed the 212°F boiling point.

Photo Opportunity

and viewing platforms around the crowd-pleasing Echinus Geyser. ▶15 Pronounced e-KI-nus, it's the world's largest frequently active acid geyser (with a pH of 3.3–3.6, similar to vinegar). It erupts at intervals of one hour to four days and plays for three to five minutes.

Beyond the overlooks, turn right at the junction near Cistern Spring ▶16 and climb the stairs along-

Geothermal

side the runoff channel from Steamboat Geyser, ▶17 the tallest active geyser in the world. From the lower viewing platform and upper overlook, patient geyser gazers await frequent, minor bursts of 10–70 feet. Its name comes from its powerful steam phase, which follows major eruptions for up to 24 hours.

The last stop on the Back Basin Loop is the vibrant Emerald Spring, ▶18 a deep, clear-blue pool that is lined with yellow sulfur deposits and often appears green. Continue back up the hill and turn right at the museum and bookstore to return to the parking area. ▶19

🚶 MILESTONES

►1   0.0 Start at Norris Geyser Basin parking area
►2   0.1 Bookstore and Norris Museum
►3   0.15 Right at Porcelain Terrace overlook
►4   0.2 Congress Pool
►5   0.3 Porcelain Springs overlook
►6   0.4 Right at junction near Hurricane Vent
►7   0.45 Whirligig Geyser
►8   0.6 Crackling Lake
►9   0.65 Black Growler Steam Vent
►10 0.7 Begin Back Basin Loop
►11 0.8 Minute Geyser
►12 0.9 Straight at junction near Tantalus Creek
►13 1.0 Pearl Geyser and Porkchop Geyser
►14 1.2 Gray Lakes and Green Dragon Spring
►15 1.5 Echinus Geyser
►16 1.6 Right up stairs near Cistern Spring
►17 1.65 Steamboat Geyser
►18 1.8 Emerald Spring
►19 2.0 Return to parking area

Southeast Yellowstone: Lake Country

Southeast Yellowstone: Lake Country

Visitor activity in the park's southeast quadrant is concentrated around the impressive, 136-square-mile Yellowstone Lake (7,732 feet), the world's second-largest freshwater alpine lake, after South America's Lake Titicaca. (For context, that's bigger than Lake Tahoe but not as deep.) The region's day-hiking trails tend to be either short and flat or steep and very scenic.

Even though it has well over a hundred miles of shoreline, Yellowstone Lake's surface typically remains frozen from late December through late May or early June. A thriving population of native cutthroat trout attracts hordes of grizzly bears in spring and anglers in summer to the lake's tributaries. The lake's average temperature of 45°F precludes swimming year-round. As with most lakes, the water is calmest in the morning and becomes increasingly turbulent in the afternoon. More than 100 people have lost their lives while boating the park's lakes and streams, making the cold water a dozen times more deadly than the park's entire grizzly population.

When combined with adjacent U.S. Forest Service lands, the remote Two Ocean Plateau and Thorofare region in the park's southeastern corner compose the largest roadless wilderness in the Lower 48 and the farthest you can get from a road in the Lower 48, a veritable long-haul backpacker wonderland.

The rugged Buffalo Bill Scenic Highway (US 14/16/20), called "the most scenic 52 miles in the USA" by Teddy Roosevelt, links Cody to Yellowstone's East Entrance via the scenic Wapiti Valley. Seven miles inside the park, Sylvan Pass (8,530 feet) usually opens in early May and closes in early November but reopens for winter snowmobile use December–April. This is possible thanks to a National Park Service (NPS) avalanche-control program, which involves helicopters dropping explosive charges and howitzers launching 105mm artillery rounds into 20 avalanche passes.

Overleaf and Opposite: *Looking west from Avalanche Peak (Trail 20)*

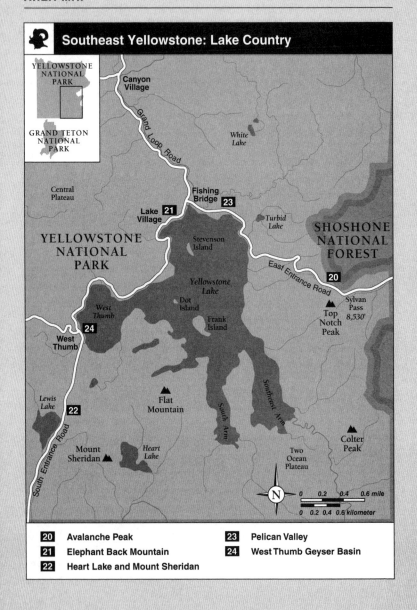

Southeast Yellowstone: Lake Country

YELLOWSTONE
NATIONAL
PARK

GRAND TETON
NATIONAL
PARK

Canyon
Village

Grand Loop Road

White
Lake

Central
Plateau

Fishing
Bridge

23

Lake
Village

21

YELLOWSTONE
NATIONAL
PARK

Stevenson
Island

Turbid
Lake

SHOSHONE
NATIONAL
FOREST

East Entrance Road

Yellowstone
Lake

20

West
Thumb

Dot
Island

Frank
Island

Sylvan
Pass
8,530'

Top
Notch
Peak

24

West
Thumb

Lewis
Lake

22

Flat
Mountain

South Arm

Southeast Arm

Colter
Peak

Mount
Sheridan

Heart
Lake

Two
Ocean
Plateau

South Entrance Road

N

0   0.2   0.4   0.6 mile

0   0.2 0.4 0.6 kilometer

20 Avalanche Peak	**23** Pelican Valley	
21 Elephant Back Mountain	**24** West Thumb Geyser Basin	
22 Heart Lake and Mount Sheridan		

Southeast Yellowstone: Lake Country

TRAIL	DIFFICULTY	LENGTH	TYPE	USES & ACCESS	TERRAIN	FLORA & FAUNA	EXPOSURE	OTHER
20	4	4.0	Out-and-back	Day Hiking	Mountain, Summit	Wildflowers	Great Views, Photo Opportunity	Swimming, Steep
21	3	3.5	Loop	Day Hiking, Child-Friendly	Mountain, Summit	Autumn Colors, Wildflowers, Wildlife	Cool & Shady, Great Views, Photo Opportunity	Swimming
22	5	15.0	Out-and-back	Day Hiking, Backpacking, Permit	Mountain, Summit, Lake, Stream	Birds, Wildlife	Great Views, Photo Opportunity	Camping, Geothermal
23	4	15.3	Loop	Day Hiking, Horses	Stream	Wildflowers, Birds, Wildlife	Great Views, Photo Opportunity	Swimming, Geothermal
24	1	0.6	Loop	Day Hiking, Child-Friendly, Wheelchair Access	Lake	Wildlife	Great Views, Photo Opportunity	Geothermal, Moonlight

USES & ACCESS
- Day Hiking
- Bicycling
- Horses
- Backpacking
- Child-Friendly
- Wheelchair Access
- Permit

TYPE
- Loop
- Out-and-back
- Point-to-point

DIFFICULTY
- 1 2 3 4 5 +
less   more

TERRAIN
- Canyon
- Mountain
- Summit
- Lake
- Stream
- Waterfall

FLORA & FAUNA
- Autumn Colors
- Wildflowers
- Birds
- Wildlife

EXPOSURE
- Cool & Shady
- Great Views
- Photo Opportunity

OTHER
- Camping
- Swimming
- Historic/Secluded
- Geologic Interest
- Geothermal
- Moonlight
- Steep

Xanterra manages three large, RV-dominated campgrounds around Yellowstone Lake. Bridge Bay Campground ($23.50, open late May–mid-September) is near Bridge Bay Marina, 3 miles southwest of Lake Village. The drive-in sites mostly attract boaters and anglers, while the two tent-only loops have the most shade and good lake views. Due to frequent ursine visits, the controversial Fishing Bridge RV Park ($50, open mid-May–early November), on the lake's north shore just east of Fishing Bridge Junction, allows only hard-sided vehicles—no pop-top campers.

On the lake's southwest shore, lakefront Grant Village Campground ($28, including two showers) has the most tent-only sites and the region's best shower and laundry facilities. It only opens around June 20, due to bears' use of nearby spawning streams, and closes by early October. At 20 miles from Old Faithful, it's the second-closest frontcountry campground to the landmark, but you have to cross Craig Pass and the Continental Divide to get there; the campground at Madison Junction is closer.

The region's less developed, NPS-run alternative is forested Lewis Lake Campground ($15, open mid-June–early November), 13 miles north of the park's South Entrance (open early May–early November). Despite the fact that it's a favorite of Shoshone Lake–bound boaters, it is often the last campground in the park to fill. There are walk-in and tent-only sites, and generators are banned. An additional 40 boat-in and backcountry campsites are spread around the southern and eastern lakeshores.

The charming, 19th-century Lake Yellowstone Hotel (open mid-May–early October; $162–$711) is listed on the National Register of Historic Places. Cabins at the nearby Lake Lodge (open early June–late September) come in two flavors: basic 1920s ($90) or motel-style ($140–$209). Even if you aren't a guest, either place is an atmospheric spot to hang out and enjoy the lake views over a snack, meal, or drink.

The modern (circa 1984) cookie-cutter hotel rooms at Grant Village (open late May–late September; $237) are hopelessly sterile but mostly wheelchair accessible.

Permits and Maps

The only trip in this chapter that requires an overnight backcountry permit is Trail 22, if you take advantage of the appealing overnight options around Heart Lake. Fishing permits are available at all of the region's ranger stations, visitor centers, and general stores. Boating permits are issued at the South Entrance, Lewis Lake Campground, Grant Village Visitor Center, Bridge Bay Ranger Station, and Lake Ranger Station.

Near the outlet of Yellowstone Lake, on the lake's north shore, the Fishing Bridge Visitor Center has a bookstore and exhibits on birds and wildlife. Call 307-242-2450; open daily, 8 a.m.–7 p.m., in summer.

On the lake's southeast shore near West Thumb, the Grant Visitor Center also has a bookstore, natural history exhibits, and a video on the role fire has played in the park. Call 307-242-2650; open daily, 8 a.m.–7 p.m., in summer. The smaller West Thumb Information Station also has a good bookstore (open daily, 9 a.m.–5 p.m., in summer).

The seasonal Lake Clinic is near the Lake Hotel. Call 307-242-7241; open daily, 8:30 a.m.–8:30 p.m., on call via 911 after hours mid-May–September).

With the exception of the first few miles of the Heart Lake Trail—which barely appears on the Old Faithful map (no. 302)—it's on the bottom-right corner of the north side—all trails described in this chapter appear on National Geographic's *Trails Illustrated* Yellowstone Lake map (no. 305, scale 1:63,360).

Southeast Yellowstone: Lake Country

Attaining some of Yellowstone's best panoramic views makes this relentless ascent worth every ounce of exertion. The route traverses whitebark pine forest, old avalanche slides, and scree slopes adjacent to the pristine North Absaroka Wilderness.

TRAIL 20

Hike
4 miles, Out-and-back
Difficulty: 1 2 3 **4** 5

For an impressive overview of Yellowstone Lake and environs, follow this rewarding, family-friendly loop through old-growth forest to a panoramic picnic overlook near Lake Village.

TRAIL 21

Hike
3.5 miles, Loop
Difficulty: 1 2 **3** 4 5

Part of the Continental Divide National Scenic Trail, this demanding day hike is popular thanks to its varied attractions.

TRAIL 22

Hike, Backpack
15.0 miles, Out-and-back
Difficulty: 1 2 3 4 **5**

This trail receives relatively light use as it loops around a wildlife-rich valley. There are several unbridged creek crossings. For experienced hikers only.

TRAIL 23

Hike, Horse
15.3 miles, Loop
Difficulty: 1 2 3 **4** 5

Experience the meeting of hot and cold liquid during this boardwalk loop around a lakeside geyser basin. It's easily accessible and home to some of the park's deepest and most colorful hot springs.

TRAIL 24

Hike
0.6 mile, Loop
Difficulty: **1** 2 3 4 5

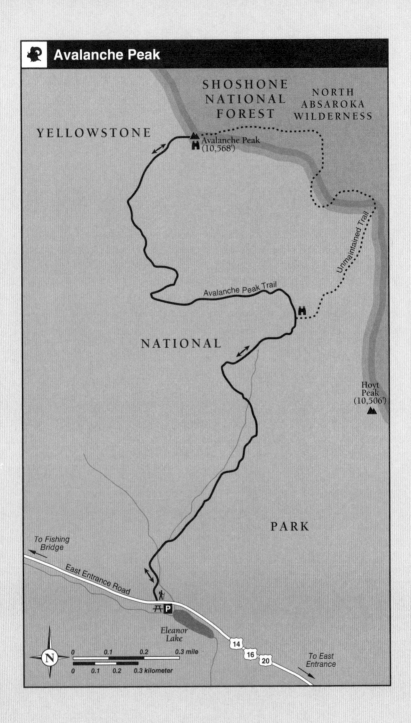

Avalanche Peak

SHOSHONE NATIONAL FOREST

NORTH ABSAROKA WILDERNESS

YELLOWSTONE

Avalanche Peak
(10,568')

Avalanche Peak Trail

Unmaintained Trail

NATIONAL

Hoyt
Peak
(10,506')

PARK

To Fishing
Bridge

East Entrance Road

Eleanor
Lake

14
16
20

To East
Entrance

N

0   0.1   0.2   0.3 mile

0   0.1   0.2   0.3 kilometer

Avalanche Peak

This quick but steep and relentless ascent skips the switchbacks. The solitude and some of Yellowstone's best panoramic views are worth every ounce of exertion. The lightly traveled route traverses whitebark pine forest, old avalanche slides, and scree slopes adjacent to the North Absaroka Wilderness.

Best Time

July–September is the best time here. Even on the steep south-facing slopes, snowfields persist above treeline well into July. Subalpine wildflowers peak soon after the late-spring snowmelt. Aside from seasonal snowmelt, there are no water sources above treeline. In the fall, grizzlies flock here to feed on whitebark pine nuts.

Finding the Trail

From the west, head 19 miles east from Fishing Bridge on the East Entrance Road and turn right into the paved parking area on the south side of the road, near the picnic area at the west end of Eleanor Lake. From the East Entrance, go 8 miles west, less than a mile past Sylvan Pass, and turn left into the parking area. The signed trailhead is across the road to the right (east) of the small creek.

Trail Description

From the trailhead (8,470 feet), ▶1 the unmarked but frequently blazed and well-maintained trail winds through unburned spruce–fir forest and

TRAIL USE
Hike

LENGTH
4 miles, 3–4 hours

VERTICAL FEET
±2,100

DIFFICULTY
– 1 2 3 **4** 5 +

TRAIL TYPE
Out-and-back

SURFACE TYPE
Dirt

FEATURES
Mountain
Summit
Steep
Wildflowers
Great Views
Photo Opportunity
Secluded

FACILITIES
None

OPTIONS

Summit Loop Trail

If you're up for a bit more of an adventure coming off the summit, look for an unmarked and unmaintained talus trail that drops precipitously down the peak's northeast arm to a saddle shared with Hoyt Peak (10,506 feet), on the park's eastern boundary. If you are comfortable negotiating this type of trail, you can descend through sparsely forested rolling hills to rejoin the main trail at the foot of the southeast bowl.

Steep   begins to climb steeply as it traces the drainage of an unnamed stream.

About half an hour from the trailhead, the official trail cuts left across the stream ▶2 and traverses west through an old avalanche chute. Avoid the temptation to follow the steeper route straight up the gulch: it's off-limits due to ongoing rehabilitation work. Next, the trail swings northeast and ducks back into mature whitebark pine stands; beware bears here in season.

Viewpoint   A bit more than halfway up the mountain, the trail flattens out as it emerges from the forest at the base of a huge, amphitheater-like bowl ▶3 where you get your first glimpse of Avalanche Peak. Above timberline, the main trail climbs left along an open scree slope to the shoulder of the peak's

Summit south ridge.

Take a break and savor the views back south and west over the Teton Wilderness and Yellowstone Lake before the final blustery ascent. The true

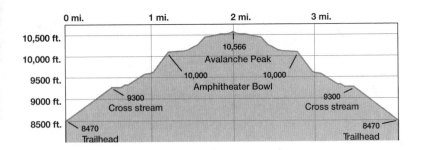

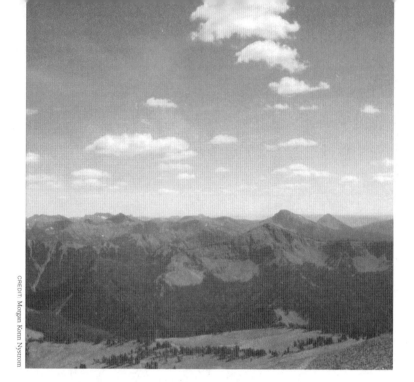

View *from the Avalanche Peak Trail*

summit ▶4 (10,568 feet) is along the narrow ridge to the northeast, beyond a series of talus wind shelters.

Photo Opportunity

From the peak, take in views of the Teton Range, Mount Washburn, and Mount Sheridan to the south, and the vast, roadless North Absaroka Wilderness in the Shoshone National Forest directly to the east.

After enjoying a hard-earned picnic lunch, retrace your steps back to the parking area. ▶5

🚶 MILESTONES

▶1	0.0 Start at Eleanor Lake parking area
▶2	0.5 Cross unnamed stream
▶3	1.2 Amphitheater bowl
▶4	2.0 Avalanche Peak
▶5	4.0 Return to parking area

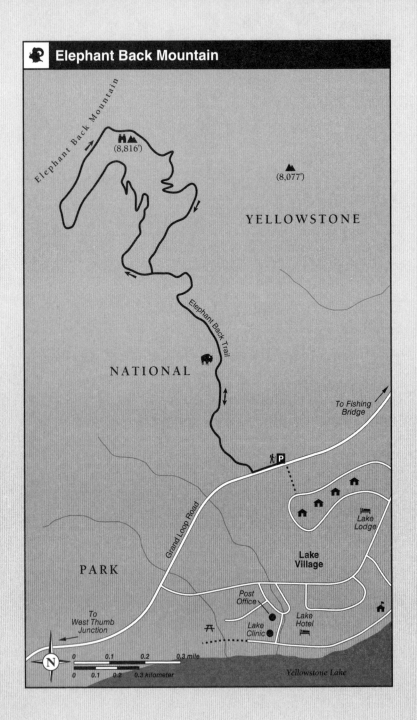

Elephant Back Mountain

(8,816')

(8,077')

YELLOWSTONE

Elephant Back Mountain

Elephant Back Trail

NATIONAL

To Fishing Bridge

P

Grand Loop Road

PARK

Lake Lodge

Lake Village

Post Office

Lake Clinic

Lake Hotel

To West Thumb Junction

N

0   0.1   0.2   0.3 mile

0   0.1   0.2   0.3 kilometer

Yellowstone Lake

Elephant Back Mountain

A popular family outing from Lake Village, this rewarding trail climbs gently through old-growth lodgepole pine forest, then loops around steeply to a picnic-worthy overlook with a panoramic view of Yellowstone Lake and beyond to the Absarokas.

Best Time

Bear activity is a possibility in spring due to the proximity to the lake's spawning streams. In 2015 a park employee was killed by a grizzly while walking off-trail in this region. After snowmelt in June, any time of day is fine, as most of the route is cool and shady.

Finding the Trail

If walking from Lake Village, follow signs and a paved path from the Lake Lodge through Section J of the cabins for 0.25 mile to Grand Loop Road opposite the trailhead. If driving from the north, go 1 mile south of Fishing Bridge Junction on Grand Loop Road and park in a turnout on either side of the road. From the south, go 20 miles north of West Thumb Junction, or 0.5 mile north (right) from Lake Junction.

Trail Description

From the parking turnout and signed trailhead (7,800 feet) on the north side of the road, ▶1 the well-maintained trail parallels the road to the south briefly before entering an impressive old-growth lodgepole pine forest.

TRAIL USE
Hike

LENGTH
3.5 miles, 1.5–2 hours

VERTICAL FEET
±800

DIFFICULTY
– 1 2 **3** 4 5 +

TRAIL TYPE
Loop

SURFACE TYPE
Dirt

FEATURES
Child Friendly
Mountain
Summit
Steep
Autumn Colors
Wildflowers
Wildlife
Cool & Shady
Great Views
Photo Opportunity

FACILITIES
Ranger Station
Restrooms
Picnic Tables
Phone

Wildlife

You soon pass by the former Lake Village waterworks and cross under a power line ▶2 before starting an easy climb. Keep an eye out here for deer and moose—and grizzlies in the spring—browsing on the abundant mushrooms and wild berries that thrive on the unburned forest floor among the wildflowers.

Wildflowers

After nearly a mile and 400 feet of gradual elevation gain, the trail forks at the loop junction. ▶3 Take the slightly shorter and marginally steeper left route 0.8 mile via a short series of switchbacks to the Elephant Back Mountain overlook (8,600 feet), ▶4 where wooden benches and pleasant picnic spots await in a clearing.

Viewpoint

The impressive views to the east include the Yellowstone River outlet to the extreme left; the meadows of Pelican Valley and Storm Point to your left just beyond Fishing Bridge; Stevenson Island in the middle of Yellowstone Lake; the lake's South and Southeast Arms to your right; and the Absaroka Range defining the horizon in the background, beyond the park's rugged eastern boundary.

Photo Opportunity

Return downhill via the gentler half of the loop 0.9 mile to rejoin the main trail at the junction, ▶5 where the left fork continues 0.9 mile back to the parking area. ▶6

MILESTONES

- ▶1 0.0 Parking area and trailhead
- ▶2 0.3 Old waterworks and power line
- ▶3 0.9 Left at loop junction
- ▶4 1.7 Elephant Back Mountain overlook
- ▶5 2.6 Left at junction
- ▶6 3.5 Return to parking area

Heart Lake and Mount Sheridan

This demanding day hike or more relaxed overnight trip is popular due to its wide range of attractions, including intriguing geysers and hot springs; the chance to bag a major peak; and inviting lakefront, hiker-only campsites. It's also a well-maintained stretch of the Continental Divide National Scenic Trail.

Best Time

The Heart Lake Bear Management Area is closed from April 1 through at least June 30 due to heavy grizzly activity. Snowfields remain on the slopes of Mount Sheridan until mid-July or later. Confirm current conditions with a ranger station or backcountry office before heading out; the closest rangers on duty are at the South Entrance and at Lake Village.

Finding the Trail

From the north, go 7 miles south on South Entrance Road from West Thumb Junction (or 5.3 miles south of Grant Village) and turn left into the signed trailhead parking area on the east side of the road. From the park's South Entrance, go 15 miles north on South Entrance Road, just beyond Lewis Lake, and turn right into the parking area.

Trail Description

From the trailhead parking area (7,785 feet), ▶1 the sandy, singletrack route—a well-maintained part of the Continental Divide National Scenic Trail—climbs subtly to the southeast through a patchwork of rolling meadows and lodgepole pine forest.

TRAIL USE
Hike, Backpack
LENGTH
15.0 miles, 1–2 days
VERTICAL FEET
±3,500, including
Mount Sheridan
DIFFICULTY
– 1 2 3 4 **5** +
TRAIL TYPE
Out-and-back
SURFACE TYPE
Dirt

FEATURES
Backcountry Permit
Stream
Mountain
Summit
Lake
Birds
Wildlife
Great Views
Photo Opportunity
Geothermal
Camping

FACILITIES
Patrol Cabin
Restrooms

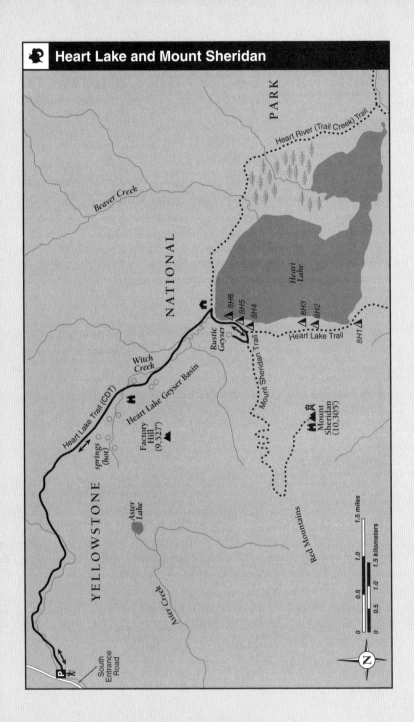

PARK

Heart River (Trail Creek) Trail

NATIONAL

Beaver Creek

Heart Lake

8H6
8H5
8H4
8H3
8H2

Rustic Geyser

Heart Lake Trail

8H1

Witch Creek

Mount Sheridan Trail

Heart Lake Trail (CDT)

Heart Lake Geyser Basin

Factory Hill (9,527')

Mount Sheridan (10,305')

springs (hot)

YELLOWSTONE

Aster Lake

Red Mountains

Aster Creek

1.5 miles

1.0

1.5 kilometers

0.5

1.0

0.5

0

0

South Entrance Road

P

N

Around 4.25 miles, after passing through a small burn area left over from the 1988 fires, the trail crests a minor rise and opens up near the head of the hydrothermally fueled Witch Creek drainage. ▶2 Below to your right are steaming fumaroles at the foot of the bald-as-an-eagle Factory Hill (9,607 feet). You also get your first tantalizing view of the lake from here on high, but it's still a couple of miles and 700 feet below.

The trail winds down along the creek through the middle of a burn area and the animated Heart Lake Geyser Basin, crossing the warm creek a couple of times via sturdy footbridges. Keep an eye out for spouting thermal features on the creek's south bank while you drop down toward the junction of the Heart Lake–Heart River Trail junction. ▶3

The Heart River Trail, along the north shore of the lake, is often also called the Trail Creek Trail, after its distant destination near the South Arm of Yellowstone Lake. Nearby, the lakefront Heart Lake Patrol Cabin is typically staffed all summer and usually has the current weather and fishing report for Heart Lake (7,455 feet).

Mount Sheridan and the Red Mountains mark the approximate southern boundary of Yellowstone's 600,000-year-old volcanic caldera.

 Geothermal

 Lake

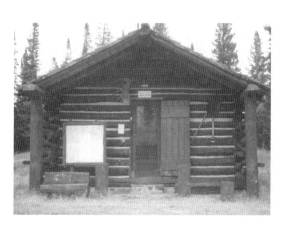

Heart Lake *Patrol Cabin*

Mount Sheridan and Overnight Camping

The laborious, spiraling 2,800-foot ascent of Mount Sheridan (10,305 feet; 6 miles and 4–5 hours round-trip) is really only feasible if you can score a reservation for a night or two at one of the six hiker-only 8H campsites. Even if you're not climbing Mount Sheridan, it's worth staying here just to see the sun rise over the lake. Only 8H2 and 8H3 (the most desirable sites) permit wood fires; all sites have a two-night-per-trip limit July 1–September 1 due to heavy demand. The 8H1 site is the farthest away and least desirable, a few hundred yards off the lake. These are some of the most popular backcountry sites in the park, so make a reservation before May 15, or come equipped with a backup plan.

At Mount Sheridan's talus-covered summit, there's a fire lookout that's staffed in summer. The awesome panorama takes in the Pitchstone Plateau to the west, Shoshone Lake to the northwest, Yellowstone Lake to the northeast, and the jagged Tetons to the south. Carry extra water as there's only snowmelt along the trail.

If you're staying overnight at one of the six 8H campsites, turn right at the patrol cabin to follow the trail a few hundred yards across the Witch Creek inlet on a log bridge, then south along the lake's sandy western shore past the informal spur path to the thermal area around Rustic Geyser. ▶4

Camping ⚠

The Mount Sheridan Trail junction and spur trails leading to campsites 8H4, 8H5, and 8H6 are a few hundred yards farther south.

After exploring the fragile, marshy thermal areas, most day hikers turn around here and retrace their steps to the trailhead parking area. ▶5

🚶 MILESTONES

▶1 0.0 Start at trailhead parking area
▶2 4.25 Witch Creek thermal area
▶3 7.25 Right at Heart Lake–Heart River Trail junction
▶4 7.5 Spur route to Rustic Geyser
▶5 15.0 Return to trailhead parking area

Pelican Valley

As it loops gently around the broad, wildlife-rich Pelican Valley, this lightly used trail provides good backcountry fishing access and a close-up look at some of the best grizzly habitat in the Lower 48. Herds of elk and bison have attracted a dynamic, denning wolf pack. Three creek fords can make completing the loop a challenge early in the season.

Best Time

Because of heavy grizzly bear activity, camping is prohibited year-round, and the trail is off-limits April 1–July 3. From July 4 through November 10 the area is open only for day use 9 a.m.–7 p.m. The opening holiday weekend is the busiest day in the valley and thus probably the least likely time to catch a glimpse of the big animals.

Due to the camping prohibition and time restrictions, you have no choice but to hike through the shadeless valley during the midday heat. Head out early, bring plenty of water, and—if you can—wait for an overcast, rainy, or even snowy day for the best chance at spotting wildlife.

Finding the Trail

From the west, go 3.5 miles east from Fishing Bridge Junction on the East Entrance Road. Turn left near the Storm Point trailhead and Indian (ex-Squaw) Pond onto an old gravel service road on the north side of the road, which leads 0.5 mile to the signed Pelican Valley trailhead (5K3) parking lot. From the east, go 23.5 miles west from the East Entrance on

TRAIL USE
Hike, Horse

LENGTH
15.3 miles, 2.5 hours

VERTICAL FEET
±450

DIFFICULTY
– 1 2 3 **4** 5 +

TRAIL TYPE
Loop

SURFACE TYPE
Dirt

FEATURES
Stream
Wildflowers
Birds
Wildlife
Great Views
Photo Opportunity
Swimming
Geothermal

FACILITIES
Horse Staging

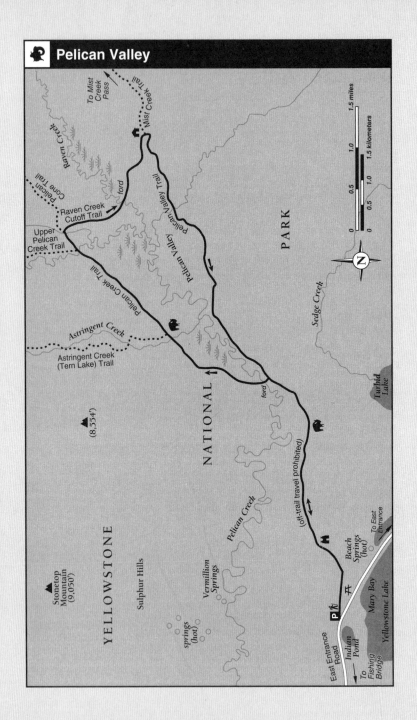

Pelican Valley

the East Entrance Road, past the Beach Springs picnic area, and turn right into the parking lot.

Logistics

Due to bear-management restrictions, the National Park Service strongly recommends a minimum of four hikers per group. Every hiker should carry bear spray. Off-trail travel is prohibited year-round along the first 2.5 miles of the Pelican Valley trail. The closest backcountry campsites are 3T3 and 3T2, east of Mist Creek Pass (8,500 feet), 10 and 11 miles from the trailhead.

Trail Description

From the trailhead parking area (7,800 feet), ▶1 the abandoned Turbid Lake service road makes a beeline straight east 0.5 mile. Where the old, off-limits road continues straight ahead, the trail forks ▶2 left (north) to follow the forest edge to an overlook. Here you get your first tempting glimpse of the wide-open Pelican Valley, ▶3 which is 1.5 miles beyond the trailhead.

The trail passes through several boggy sections—which are covered with wildflowers in midsummer—as it descends gently through open meadows to the valley floor. As you approach the usually unsigned (and off-limits) Turbid Lake Trail junction around 2 miles, make plenty of noise, keep alert, and monitor the forest edges—and the trail—for signs of elk, bison, coyote, and grizzly activity.

After 3.0 miles, you reach the south bank of Pelican Creek, ▶4 near the deteriorating remains of an old fire-road bridge.

Watch for fishing birds and cutthroat trout as you make the easy, ankle- to knee-high ford of the relatively warm, slow-moving creek. Here Pelican Creek Trail climbs gently up above the north bank

The fire lookout atop the 4-mile trail to Pelican Cone (9,643 feet) was used during the mid-1980s as a safe vantage point from which to study human impact on grizzly bear movements and habitat.

Photo Opportunity

Wildflowers

Wildlife

of the meandering creek 1.5 miles to an easy ford of Astringent Creek. ▶5 Continue straight ahead to just beyond the creek, where Astringent Creek Trail (also known as Tern Lake Trail) forks north (left) up the Astringent Creek drainage to the closest back-country campsites, beyond Fern Lake, in the Broad Creek drainage.

The trail contours along above some springs and minor marshy thermal areas: more good spots to survey the valley for wildlife. Keep one eye on the abundant clover patches here for signs of bear activity as you continue northeast along the forest edge 1.7 miles, then drop down to another uncomplicated ford of Pelican Creek, just before the Upper Pelican Creek Trail ▶6 junction. Stay in the open meadows to the right where the trail forks left (north) along the east side of Pelican Creek toward Wapiti Lake—more prime grizzly habitat.

A small, unnamed stream 0.4 mile farther along, just before the Pelican Cone Trail ▶7 junction, provides the valley's best drinking water; it's cool and clear, but purification is always advisable.

The ill-defined Raven Creek Cutoff Trail wends its way southeast across the rolling meadows in the middle of Pelican Valley. Halfway across, it often requires a bit of scouting around to find a shallow ford among the meandering oxbows of Raven Creek. ▶8 On the positive side, there are plenty of angling pools and waist-deep swimming holes here to cool off in the middle of a hot summer day.

Beyond Raven Creek, the faint trail can be difficult to follow as it continues through sagebrush-interspersed meadows, past a pond that reeks of sulfur and attracts flocks of waterfowl. Mount Chittenden (10,181 feet) and other peaks in the Absaroka Range define the park's rugged eastern boundary.

The trail drops down to a dormant thermal area, ducks into a patch of unburned forest, and rollercoasters over some sagebrush rises en route to the

Stream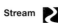

Swimming

Pelican Springs Patrol Cabin, ▶9 where there's a freshwater spring near the Mist Creek Trail junction.

Turn right to loop back southwest along the forested southern fringe of the valley toward the trailhead. It's 4 miles of ups and downs along the well-defined trail to reach the Pelican Bridge junction, ▶10 then another 3 miles on the now-familiar lollipop stretch of the loop to return to the trailhead parking area. ▶11

If you only want to do an easy 6-mile day hike, turn around at Pelican Creek after a picnic lunch.

🚶 MILESTONES

▶1	0.0 Start at trailhead parking area
▶2	0.5 Left at first fork
▶3	1.5 Pelican Valley
▶4	3.0 Pelican Creek ford and old bridge
▶5	4.5 Ford Astringent Creek
▶6	6.2 Right at Upper Pelican Creek Trail junction
▶7	6.6 Right at Pelican Cone Trail junction
▶8	7.3 Raven Creek ford
▶9	8.3 Right on Mist Creek Trail junction at Pelican Springs Patrol Cabin
▶10	12.3 Straight at Pelican Creek ford junction
▶11	15.3 Return to trailhead parking area

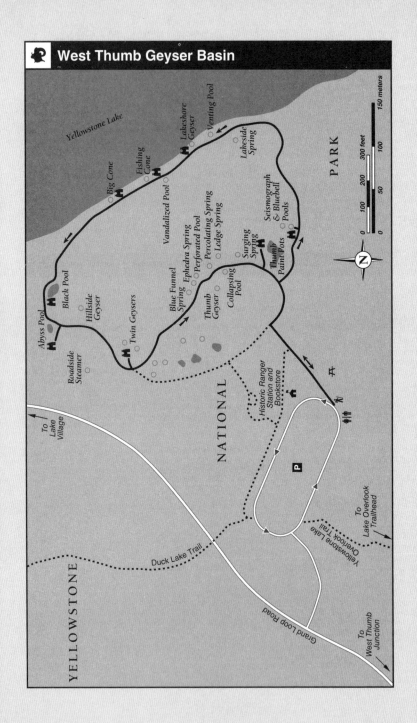

West Thumb Geyser Basin

Yellowstone Lake

Venting Pool

Lakeshore Geyser

Lakeside Spring

Fishing Cone

Big Cone

Vandalized Pool

Seismograph & Bluebell Pools

Ephedra Spring

Percolating Spring

Ledge Spring

Black Pool

Blue Funnel Spring

Perforated Pool

Surging Spring

Hillside Geyser

Twin Geysers

Thumb Paint Pots

Abyss Pool

Thumb Geyser

Collapsing Pool

Roadside Steamer

PARK

150 meters

300 feet

100

200

100

50

0

Historic Ranger Station and Bookstore

NATIONAL

To Lake Village

P

To Lake Overlook Trailhead

Yellowstone Lake Overlook Trail

Duck Lake Trail

YELLOWSTONE

Grand Loop Road

To West Thumb Junction

West Thumb Geyser Basin

This relatively flat boardwalk loops around a varied geyser basin, a volcanic caldera within a caldera, and past some of the park's most colorful hot springs. Though they aren't the most volatile or dynamic attractions, it's an intimate and usually uncrowded look at some unique hydrothermal features. For the bigger picture, add a short climb to an overlook of the lake.

Best Time

Rain and snow tend to dilute the vibrant colors in many hydrothermal features. Therefore, the geyser basin is at its most brilliant in the middle of summer, especially July and August. It's also a popular winter destination. There's no shade, so it can get hot at midday. The overlook extension is worth the effort only on clear days.

Finding the Trail

From Old Faithful, drive east 17 miles on Grand Loop Road over Craig Pass (8,262 feet), turn left at West Thumb Junction, and then immediately turn right into the Geyser Basin parking area on the southeast side of the road. From Lake Village, go 21 miles southwest along the lakeshore on Grand Loop Road and turn left into the parking area. From the south, go north 22 miles on the South Entrance Road and turn right at West Thumb Junction. The Geyser Basin loop starts near the bookstore in the parking lot's southeast corner. The Lake Overlook trailhead is in the southwest corner.

TRAIL USE
Hike
LENGTH
0.6 mile, less than 1 hour
VERTICAL FEET
Negligible
DIFFICULTY
− **1** 2 3 4 5 +
TRAIL TYPE
Loop
SURFACE TYPE
Boardwalk

FEATURES
Child Friendly
Handicap Access
Lake
Wildlife
Great Views
Photo Opportunity
Geothermal
Moonlight Hiking

FACILITIES
Ranger Station
Bookstore
Restrooms
Picnic Tables
Phone

189

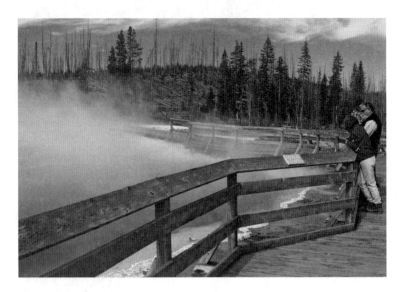

Hikers *check out the Abyss Pool.*

Trail Description

Before leaving the parking lot, ►1 stop at the historic 1925 Ranger Station ►2 to browse some books, chat with the friendly Yellowstone Association staffers, and warm up by the woodstove. Head out counterclockwise (right) on the wheelchair-accessible boardwalk. ►3

Geothermal

Depending on the season, you may find miniature acidic mud volcanoes known as the Thumb Paint Pots ►4—called "mud puffs" by the 1871 Hayden Expedition—plopping and sputtering away (if there's been recent precipitation, they might be washed out).

Photo Opportunity

Nearby, the ultra-blue Seismograph and Bluebell Pools receive runoff from the mud pots; the former is thought to perhaps have been altered by the 1959 Hebgen Lake earthquake, which registered 7.5 on the Richter scale.

Near the lakeshore, Lakeside Spring and Lakeshore Geyser ►5 contribute to the average of 3,100 gallons of superheated water that overflows from the geyser basin into the lake every day. One of the geyser's vents usually remains submerged until the end of August. Though spouts of up to 50 feet were reported in the 1920s and 1930s, the last major eruption was in 1970.

The basin's most famous feature is Fishing Cone, ▶6 where tall tales grew out of the legends of mountain men "hooking and cooking" trout in one swift motion in the boiling natural stew pot. Today, fishing is not allowed here, and the cone stays underwater until early summer.

 Viewpoint

Black Pool and Abyss Pool ▶7 are the basin's most striking, and most photographed, springs. Abyss, one of the park's deepest pools, is a real looker and is said to have a seemingly endless bottom; wait for a steam-free moment before snapping a photo. Black Pool is so named because it once harbored a thick, dark mat of thermophile bacteria, but now it's kaleidoscopically colorful. The pool erupted several times in 1991 and 1992, and subsequent rising water temperatures killed off the original black hue.

 Photo Opportunity

Turn left just before the inner boardwalk loop ▶8 to reach a spur platform out to the Twin Geysers. Though its eruptions are infrequent and unpredictable, when they last blew in 1999 the twin vents spouted in succession, 70 feet in the west, followed by more than 100 feet in the east.

The highlights of the dynamic Central Basin ▶9 area between the two boardwalks are the brilliantly tinted Blue Funnel Spring; the overflowing, 167°F Surging Spring ▶10; and the Collapsing Pool, which is constantly in flux.

 Geothermal

Following the inner loop, you'll end up back where you started on the outer boardwalk, ▶11 a short distance from the Ranger Station and parking lot. ▶12

If you aren't ready to jump back on the road, cross the parking lot to pick up the Lake Overlook Trail near the exit for West Thumb Junction.

Yellowstone Lake Overlook

For a superb view of Yellowstone Lake and the park's entire eastern half, hike the Lake Overlook Trail loop (2 miles round-trip, 1 hour, 200-foot elevation gain). It starts from the southwest corner of the parking lot and passes through meadows, a 1988 burn area, and regenerating forest before reaching the overlook. Highlights include a decent chance of spotting deer, elk, and bison—plus a minor possibility of encountering bears—and expansive views across the lake to the park's eastern boundary in the Absaroka Range. July is the best time for wildflowers.

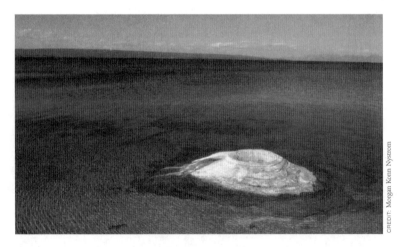

CREDIT: Morgan Konn Nystrom

Cookin' on the hook *is no longer allowed at Fishing Cone, on the edge of Yellowstone Lake.*

MILESTONES

▶1   0.0 Start at West Thumb Geyser Basin parking area

▶2   0.0 Historic Ranger Station: bookstore and warming hut

▶3   0.1 Right on outer boardwalk

▶4   0.15 Thumb Paint Pots and Seismograph and Bluebell Pools

▶5   0.2 Lakeside Spring and Lakeshore Geyser

▶6   0.25 Fishing Cone

▶7   0.3 Black Pool and Abyss Pool

▶8   0.35 Left onto Twin Geysers platform just before inner boardwalk loop

▶9   0.4 Central Basin: Blue Funnel Spring and Ephedra Spring

▶10   0.45 Thumb Geyser, Surging Spring, and Collapsing Pool

▶11   0.5 Right at outer boardwalk

▶12   0.6 Return to parking area

Hot-Spring Organisms and Chemosynthesis

NOTES

After five years of field research, University of Colorado scientists have theorized that the primary energy source for primitive organisms living in the park's hot springs at temperatures above 158°F (where photosynthesis isn't possible) is not sulfur, as is widely assumed, but hydrogen—the most abundant element in the universe.

The colors visible in hot springs are radiated by thermophile (heat-loving) organisms; they correspond roughly to temperature ranges: Green and brown are the coolest; yellow and orange are hotter; and the whitish blue of near-boiling waters indicates the hottest pools, where only the hardiest organisms, called extremophiles, can survive.

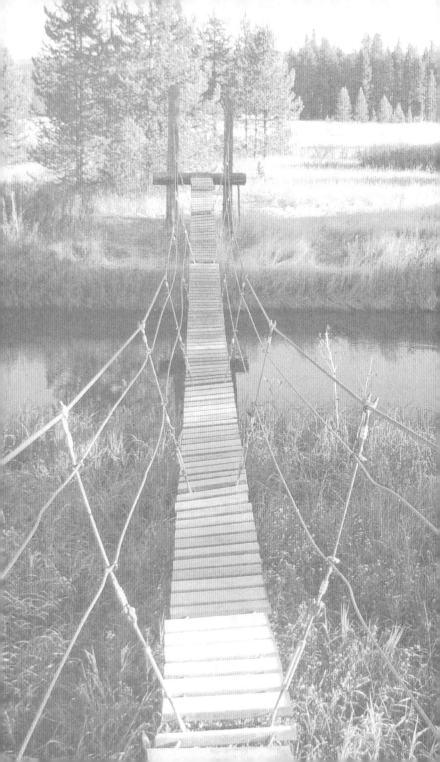

CHAPTER 5

Southwest Yellowstone: Cascade and Geyser Country

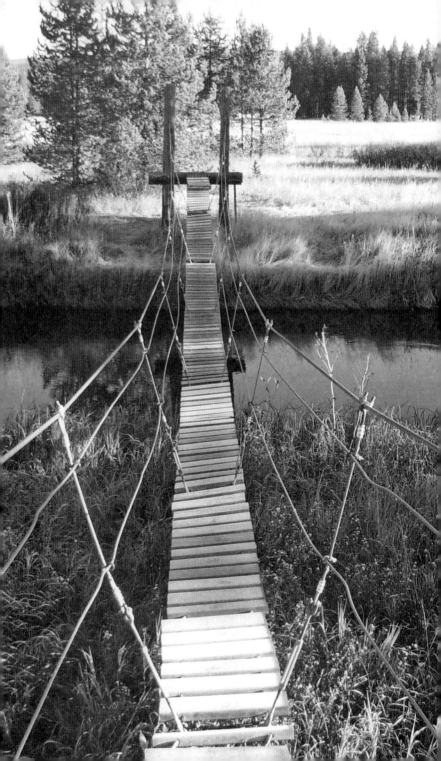

Southwest Yellowstone: Cascade and Geyser Country

Yellowstone's southwest corner exemplifies why one of the earliest nicknames for the park was America's Wonderland. Before the park was established in 1872, explorers queried respected periodicals back east about publishing their accounts of encounters with the region's astounding geysers, wildlife, and thermal features. The response was unanimous: "Sorry, we don't publish fiction."

Today, the region's world-famous geothermal features are as active and popular as ever. The pilgrimage to the Old Faithful is obligatory for first-time visitors, and a wander through the gushing surrounding Upper Geyser Basin never fails to impress. Beyond the frontcountry boardwalks, several of the park's most spectacular geysers and waterfalls await only short distances from roadside trailheads.

The Lamar Valley and Old Faithful aside, many frequent visitors claim that the Cascade Corner is Yellowstone's most captivating region. For those with a few days to spare, overnight backpacking and boating around Shoshone Lake offer enticing escapes from the crowds. Accessing the relative solitude of the 200-square-mile Bechler backcountry (pronounced BECK-ler; also known as the Cascade Corner thanks to its many waterfalls) requires some dedication, since it's a long drive outside the park—from either West Yellowstone or the South Entrance.

The nearest developed campground to Old Faithful is at Madison Campground ($23.50), 16 miles north of Old Faithful, at which you can (and should) reserve sites in advance. There are also several easy overnight options at nearby backcountry campsites, most of them discussed in this chapter's trail descriptions.

Overleaf and opposite: *Hiking in the Bechler region requires wading across several rivers; this suspension bridge offers a rare dry crossing (Trail 25).*

CREDIT: Bradley Mayhew

197

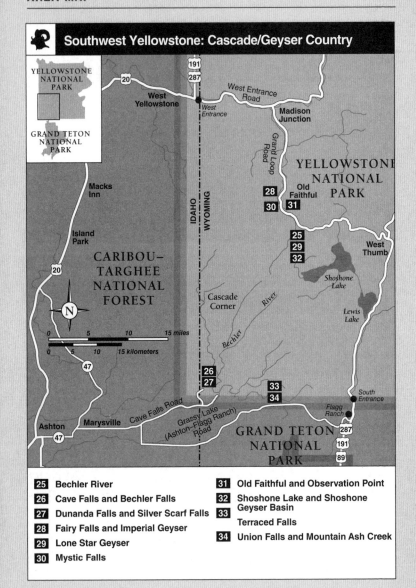

Southwest Yellowstone: Cascade/Geyser Country

25 Bechler River	**31** Old Faithful and Observation Point
26 Cave Falls and Bechler Falls	**32** Shoshone Lake and Shoshone Geyser Basin
27 Dunanda Falls and Silver Scarf Falls	**33** Terraced Falls
28 Fairy Falls and Imperial Geyser	**34** Union Falls and Mountain Ash Creek
29 Lone Star Geyser	
30 Mystic Falls	

TRAIL FEATURES TABLE

Southwest Yellowstone: Cascade and Geyser Country

TRAIL	DIFFICULTY	LENGTH	TYPE	USES & ACCESS	TERRAIN	FLORA & FAUNA	EXPOSURE	OTHER
25	5	29.7	Point-to-point	Day Hiking, Horses, Backpacking, Permit	Canyon, Mountain, Stream, Waterfall	Autumn Colors, Wildflowers, Birds, Wildlife	Cool & Shady, Great Views, Photo Opportunity	Camping, Swimming, Historic/Secluded, Geothermal
26	3	7.3	Loop	Day Hiking, Horses, Child-Friendly	Stream, Waterfall	Autumn Colors, Birds, Wildlife	Photo Opportunity	Swimming
27	5	16.4	Out-and-back	Day Hiking, Horses, Backpacking, Permit	Stream, Waterfall	Autumn Colors, Birds, Wildlife	Photo Opportunity	Camping, Swimming, Historic/Secluded, Geothermal
28	3	6.8	Out-and-back	Day Hiking, Bicycling, Backpacking, Child-Friendly	Waterfall	Wildflowers, Birds	Great Views, Photo Opportunity	Camping, Swimming, Geothermal
29	2	5.0	Out-and-back	Day Hiking, Bicycling, Backpacking, Child-Friendly, Wheelchair Access	Stream	Wildlife	Cool & Shady, Photo Opportunity	Camping, Geothermal, Moonlight
30	3	4.0	Loop	Day Hiking, Child-Friendly	Canyon, Stream, Waterfall	Wildflowers	Great Views, Photo Opportunity	Geothermal, Steep
31	2	2.4	Loop	Day Hiking, Child-Friendly, Wheelchair Access			Great Views, Photo Opportunity	Geothermal, Moonlight, Steep
32	5	17.0	Out-and-back	Day Hiking, Backpacking, Permit	Lake, Stream	Autumn Colors, Wildflowers, Birds, Wildlife	Great Views, Photo Opportunity	Camping
33	2	3.6	Out-and-back	Day Hiking, Child-Friendly	Canyon, Stream, Waterfall	Autumn Colors	Cool & Shady, Great Views, Photo Opportunity	Historic/Secluded, Geologic Interest
34	5	15.8	Out-and-back	Day Hiking, Horses, Backpacking, Permit	Canyon, Stream, Waterfall	Autumn Colors	Photo Opportunity	Camping, Swimming, Historic/Secluded, Geologic Interest

USES & ACCESS
- Day Hiking
- Bicycling
- Horses
- Backpacking
- Child-Friendly
- Wheelchair Access
- Permit

TYPE
- Loop
- Out-and-back
- Point-to-point

DIFFICULTY
- 1 2 3 4 5 +
less   more

TERRAIN
- Canyon
- Mountain
- Summit
- Lake
- Stream
- Waterfall

FLORA & FAUNA
- Autumn Colors
- Wildflowers
- Birds
- Wildlife

EXPOSURE
- Cool & Shady
- Great Views
- Photo Opportunity

OTHER
- Camping
- Swimming
- Historic/Secluded
- Geologic Interest
- Geothermal
- Moonlight
- Steep

The century-old Old Faithful Inn (open early May–early October; doubles $115–$268, suites $503–$572), a National Historic Landmark built in 1903–04 with native logs, is worth a visit to see the spectacular architecture even if you aren't able to reserve a room or dine there. The original "Old House" rooms in both the east and west wings completed an $11 million restoration in late 2008, but some still have shared bathrooms down the hall. You'll need to book six months in advance to get a room at the inn.

Nearby, the less atmospheric Old Faithful Lodge (open mid-May–late September) has basic cabins ($88) with shared toilets, and motel-style units ($148) with private bathrooms. The shared showers ($4) in the lodge are available to nonguests; pick up a towel at the reception desk.

The modern Old Faithful Snow Lodge (open early May–mid-October and mid-December–mid-March; cabins $114–$163, rooms $264–$284) is a hive of activity, particularly in winter. The West Entrance Road between West Yellowstone, Montana; Madison Junction; and Old Faithful typically opens for oversnow travel (including cross-country skiing, snow coaches, and snowmobiles) in mid-December and is groomed until mid-March.

Depending on the weather, the vehicle-free period in early spring—before the road opens around the third week in April—can be a magical time to explore Grand Loop Road. While park service crews perform spring road maintenance, visitors can bicycle, jog, in-line-skate, or explore via other nonmotorized means between the West Entrance and Mammoth, and sometimes between Norris Geyser Basin and Canyon Village. Contact the National Park Service at 307-344-2117 to verify seasonal opening schedules. (See page 16 for more details on the spring bicycling period.)

Permits and Maps

The only permits required for hikes in this chapter are for fishing, boating, and overnight stays at the region's numerous and popular backcountry campsites.

The recently remodeled Old Faithful Visitor Center is the park's busiest information center, receiving upwards of 25,000 visitors per day. Besides answering the million-dollar question (Q: When is Old Faithful scheduled to erupt? A: There's no "schedule."), rangers issue permits and lead free interpretive walks through the geyser basins. There's also a good bookstore and a theater that screens short films timed to start just after an eruption of Old Faithful. Call 307-545-2750; open daily, 8 a.m.–8 p.m. in summer; hours are reduced in fall and winter.

The remote, summer-only Bechler Ranger Station also issues permits, but it's best to arrange for permits and campsite reservations at another backcountry office (see the Appendix, page 348, for a complete list) before trekking all the way out to the park's bottom-left corner. For the Bechler Ranger Station, call 406-581-7074; open daily, 8 a.m.–4:30 p.m., in summer.

National Geographic's *Trails Illustrated* Old Faithful (no. 302, scale 1:63,360) map shows all the hikes, trailheads, and campgrounds described in this chapter.

Southwest Yellowstone: Cascade and Geyser Country

Bechler River 204

The Cascade Corner comes as close as any region in Yellowstone to having it all—prime fishing, soakable hot springs, and lots of wildlife. This three- to five-day backcountry route passes by many of the region's highlights. And with a car shuttle, it's downhill most of the way.

TRAIL 25

Hike, Backpack, Horse
29.7 miles, Point-to-point
Difficulty: 1 2 3 4 **5**

Cave Falls and Bechler Falls 215

This easy loop avoids river fords and provides a sample of what the remote Bechler region has to offer. It's not worth the drive by itself, but it is a nice easy hike if you already happen to be in the area.

TRAIL 26

Hike, Horse
7.3 miles, Loop
Difficulty: 1 2 **3** 4 5

Dunanda Falls and Silver Scarf Falls 220

This long but rewarding route offers a good sample of the Cascade Corner's varied delights: lush riparian zones; vast, wildlife-rich meadows; sublime hot pots; mesmerizing waterfalls; and invigorating stream crossings. And it is easily extended into a moderate overnight trip.

TRAIL 27

Hike, Backpack, Horse
16.4 miles, Out-and-back
Difficulty: 1 2 3 4 **5**

Fairy Falls and Imperial Geyser 226

This family-friendly outing is a perfect length to take a sack lunch on the trail, and it affords a tantalizing taste of what's so wonderful about Yellowstone's backcountry. One of the park's tallest waterfalls, intriguing geothermal features, and easy camping options await surprisingly close to the Grand Loop Road.

TRAIL 28

Hike, Bike, Backpack
5.2 or 6.8 miles
Out-and-back
Difficulty: 1 2 **3** 4 5

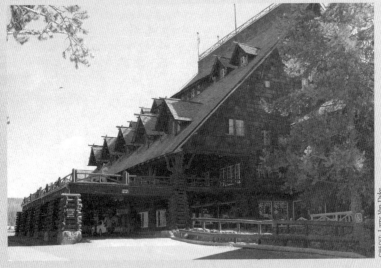

Old Faithful Inn is a classic example of National Park Service "parkitecture."

Shoshone Lake and Shoshone Geyser Basin 251

With no road access and no motorized boats allowed, forest-lined Shoshone Lake is the largest backcountry lake in the Lower 48 US states. It's home to an amazing geyser basin and good fishing—and with the option of boat-in camping, it's no surprise that it's one of Yellowstone's most popular overnight destinations.

TRAIL 32

Hike, Backpack
17.0 miles, Out-and-back
Difficulty: 1 2 3 4 **5**

Terraced Falls 258

This remote, lightly used trail is difficult to access but provides an up-close look at a large, multitier waterfall, set in a dramatic, volcano-forged canyon. It's a great late-season choice and combines nicely with an overnight trip to Union Falls.

TRAIL 33

Hike, Horse
3.6 miles, Out-and-back
Difficulty: 1 **2** 3 4 5

Union Falls and Mountain Ash Creek 263

Greater Yellowstone's most impressive backcountry waterfall and a sublime swimming hole are the rewards at the end of this hearty hike alongside lovely streams. Scoring a reservation at one of the popular campsites near the falls will allow you to extend this long dayhike into an easygoing overnight trip.

TRAIL 34

Hike, Backpack, Horse
15.8 miles, Out-and-back
Difficulty: 1 2 3 4 **5**

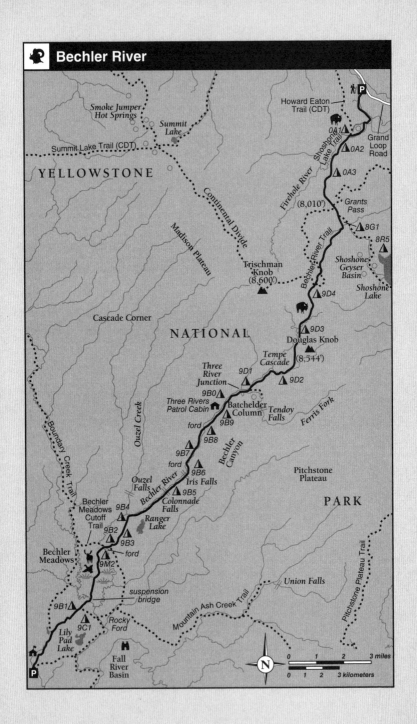

Smoke Jumper
Hot Springs

Summit
Lake

Summit Lake Trail (CDT)

YELLOWSTONE

Continental Divide

Madison Plateau

Cascade Corner

Trischman
Knob
(8,600')

NATIONAL

Howard Eaton
Trail (CDT)

0A1

0A2

Grand
Loop
Road

Shoshone Lake Trail

Firehole River

0A3

(8,010')

Grants
Pass

8G1

8R5

Bechler River Trail

Shoshone
Geyser
Basin

Shoshone
Lake

9D4

9D3

Douglas Knob
(8,544')

Tempe
Cascade

Three
River
Junction

9D1

9D2

9B0

Three Rivers
Patrol Cabin

Batchelder
Column

Tendoy
Falls

Ferris Fork

ford

9B9

9B8

Ouzel Creek

9B7

ford

Bechler Canyon

Pitchstone
Plateau

9B6

Ouzel
Falls

Iris Falls

Bechler River

9B5

Colonnade
Falls

PARK

Boundary Creek Trail

Bechler
Meadows
Cutoff
Trail

9B4

Ranger
Lake

9B2

9B3

ford

Bechler
Meadows

9M2

suspension
bridge

Union Falls

Pitchstone Plateau Trail

9B1

9C1

Rocky
Ford

Lily
Pad
Lake

Fall
River
Basin

Mountain Ash Creek Trail

N

| 0 | 1 | 2 | 3 miles |

| 0 | 1 | 2 | 3 kilometers |

Bechler River

The Cascade Corner comes as close as any part of Yellowstone to having it all. This three- to five-day route passes by many of the region's highlights. It's tough to argue with good catch-and-release fishing, soakable five-star hot pots, lovely backcountry campsites, and wildlife galore in the lower stretches—especially when the majority of the trail is downhill.

Best Time

Grants Pass (8,010 feet), between Lone Star Geyser and the west end of Shoshone Lake, typically isn't free of snow until late June or early July. In Bechler Meadows, high water and pesky mosquitoes typically don't subside until late July or early August. For these reasons, this trip is most popular in August and September, when advance reservations are essential. October conditions can be glorious, but snaps of foul weather are also quite possible.

Finding the Trail

From the north, head south from Old Faithful 2.7 miles on Grand Loop Road. Turn right into the parking area just past the Kepler Cascades turnout, signed for the Lone Star trailhead, on the south side of the road. From Grant Village, go west on Grand Loop Road from West Thumb Junction 14.5 miles over Craig Pass (8,262 feet), and turn left into the trailhead parking area.

TRAIL USE
Hike, Backpack, Horse

LENGTH
29.7 miles, 3–5 days

VERTICAL FEET
+1,300/–2,100

DIFFICULTY
– 1 2 3 4 **5** +

TRAIL TYPE
Point-to-point

SURFACE TYPE
Dirt

FEATURES
Backcountry Permit
Canyon
Mountain
Stream
Waterfall
Autumn Colors
Wildflowers
Birds
Wildlife
Cool & Shady
Great Views
Camping
Swimming
Secluded
Geothermal

FACILITIES
None

Logistics

Check the predicted eruption schedule for Lone Star Geyser at the Old Faithful Ranger Station so you can plan your departure time accordingly. Seeing this impressive geyser in action is worth fitting into your trip schedule.

Bechler's backcountry campsites aren't available for advance reservation until after July 15; some sites may be available earlier for in-person reservations, depending on weather conditions. During summer, it's a good idea to reserve Bechler's limited backcountry campsites as far in advance as possible. Most Bechler campsites may be reserved for only one or two nights. Contact the Bechler Ranger Station for an update on current weather, river-ford, and trail conditions.

The only nearby frontcountry camping option is the riverside U.S. Forest Service Cave Falls Campground (with water and restrooms), 1 mile east of the turnoff for the Bechler Ranger station ($10), in the Caribou-Targhee National Forest. There's also plenty of room for dispersed camping in the surrounding national forests.

A car shuttle is necessary for this hike, and be prepared for a long drive. From the Lone Star trailhead, the easiest way to reach the Bechler Ranger Station is via the West Entrance and West Yellowstone. The winding, 105-mile drive takes at least four hours each way in favorable conditions. From Ashton, Idaho (60 miles and 1.5 hours south of West Yellowstone, Montana, via US 20), drive 10 miles east past

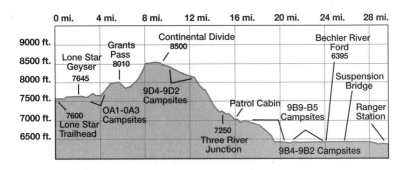

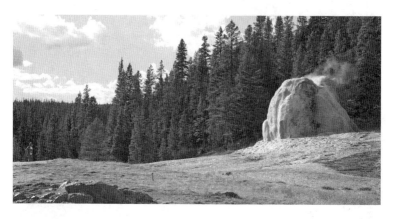

Lone Star Geyser *(Trails 25, 29, and 32)*

Marysville, and jog left at the turnoff for Mesa Falls (ID 47) to reach Cave Falls Road. Continue 10 miles on the graded gravel road past the Idaho–Wyoming state line, and then turn left for the Bechler Ranger Station at the signed junction for Cave Falls.

The alternative route, via the South Entrance and the unpaved Grassy Lake Road, is only slightly shorter but is much rougher and takes even longer. From 2 miles south of Yellowstone's South Entrance at Flagg Ranch, it's possible to head 50 miles west on the unpaved Grassy Lake Road (variously called Ashton–Flagg Ranch Road, Reclamation Road, and USFS Road 261 on older maps) to reach a cutoff for Cave Falls Road. At the trailhead, park adjacent to the barn (if day hiking) or in the horse staging area (if staying overnight).

To arrange a commercial shuttle drop, contact a company like Yellowstone Roadrunner in West Yellowstone; call 406-640-0631 or visit yellowstoneroadrunner.com. Don't leave any valuables in your vehicles at the trailheads, display your backcountry permit inside your windshield, and register your plans with the Bechler Ranger Station. If you're

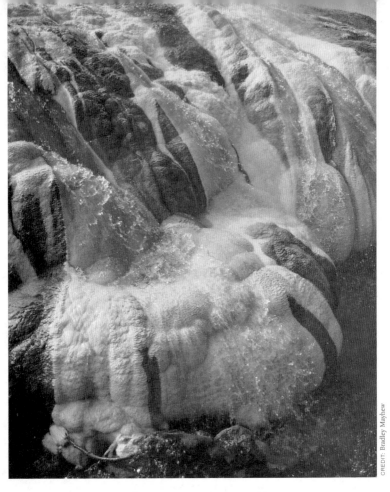

The Ferris Fork *has plentiful waterfalls and intriguing thermal features*

concerned about the security of your vehicle, park at the nearby Kepler Cascades turnout, which sees less traffic.

You definitely need to bring hiking sandals or wading shoes, plus trekking poles for added stability, and you need to be prepared to cross thigh-high rivers with your pack on. A camp towel and some kind of swimming attire are useful if visiting the Mr. Bubbles hot spring. Unless otherwise noted, campsites described here are hiker-only, allow wood campfires, and have a one-night limit.

Trail Description

From the Lone Star trailhead, ►1 an abandoned service road heads south along the upper Firehole River. After passing the remains of an old waterworks, the paved road traces the east bank of the river as it heads upstream.

Geothermal

After passing the Spring Creek Trail ►2 junction at 1.6 miles, you may hear Lone Star Geyser ►3 before you see it. During its steam phase, it can be heard up to a mile away. Major eruptions occur like clockwork, every three hours on average, with significant preplay in between active phases. Allow about an hour to reach the geyser on foot from the trailhead. (For details about Lone Star Geyser, see Trail 29, page 233.)

Wildlife

A few hundred yards beyond the geyser basin, take a left at the well-signed Shoshone Lake Trail ►4 junction, where bison are often spotted grazing and wallowing around thermal areas adjacent to the trail. If you are doing a five-day trip, you have three decent trailside options for first-night campsites in the next 1.5 miles.

Camping

First up, the wide-open campsite OA1 ►5 is the only one that also allows stock parties. Watch out for bison barging through in the middle of the night. Four hundred yards down-trail, across the Upper Firehole River, campsite OA2 ►6 is your best choice. Almost a mile farther upstream, campsite OA3 ►7 is near Firehole Springs. Beyond here, the trail leaves the river and starts to climb up to cross the Continental Divide.

If you choose not to linger here for fishing or geyser-gazing on your first day, you'll have to contend with a 300-foot climb through unburned forest to unsigned Grants Pass (8,010 feet) ►8 and a similar descent to the signed Bechler River Trail junction, ►9 at 6.4 miles. The hiker- and llama-only campsite 8G1 (no wood fires) is a hundred yards to the left, off the Shoshone Lake Trail in Shoshone

Camping Meadows. If you can't reserve a spot here, it's a 2.5-mile detour down to the lovely campsite 8R5 (no wood fires), which fronts Basin Point Bay on the west shore of Shoshone Lake. If you stay here, don't miss the opportunity to explore the Shoshone Geyser Basin, detailed in Trail 32, page 251.

If you have opted for the three-night plan, the absolute farthest you can comfortably go during your first day is 9.5 miles, crossing the Continental Divide (8,500 feet) again, to campsite 9D4. ►10 The last first-night resort is the rocky campsite 9D3, ►11

Wildlife a popular stock-grazing site 1.2 miles farther along through meadows and prime moose habitat below Douglas Knob ►12 (8,544 feet). Neither of these sites allows wood fires.

It's all downhill beyond 9D4. Below 9D3, the trail drops into the Littles Fork drainage, then crosses the Gregg Fork of the Upper Bechler River just before campsite 9D2, ►13 a decent overnight

Waterfall option at 13.5 miles. Just downstream is the 55-foot Twister Falls cascade, out of sight but visible from a short spur trail. From here on down, you're in the thick of the Waterfall Wonderland, first mapped in 1872 by the Hayden Survey's chief topographer, Gustavus R. Bechler.

The trail descends gradually through lush, unburned forest, along the east side of the Gregg Fork for another 1.5 miles to a typically unsigned (but well-beaten) 0.5-mile side trail that heads east (left), past a hitch rail and upstream along the north bank of the Ferris Fork. The main attraction here is the huge, circular hot-spring soak known as "Mr. Bubbles," which easily ranks as the park's finest backcountry soak, but there are also several hot springs and calcite terraces that warrant exploration. Intrepid bushwhackers may discover several seldom-seen waterfalls upstream.

Back on the main route, the trail switchbacks down across the Gregg Fork, past 45-foot Ragged Falls to the ideal campsite 9D1, ►14 (no wood fires) perched above Three River Junction, the captivating confluence of the Phillips, Gregg, and Ferris Forks, forming the headwaters of the Bechler River. The Three Rivers Patrol Cabin ►15 and stock-party campsite 9B0 (two-night limit, no wood fires) are a mile below the junction, in a meadow riddled with algae-laden thermal features.

The better overnight option, campsite 9B9 (two-night limit, no wood fires), awaits a few hundred yards downstream, tucked away on the left side of the trail below the towering Batchelder Column. ►16 The impressive, roaring, 260-foot Albright Falls cascade is visible (and audible) from the stellar campsite. Fishing can be good below the falls.

A mile downstream, the trailside campsite 9B8 ►17 (with a pit toilet) is below a patch of burned forest, just before the first of two substantial fords of the Bechler River. Orange blazes usually mark the best places to cross, but don't hesitate to scout upstream and downstream options if you don't like the looks of things where the trail hits the water.

Albright Falls was named in 1986 in honor of Horace Marden Albright, who helped to found the National Park Service in 1916 and who served as Yellowstone's superintendent from 1919 to 1929.

 Camping

 Waterfall

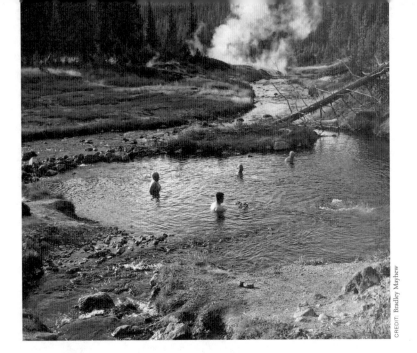

Hikers *enjoying the remote hot spring waters of Mr. Bubbles*

Canyon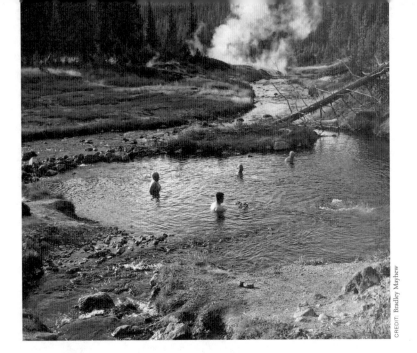

Another mile down-canyon, just after a more serious 50-foot-wide ford (up to hip-deep in August), is campsite 9B7, ▶18 set back well off the trail, up against the sheer canyon walls.

There's plenty more mud here, as cold feeder streams tumble across the trail. Less than a mile downstream is the nice trailside campsite 9B6. ▶19 The trail gets a bit steeper and rockier as it approaches the first of several cascades above the forested Treasure Island islet, in the middle of the river. To your left in the wet season, a series of unnamed cataracts plunge down from the Pitchstone Plateau.

The damp, less desirable campsite 9B5 ▶20 is between the 40-foot, rainbow-producing Iris Falls and the spectacular, two-tiered Colonnade Falls, ▶21

Viewpoint

which is visible from a signed, 300-yard side trail that dead-ends at a viewpoint and picnic spot.

The lower stretch of trail alternates between meadows, fir–spruce forest, and boulder fields festooned with edible raspberries, huckleberries, and thimbleberries. Angler alert: A couple of miles downstream, just before leaving the canyon, there's an opportunity to bushwhack up to your left—to Ranger Lake, where rainbow trout are rumored to lurk.

At the mouth of Bechler Canyon, trailside campsite 9B4 ▶**22** awaits below Ouzel Falls, which is 0.5 mile north of the trail and visible for miles around.

Less than a mile farther along, fronting the eastern edge of the vast meadows, campsite 9B3 ▶**23** (two-night limit) is reserved for stock parties. The popular trailside campsite 9B2 ▶**24** (two-night limit, no wood fires) is just before the knee- to thigh-high Bechler River ford, 5.7 miles from the exit trailhead.

Depending on the season and water level, you can opt to turn left here and stay on the east side of the Bechler River for a slightly longer but more scenic route back to the ranger station, via the wider but shallower Rocky Ford.

Our route continues straight ahead beyond the Bechler River ford. It passes the 9M2 stock campsite (two-night limit, no wood fires) before crossing a boggy section on a footbridge, just before the signed Bechler Meadows Cutoff Trail junction. ▶**25**

Again, depending on the season and prevailing conditions, it can be a soggy slog for the next 1.5 miles through the wildlife-rich meadows to the Boundary Creek suspension bridge. ▶**26**

Just beyond Boundary Creek is the exposed trailside campsite 9B1. ▶**27** Keep straight on the Bechler Meadows Trail as the alternate River Trail rejoins from the left, unless you have reserved the riverfront campsite 9C1 (two-night limit) 0.5 mile downstream (to your left at the junction). After a long stretch across a forested upland island, stay left at the Boundary Creek Trail junction. ▶**28** From here, it's 1.6 miles to a signed junction ▶**29** and, finally, the pit toilets and drinking-water spigot near the Bechler Ranger Station. ▶**30**

At 230 feet, Ouzel Falls is one of Yellowstone's tallest cascades, though it's hardly the most impressive. It's most striking early in the season, as it loses much of its oomph by the end of August.

 Camping

▶1   0.0 Start at Lone Star trailhead

▶2   1.6 Right at Spring Creek Trail junction

▶3   2.5 Lone Star Geyser

▶4   2.7 Left at Shoshone Lake Trail junction

▶5   2.9 Campsite OA1

▶6   3.3 Campsite OA2

▶7   4.1 Campsite OA3

▶8   6.0 Grants Pass

▶9   6.4 Right at Bechler River–Shoshone Lake Trail junction

▶10   9.5 Campsite 9D4

▶11   10.7 Campsite 9D3

▶12   12.0 Douglas Knob

▶13   13.5 Campsite 9D2

▶14   15.9 Three River Junction and campsite 9D1

▶15   16.8 Three Rivers Patrol Cabin and campsite 9B0

▶16   17.0 Campsite 9B9 and Batchelder Column

▶17   17.9 Campsite 9B8

▶18   18.9 Campsite 9B7

▶19   19.6 Campsite 9B6

▶20   20.8 Campsite 9B5

▶21   20.9 Colonnade Falls

▶22   22.6 Campsite 9B4

▶23   23.3 Campsite 9B3

▶24   24.0 Campsite 9B2 and Bechler River ford

▶25   24.5 Left at Bechler Meadows Cutoff Trail junction

▶26   26.0 Boundary Creek suspension bridge

▶27   26.3 Straight on Bechler Meadows Trail past campsite 9B1

▶28   28.0 Left at Boundary Creek Trail junction

▶29   29.6 Straight to Bechler Ranger Station

▶30   29.7 Arrive at Bechler Ranger Station parking area

Cave Falls and Bechler Falls

Wider than they are tall, Bechler and Cave Falls are the most accessible cascades in the remote Bechler region. This easy loop provides a sample of what the area has to offer while avoiding river fords.

Best Time

Runoff is highest from May on, but access to the region is difficult, and trails remain wet and muddy until mid-July. Of course, by the time the trails have dried out in August and September, the volume of the waterfalls is greatly diminished. Throughout October, the weather can be good but is very unpredictable.

Finding the Trail

From the West Entrance at West Yellowstone, Montana, head south 60 miles (1.5 hours) on US 20 to Ashton, Idaho. Turn east on ID 47 for 6 miles, past Marysville, and just after the road jogs to the left take a right onto Cave Falls Road. Continue 17 miles, past the Idaho–Wyoming state line, and then turn left for the Bechler Ranger Station at the signed junction for Cave Falls.

An alternate but very rough route from Yellowstone's South Entrance heads 50 miles west from Flagg Ranch to a cutoff for the Bechler Ranger Station via the unpaved Grassy Lake Road (called Ashton–Flagg Ranch Road, Reclamation Road, or USFS Road 261 on some older maps).

TRAIL USE
Hike, Horse

LENGTH
7.3 miles, 2.5–3 hours

VERTICAL FEET
Negligible

DIFFICULTY
– 1 2 **3** 4 5 +

TRAIL TYPE
Loop

SURFACE TYPE
Dirt

FEATURES
Child Friendly
Stream
Waterfall
Autumn Colors
Birds
Wildlife
Photo Opportunity
Swimming

FACILITIES
Ranger Station
Restrooms
Picnic Tables
Horse Staging

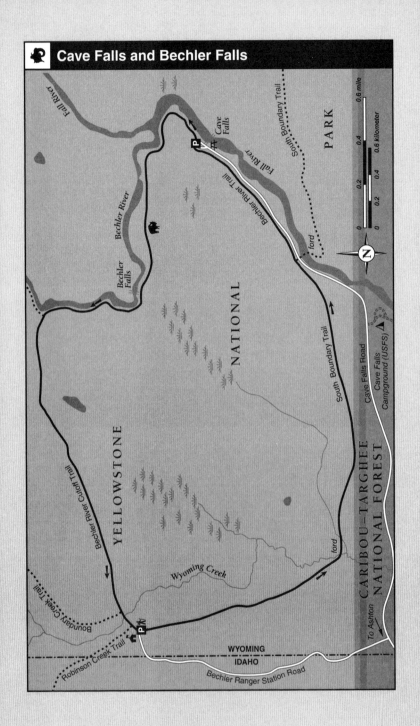

Cave Falls and Bechler Falls

Fall River

Cave Falls

Fall River

South Boundary Trail

PARK

0.6 mile

0.4

0.2

0

0.6 kilometer

0.4

0.2

0

N

Bechler River Trail

ford

Bechler River

Bechler Falls

NATIONAL

South Boundary Trail

Cave Falls Road

Cave Falls Campground (USFS)

CARIBOU–TARGHEE NATIONAL FOREST

YELLOWSTONE

Bechler River Cutoff Trail

ford

Wyoming Creek

To Ashton

Boundary Creek Trail

Robinson Creek Trail

WYOMING

IDAHO

Bechler Ranger Station Road

Trail Description

From the day-hiking parking area near the Bechler Ranger Station, ▶1 look just south for the South Boundary Trail trailhead. ▶2 The trail heads out southeast through lodgepole pines on a different route than the other trails that leave from the northwest side of the barn.

There's an easy ford of Wyoming Creek 0.5 mile from the trailhead, after which the trail parallels the park's southern boundary and paved Cave Falls Road for a mile. After passing the U.S. Forest Service Cave Falls Campground on the opposite side of the road, ▶3 the trail enters the Cave Falls parking lot and picnic area at the end of the road, 3.8 miles from the trailhead. ▶4

Cave Falls' name comes from the large cavern near its base on the river's west bank. Depending on the flow of the wide, two-tiered plunge, it's sometimes possible to wade upstream and swim near the base of the falls.

Beyond the falls, the trail continues upstream 0.2 mile along the west side of the Fall River past some rapids to the Bechler River confluence. ▶5 Less than a mile farther upstream, Bechler Falls ▶6 cascades over 15 feet. The understory vegetation here is a lush mix of mosses, ferns, and thickets of berry bushes beneath a crowded spruce–fir canopy. Monitor the banks above the river for moose, deer, and other berry-loving browsers.

The trail leaves the river a mile beyond the falls at the Bechler River Cutoff Trail junction, ▶7 where it loops back around through unburned forest to the Bechler Ranger Station parking area. ▶8

South of the park, below the Cave Falls Campground, the Fall River features a 14-mile, Class III whitewater kayak run through prime grizzly bear and bald eagle habitat.

 Waterfall

 Swimming

 Wildlife

Above Cave Falls, the cutthroat and rainbow trout get bigger, and upstream the fishing gets better the farther you hike off-trail. Aquatic insects begin to hatch in July.

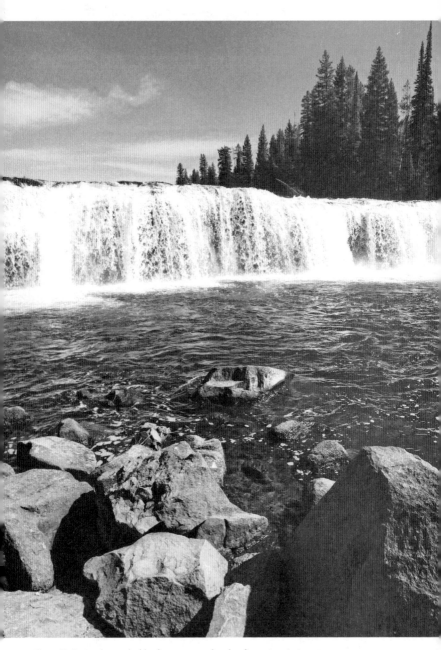

Cave Falls *can be reached by foot or car and makes for a nice picnic spot.*

CREDIT: Bradley Mayhew

🚶 MILESTONES

▶1   0.0 Start at Bechler Ranger Station trailhead

▶2   0.1 Southeast on South Boundary Trail

▶3   2.8 Straight past Fall River ford parking area

▶4   3.8 Cave Falls overlook and picnic area

▶5   4.0 Bechler River–Fall River confluence

▶6   4.8 Bechler Falls

▶7   5.8 Left at Bechler River Cutoff Trail junction

▶8   7.3 Return to Bechler Ranger Station parking area

OPTIONS

Save the Best for Last?

The loop can be done in either direction with no change in difficulty. As described, the route leaves the best for the second half of the hike. You can cut out the part along the road by doing the trip clockwise and turning around at either Bechler or Cave Falls and retracing your steps.

Alternatively, you can start at the Cave Falls trailhead parking area and do an easy 2-mile, one-hour out-and-back jaunt to Bechler Falls.

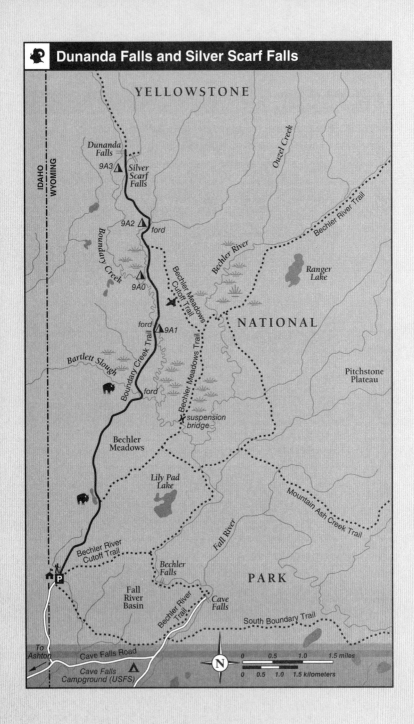

Dunanda Falls and Silver Scarf Falls

YELLOWSTONE

IDAHO
WYOMING

Dunanda
Falls
9A3
Silver
Scarf
Falls

Ouzel Creek

Boundary Creek

9A2   ford

Bechler River Trail

Bechler River

Ranger
Lake

9A0

Bechler Meadows Cutoff Trail

ford   9A1

NATIONAL

Boundary Creek Trail

Bartlett Slough

Bechler Meadows Trail

Pitchstone
Plateau

ford

suspension
bridge

Bechler
Meadows

Lily Pad
Lake

Mountain Ash Creek Trail

Bechler River
Cutoff Trail

Bechler
Falls

PARK

Fall River

P

Fall River
Basin

Bechler River Trail

Cave
Falls

South Boundary Trail

To
Ashton

Cave Falls Road

Cave Falls
Campground (USFS)

N

| 0 | 0.5 | 1.0 | 1.5 miles |
| 0 | 0.5 | 1.0 | 1.5 kilometers |

Dunanda Falls and Silver Scarf Falls

Highlights include lush riparian zones; vast, wildlife-rich meadows; sublime hot pots; invigorating stream crossings; and mesmerizing waterfalls. Because there are several good campsites en route, the trip is easily extended into a moderate overnighter.

Best Time

The Bechler is wet and buggy through the end of July. River fords can be tricky and run high until mid-July, but waterfalls are at their most spectacular early in the season. August and September are the classic times to hike the Bechler. October is bug-free and can be glorious or a real boondoggle if an early winter storm sweeps through. The lowest-lying parts of the trail can be swampy year-round. Definitely bring your hiking sandals or wading shoes, plus trekking poles for added stability.

Finding the Trail

From the West Entrance at West Yellowstone, Montana, head south 60 miles (1.5 hours) on US 20 to Ashton, Idaho. Turn east on ID 47 and travel 6 miles, past Marysville, then jog right onto Cave Falls Road. Continue 17 miles, past the Idaho–Wyoming state line, and then turn left for the Bechler Ranger Station at the signed junction for Cave Falls.

An alternate but very rough route from Yellowstone's South Entrance heads 50 miles west from Flagg Ranch to a cutoff for the Bechler Ranger Station via the unpaved Grassy Lake Road (called Ashton–Flagg Ranch Road, Reclamation Road, or USFS Road 261 on some older maps).

TRAIL USE
Hike, Backpack, Horse

LENGTH
16.4 miles, 8–10 hours

VERTICAL FEET
±400

DIFFICULTY
– 1 2 3 4 **5** +

TRAIL TYPE
Out-and-back

SURFACE TYPE
Dirt

FEATURES
Backcountry Permit
Stream
Waterfall
Autumn Colors
Birds
Wildlife
Photo Opportunity
Camping
Swimming
Secluded
Geothermal

FACILITIES
Ranger Station
Restrooms
Water
Horse Staging

221

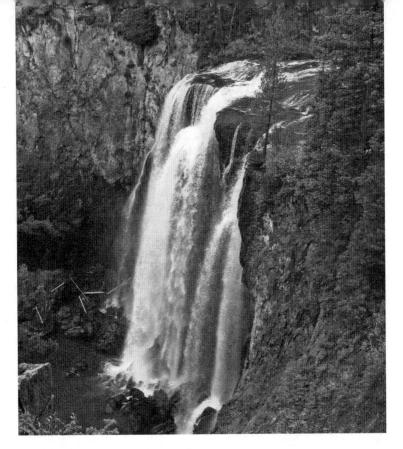

View of Dunanda Falls *from the overlook*

Trail Description

Dunanda, the name of the 150-foot plunge, comes from the Shoshone word for "straight down." For a sample of the Cascade Corner's varied delights, this rewarding, daylong hike can't be beat.

From trailhead 9K1 between the barn and the Bechler Ranger Station, ▶1 head north into unburned upland islands of lodgepole pine forest. Just beyond the Bechler Meadows Trail junction, ▶2 the trail crosses a rotting boardwalk (it may have been replaced by the time you read this).

At 1.6 miles from the trailhead, fork left onto the Boundary Creek Trail, ▶3 which continues north past several ponds and through small, marshy meadows. The forest thins out a bit as the trail crosses several boggy areas on logs.

As you approach the southern edge of the flat expanse of Bechler Meadows, you'll have to wade

through the stagnant, murky Bartlett Slough. Early
in the season it can be difficult to see the solid bottom, but by August it is usually a shallow crossing
and, if you're lucky, may be bridged by logs. On the
upside, there are good views of the Tetons in the
background, and the surrounding territory is prime
moose stomping grounds.

Wildlife

Trailside campsite 9A1, situated in a mature
island of lodgepole pine overlooking the meadows,
receives heavy stock use and is a hundred yards
before the Boundary Creek ford, ▶4 5 miles from
the trailhead. The crossing here can be knee- to
thigh-high, even after the water level drops in July.
Late in the season, the creek may be serendipitously
bridged by deadfall. Things only get damper as you
head upstream between the edge of the forest and
the east bank of Boundary Creek. Scan the meadows
for great blue herons and sandhill cranes.

Camping

Birds

At 6.4 miles, campsite 9A0 is another popular
stock site, on the opposite bank of a Boundary
Creek tributary, just beyond the Bechler Meadows
Cutoff Trail junction. ▶5 You'll encounter several
small, unbridged fords in the next mile—most
should be crossable on fallen logs. Beyond a small

OPTIONS

To Ford or Not to Ford?

By adding 0.6 mile in each direction, you can avoid the ford of
Boundary Creek: On your way to the falls, stay on the Bechler
Meadows Trail at the Boundary Creek Trail junction, and then
turn left on the Bechler Meadows Cutoff Trail to rejoin the
Boundary Creek Trail. There's no guarantee, however, that the
trail through Bechler Meadows will be any less wet than the
fords. It's always a good idea to check current ford and trail
conditions at the Bechler Ranger Station before heading out.
By taking this route in one direction, you get a loop hike that
avoids too much repetition and adds only 0.6 mile.

Overnight Options

Few backpackers (and even fewer day hikers) venture upstream above Dunanda Falls on the Boundary Creek Trail. The trail traces Boundary Creek as it climbs several hundred feet past solitary campsite 9A4 and several intriguing thermal areas. Eventually it ends up at fishless Buffalo Lake, 1 mile east of the park's western boundary.

If you can score a campsite reservation, there are many good options for extending the trip overnight.

Camping

ford and the nice hiker-only campsite 9A2, in the middle of a large meadow, the trail traverses a decade-old burn area.

A short spur trail to the hiker-only campsite 9A3 joins the main trail just before the Silver Scarf

Waterfall

Falls junction, ▶6 8 miles from the trailhead. The campsite is within earshot of Dunanda Falls and is a great base camp for exploring nearby hydrothermal wonders. It's worth exploring nearby cascades of Silver Scarf Falls.

The Dunanda Falls overlook ▶7 is just beyond the final junction, a few hundred yards up the trail's left fork.

Geothermal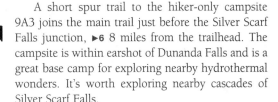

After exploring off-trail around the brink of the falls, it's a simple matter of relaxing in one of the popular riverside hot pots, formed where hot springs mix with cool river water. It's a delicious sensation to feel the cold spray of the waterfalls on your face as the rest of you soaks in bathtub-temperature waters. Eventually you'll have to pull yourself away from the hot pots before retracing your steps back to the Bechler Ranger Station. ▶8

🚶 MILESTONES

▶1 0.0 Start at Bechler Ranger Station trailhead
▶2 0.1 Left at Bechler Meadows Trail junction
▶3 1.6 Left at Boundary Creek Trail junction
▶4 5.0 Campsite 9A1 and Boundary Creek ford
▶5 6.4 Left at Bechler Meadows Cutoff Trail; campsite 9AO
▶6 8.0 Left at Silver Scarf Falls spur trail junction
▶7 8.2 Dunanda Falls overlook
▶8 16.4 Return to Bechler Ranger Station parking area

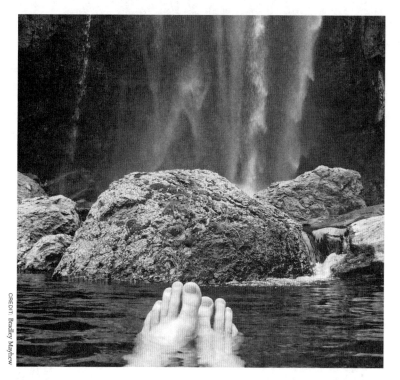

CREDIT: Bradley Mayhew

Soaking in hot springs *at the base of Dunanda Falls*

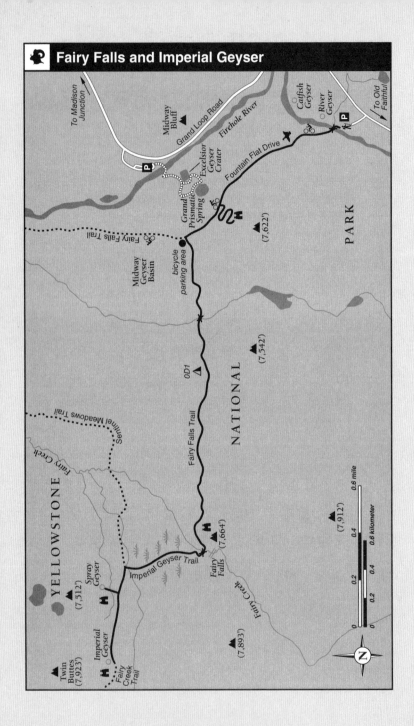

Fairy Falls and Imperial Geyser

To Madison Junction

Midway Bluff

Grand Loop Road

Firehole River

Catfish Geyser

River Geyser

To Old Faithful

P

Excelsior Geyser Crater

Fountain Flat Drive

Grand Prismatic Spring

(7,622')

PARK

Fairy Falls Trail

bicycle parking area

Midway Geyser Basin

(7,542')

NATIONAL

OD1

Fairy Falls Trail

Sentinel Meadows Trail

Fairy Creek

(7,912')

0.6 mile

0.6 kilometer

(7,664')

Fairy Falls

Imperial Geyser Trail

Fairy Creek

Spray Geyser

YELLOWSTONE

(7,512')

(7,893')

Imperial Geyser

Twin Buttes
(7,923')

Fairy Creek Trail

N

0.2   0.4   0.6 mile

0   0.2   0.4   0.6 kilometer

Fairy Falls and Imperial Geyser

This family-friendly day hike epitomizes what's so wonderful about the Yellowstone backcountry. Just a short distance off the road, you'll find one of the park's tallest waterfalls and a couple of intriguing, seldom-seen geothermal features. It's a jeans-and-tennis-shoes sort of picnic outing; you can even cycle part of the way.

Best Time

Fairy Falls is at its most spectacular in spring, and the trail is normally hikable from the end of May to October. There's little shade and no water along the trail, except at the falls. Head out early to dodge the crowds and avoid the midday heat. The entire surrounding Firehole area, including Firehole Freight Road and Firehole Lake Drive, is closed for bear management from March 10 through the Friday of Memorial Day weekend.

Finding the Trail

From the south, go 4.3 miles north from the Old Faithful overpass on Grand Loop Road and turn left into the Fairy Falls (also known as Steel Bridge) trailhead parking area, on the west side of the road. This is a very popular trailhead, so get here early to snag a parking spot. From the north, head 11.2 miles south from Madison Junction on Grand Loop Road, 1.4 miles past the Midway Geyser Basin turn-off, and turn right into the busy parking area.

TRAIL USE
Hike, Bike, Backpack

LENGTH
5.2 miles (6.8 miles including Imperial Geyser), 2–3.5 hours

VERTICAL FEET
Negligible

DIFFICULTY
– 1 2 **3** 4 5 +

TRAIL TYPE
Out-and-back

SURFACE TYPE
Dirt

FEATURES
Child Friendly
Waterfall
Wildflowers
Birds
Great Views
Photo Opportunity
Camping
Swimming
Geothermal

FACILITIES
None

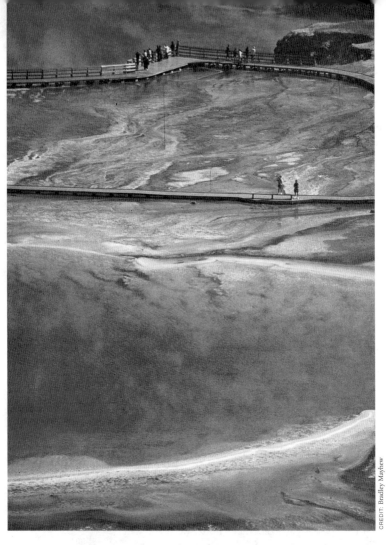

CREDIT: Bradley Mayhew

View of *Grand Prismatic Spring from the viewpoint above Fountain Flat Drive*

Logistics

Check at the Old Faithful Visitor Center or call rangers at 307-344-2750 to ask about recent Imperial Geyser activity before heading out. Rangers lead Adventure Hikes to Fairy Falls and Imperial Geyser June–August on Thursdays at 8 a.m. Check the park newspaper for details.

Trail Description

From the trailhead parking area, ▶1 the wide, gravel Fountain Flat Drive (originally known as National Park Avenue) starts on the other side of an old steel trestle bridge ▶2 that spans the Firehole River. This stretch of the Firehole is a popular catch-and-release fishing access point. The first section of the trail skirts several riverside thermal features. The road itself is popular with bicyclists heading to the Fountain Flat Drive trailhead, 3.5 miles north. If you are short on time, consider cycling to the turnoff to Fairy Falls and begin hiking from there, shaving 2 miles off the walk.

As the trail swings away from the river, look for ducks and geese in the ponds and marshes to your right. Signs of the 1988 fires abound in the open meadows and on the denuded hillsides. Straight ahead, look for the steam rising from the Midway Geyser Basin.

Before you come level with Grand Prismatic Spring after 0.6 mile, you'll see its huge, marshy runoff field. Notice how the steam reflects the rainbow colors of the spring, which are especially visible with polarized sunglasses. You can get some idea of the vibrancy and immensity of the awe-inspiring spring as the trail skirts the Midway Geyser Basin, but the best views are from the hills to your left. Hikers have long climbed unofficial trails up the hillside here, and in 2016 the park service decided to construct a formal trail up the hillside, spurred to action after a falling tree killed a Taiwanese hiker the year before. The new trail climbs a few hundred feet to offer one of the park's newest and greatest viewpoints. ▶3 Only from this height can you truly appreciate the rainbowlike multicolored bands ringing Grand Prismatic Springs.

Back on the main trail, after 1 mile, just beyond the geyser basin, the trail joins the Fairy Falls Trail (bicycles not allowed, so park yours at the junction).

Grand Prismatic Spring is one of the world's largest hot springs, comparable in size to Deildartunguhver in Iceland but smaller than the geothermal complex in New Zealand's volcanic Waimangu Valley.

 Birds

 Photo Opportunity

 Geothermal

 Viewpoint

►4 Turning left, the trail enters an alley of regenerating lodgepole pines, already well over head height. You are also in the heart of the Firehole Bear Management Area, so keep your wits about you, and obey any posted signs.

Camping

You soon cross a wooden footbridge over a stream coming out of a small, unnamed lake before reaching the well-signed 0D1 campsite ►5 turnoff at 1.7 miles. The campsite is a few hundred yards north of the trail, in a small island of mature lodgepole pines that survived the 1988 fires. It's also less than an hour from the trailhead, a good overnight option for families and first-time backpackers—but there's no water, and shade is sparse.

Wildflowers

Beyond the 0D1 spur trail junction, the main trail does a few gentle ups and downs as it hugs the base of the ridge to your left. You soon start to see signs of forest diversification, including some wildflowers and quaking aspen saplings. Check out the twisted, gnarled branches on some of the remaining snags. Stop for a moment: Can you hear the falls reverberating off the base of the hills? Straight ahead, the Twin Buttes loom, bald as eagles.

Waterfall

As you turn the corner to Fairy Falls, ►6 2.6 miles from the trailhead, you'll notice how the mist from the falls makes the lush vegetation dramatically different. With a drop of almost 200 feet, it's the tallest frontcountry waterfall in Greater Yellowstone. You can catch a brisk shower if the weather is particularly

---

Imperial Geyser and Twin Buttes

The round-trip to Imperial Geyser adds 1.6 miles, negligible elevation gain, and about an hour, depending on how much of a geyser-gazer you are. From the geyser basin, you can continue north off-trail 0.5 mile to summit the Twin Buttes and get a good overview of the Lower and Midway Geyser Basins.

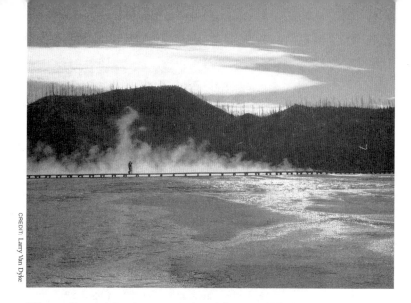

Hikers *walk around Grand Prismatic Spring with fire-scarred hillsides beyond.*

hot. The area just downstream from the falls, where raspberries shoot up between the rocks, makes a nice picnic spot (shade or sun; take your pick).

From the falls, you can either retrace your steps to the trailhead or forge ahead 0.8 mile to a couple of seldom-seen geysers for the unchoreographed antithesis of the Old Faithful experience. If you decide to press on, a trail sign for the Imperial Geyser Trail, ▶7 just beyond the bridge, points the way. It's 0.4 mile from the falls to a junction with the Sentinel Meadows Trail, ▶8 then a few hundred yards more to the geyser basin.

Geothermal

Cross a couple of long boardwalks that span damp meadows. These boardwalks may be closed to stock use. If the buffalo chips atop the walkway are any indication, apparently the bison are impervious to National Park Service management directives. From the middle of the second boardwalk, look for a steam plume off to your left. The broad trail wends its way past more aspen saplings as it heads toward the Twin Buttes. Watch here for black beetles and other winged insects that colonize burn areas after fires.

Geothermal

Photo Opportunity 📷

At the final unsigned junction, ▶9 the right fork crosses a thermal runoff channel full of orange and green thermophile strands and mats. If possible, please use the logs to cross, and tread carefully to preserve the fragile microbiology. Solitary Spray Geyser is a near-perpetual spouter, erupting frequently to a height of 6–8 feet.

Retrace your steps to a game trail that follows the runoff channel upstream through several bison wallows to reach Imperial Geyser, ▶10 which erupts frequently.

If you approach the sulfurous mud kettles around the back side of the geyser basin, take great care in the fragile area, and listen to the belching sounds for clues about how the basin's plumbing is connected.

Follow the trail downstream along the far side of the runoff channel to retrace your steps. Turn right at the Imperial Geyser Trail junction to return to the Fairy Falls trailhead parking area. ▶11

🚶 MILESTONES

▶1   0.0 Start at Fairy Falls trailhead

▶2   0.1 Cross Firehole River on Soldier Bridge

▶3   0.6 Climb new trail to viewpoint

▶4   1.0 Left at Fairy Falls Trail junction

▶5   1.7 Straight past campsite 0D1 spur trail

▶6   2.6 Fairy Falls

▶7   2.8 Left at Imperial Geyser Trail junction

▶8   3.0 Left at Sentinel Meadows Trail junction

▶9   3.2 Right at unsigned fork to Solitary Spray Geyser

▶10   3.4 Right upstream to Imperial Geyser

▶11   6.8 Return to Fairy Falls parking area

Lone Star Geyser

It's an easy stroll along an abandoned road to one of the park's most impressive and dependable geysers. The hike is justifiably popular with tour groups, and you might see a few backpackers heading out for the Bechler River Trail, which begins a day's hike down-trail, beyond Shoshone Lake. The trail also offers one of the park's few opportunities for a 10- to 15-minute, traffic-free bike ride on a paved road to the geyser. Allow at least an hour for the hike so you don't miss the eruption.

Best Time

Lone Star is a popular year-round destination, even in winter. Eruptions take place every three hours or so, meaning you could wait up to three hours for an eruption if your timing is off. If you have time to kill, consider exploring the trail headed toward Shoshone Lake, which has some interesting thermal features not far from Lone Star Geyser.

Finding the Trail

From the Old Faithful overpass, head 2.5 miles south on Grand Loop Road, and turn right into the trailhead parking lot on the south side of the road. From the southeast, go 14.5 miles west over Craig Pass (8,262 feet) from West Thumb and turn left into the parking lot. The trailhead is just south of the Kepler Cascades turnout, which is a parking alternative if the Lone Star lot is full.

TRAIL USE
Hike, Bike, Backpack
LENGTH
5.0 miles, 2.5–3 hours
VERTICAL FEET
Negligible
DIFFICULTY
− 1 **2** 3 4 5 +
TRAIL TYPE
Out-and-back
SURFACE TYPE
Paved

FEATURES
Child Friendly
Handicap Accessible
Stream
Wildlife
Cool & Shady
Photo Opportunity
Camping
Geothermal
Moonlight Hiking

FACILITIES
Restrooms

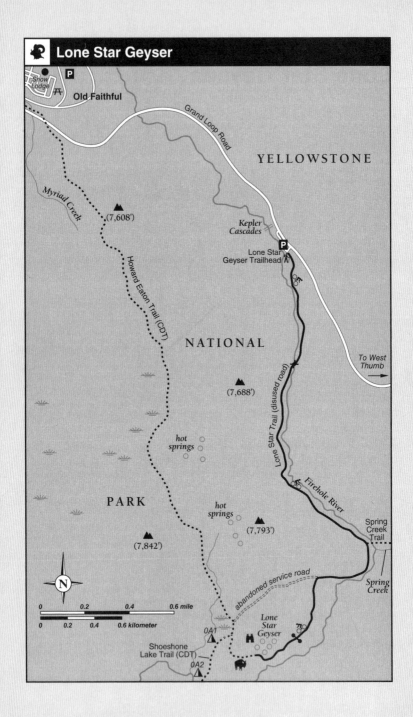

Lone Star Geyser

Old Faithful

Show Lodge

P

YELLOWSTONE

Grand Loop Road

Myriad Creek

(7,608')

Kepler Cascades

P

Lone Star Geyser Trailhead

Howard Eaton Trail (CDT)

NATIONAL

(7,688')

To West Thumb

hot springs

Lone Star Trail (disused road)

Firehole River

hot springs

(7,793')

PARK

Spring Creek Trail

(7,842')

N

0   0.2   0.4   0.6 mile

0   0.2   0.4   0.6 kilometer

abandoned service road

Spring Creek

Lone Star Geyser

0A1

Shoeshone Lake Trail (CDT)

0A2

Logistics

Rangers lead 4.5-hour hikes here in the summer every Tuesday at 8 a.m. when budgets allow; check the park newspaper for the current schedule. Regular eruptions happen about every 3 hours, with minor eruptions around 30 minutes before the main event. Splashing preplay starts up to an hour before eruptions, and there's a noisy steam phase afterward.

Trail Description

From the parking lot, ▶1 the trail starts out on a flat, abandoned service road just upstream from the Kepler Cascades. The traffic noise from Grand Loop Road quickly fades as birds twittering, chipmunks chattering, and the rush of the Firehole River take over. If you stop to listen and use your imagination, the wind here might sound like the ocean whistling through the trees.

After a few hundred yards, check out the old waterworks ▶2 on the right, where the trail joins the Firehole River. The road becomes asphalt as the trail traces the east bank of the river upstream. Mature mixed-conifer forest surrounds the route on all sides. There's a dampness in the air and green mosses in the understory as the river passes under a bridge and calms upstream. Watch for steaming thermal features off-trail in the woods to the right. Note the saplings growing up through the roadbed.

Stay on the road where the Spring Creek Trail ▶3 joins in from the left after 1.6 miles. At 2 miles, follow the road as it jogs left at an abandoned service road. ▶4

 Geothermal

You may hear Lone Star Geyser before you actually see it. During its steam phase between eruptions, it can be heard as far as a mile away. As the road ends, you'll have to park your bike and walk the last short section. Less than a hundred yards after the road ends, ▶5 you'll see the impressive,

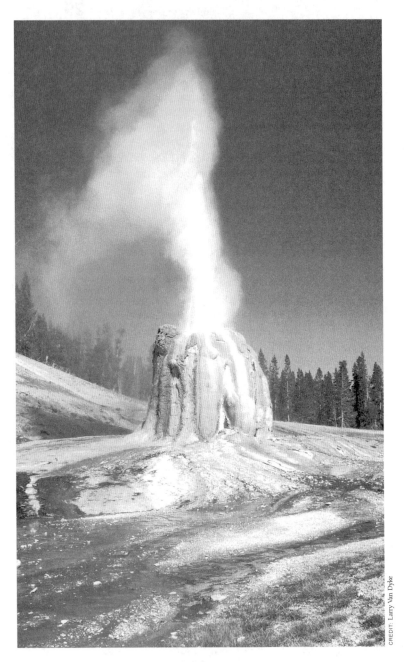

Lone Star Geyser *erupts roughly every three hours (Trails 25, 29, and 32).*

OPTIONS

Yellowstone's Moonlight-Hiking Highlights

Full moonlight is the best time to explore the following favorites, but if you pack a flashlight or headlamp and stay alert for
wildlife, most any boardwalk and geyser basin can be enjoyable to explore under a crescent moon.

- **Mammoth Hot Springs** (Trail 7, page 74) Boardwalks are
  fun to explore after dark from Liberty Cap side.

- **Grand Canyon of the Yellowstone** (Trails 14 and 15, pages
  130–140) The North and South Rims are best explored from
  the main parking areas near the Upper and Lower Falls and
  Inspiration and Artist Points. Take care when walking beside
  the canyon walls at nighttime.

- **Norris Geyser Basin** (Trail 19, page 157) The odds are steep,
  but you'll never forget seeing a geyser like Steamboat erupt
  at night.

- **West Thumb Geyser Basin** (Trail 24, page 188) Super views
  of Yellowstone Lake; be alert for wildlife.

- **Grand Prismatic Spring and Midway Geyser Basin boardwalks** (Trail 28, page 226) Awesome steam shows.

- **Lone Star Geyser** (Trail 29, page 233) A unique opportunity
  to access a backcountry geyser via a paved road, which
  makes nighttime hiking slightly safer. Go with a good-size
  group, and make plenty of noise.

- **Old Faithful and Observation Point** (Trail 31, page 243)
  Essential if you're staying at or near the geyser basin.

If you're lucky enough to be camping out near an active backcountry thermal area such as Shoshone Geyser Basin (Trail 32,
page 251) during a full moon, then you should feel obligated to
check out the natural phenomena—from a distance, mind you—
by night as well as by day.

12-foot-tall geyserite cone. ►6 Major eruptions happen like clockwork, every three hours on average, with significant preplay in between. The eruptions can reach up to 45 feet and usually last 20–30 minutes. Check the National Park Service logbook near the bridge over the runoff channel to read reports and timings of recent activity.

After the eruption, retrace your steps on the paved road back to the trailhead. ►7

MILESTONES

►1	0.0 Start at Lone Star trailhead/Kepler Cascades parking lots
►2	0.2 Old Firehole River waterworks
►3	1.6 Keep right at Spring Creek Trail junction
►4	2.0 Keep left at abandoned service road
►5	2.4 End of paved road; bicycle parking area
►6	2.5 Lone Star Geyser
►7	5.0 Return to parking area

OPTIONS

Howard Eaton Trail

You can avoid the crowds en route to Lone Star Geyser by starting out from the Old Faithful area at the Howard Eaton trailhead. The route—part of the Continental Divide National Scenic Trail—is actually less scenic and a bit longer (5.8 miles round-trip), which is why you should have it all to yourself.

Backcountry Camping

The three campsites just beyond Lone Star Geyser on the Shoshone Lake Trail are perfect places for a family to spend a first night in the backcountry. Campsite OA1 is 2.9 miles from the Lone Star trailhead; it allows stock parties. The hiker-only sites OA2 and OA3 are 0.4 and 1.2 miles farther along. All of these sites allow campfires but can be buggy in early summer.

Mystic Falls

This day hike is popular thanks to its proximity to Old Faithful, and it offers easy access to a pretty backcountry cascade. Complete the full loop to leave the crowds behind and for an expansive overview of the Upper Geyser Basin.

Best Time

The flat, out-and-back option to the base of the falls is enjoyable any time May–October. Since there's a lack of shade, on sunny days the full loop should be done outside of midday hours.

Finding the Trail

From the south, go 2 miles north on Grand Loop Road from the Old Faithful overpass and turn left into the Biscuit Basin Boardwalk parking area on the west side of the road. From the north, go 13.5 miles south from Madison Junction on Grand Loop Road and turn right. The Mystic Falls trailhead is across the Firehole River Bridge, on the far side of the boardwalk loop, 0.3 mile west of the parking lot.

Logistics

Rangers offer free, guided, 90-minute walks three times a week during summer; check the park newspaper for current schedules. Trips depart at 9 a.m. from the Firehole River Bridge, adjacent to the Biscuit Basin parking lot.

Here's a tip: You can avoid parking hassles and enjoy a fun family bike ride by cycling the 2 miles

---

TRAIL USE
Hike

LENGTH
4.0 miles, 2–3 hours

VERTICAL FEET
±500 to falls, ±1,000 for loop

DIFFICULTY
– 1 2 **3** 4 5 +

TRAIL TYPE
Loop

SURFACE TYPE
Boardwalk and Dirt

FEATURES
Child Friendly
Canyon
Stream
Waterfall
Wildflowers
Great Views
Photo Opportunity
Geothermal
Steep

FACILITIES
None

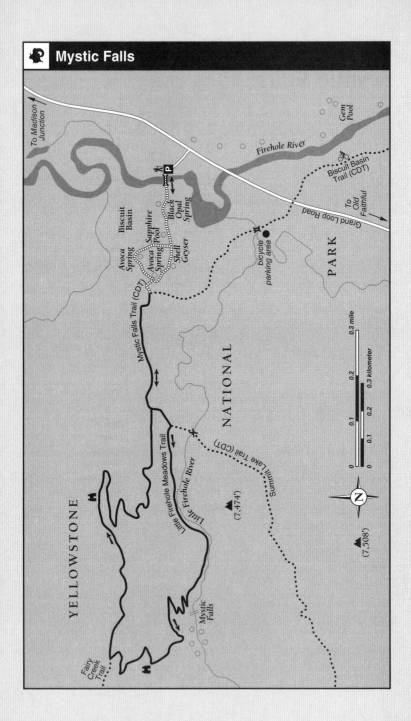

Mystic Falls

Biscuit Basin

Gem Pool

Firehole River

Biscuit Basin Trail (CDT)

To Madison Junction

P

Black Opal Spring

Sapphire Pool

Avoca Spring

Avoca Spring Pool

Shell Geyser

To Old Faithful

Grand Loop Road

bicycle parking area

PARK

Mystic Falls Trail (CDT)

NATIONAL

0.3 mile

0.2

0.1

0

0.3 kilometer

0.2

0.1

0

N

Little Firehole River

Little Firehole Meadows Trail

Summit Lake Trail (CDT)

(7,474)

(7,508)

YELLOWSTONE

Mystic Falls

Fairy Creek Trail

from Old Faithful to Grand Loop Road near the
trailhead via the Upper Geyser Basin Trail. Park
your bike on the far side of Grand Loop Road, and
start your hike from there.

**More than a quarter
of the world's geysers
are concentrated in
the Upper Geyser
Basin, which is home
to about 150 spouting
hydrothermal features.**

Trail Description

From the Biscuit Basin parking lot, ▶1 cross the
Firehole River footbridge and follow the south
side of the boardwalk loop ▶2 clockwise (left) past
several notable geysers and hot springs. Before you
reach Avoca Spring, watch for a wide, sandy trail
▶3 that heads off the boardwalk to your left, into
the regenerating lodgepole pine forest. It's often
unsigned but usually marked by orange blazes.
Wildflowers such as lupines, fireweed, and Indian
paintbrush bloom prolifically here thanks to the
1988 fires.

 Wildflowers

Beyond the boardwalk, the nearly flat route—
part of the Continental Divide National Scenic
Trail—parallels the north side of the Little Firehole
River. Stay left at 0.6 mile when the trail is met by
the return loop of the Mystic Falls Trail. ▶4 You
will return here in about an hour if you opt for the
full loop.

Soon after, head uphill (right) at the Summit
Lake/Little Firehole Meadows Trail junction, ▶5 near
the mouth of the Little Firehole River canyon; you've
missed the turnoff if you cross the river on the footbridge. The trail climbs gradually up into the canyon
above the north side of the river 0.5 mile to the base
of Mystic Falls. ▶6 Steam and orange algae blooms
indicate abundant thermal seeps in the runoff.

 Canyon

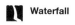 **Waterfall**

While the multitiered, 70-foot cascade is
enchanting from below, it's best admired from
above. You can either turn around here, making the
hike an hour total, or continue the loop by climbing
several hundred feet of switchbacks in a little less
than a mile to a worthwhile overlook of Old Faithful
and the Upper Geyser Basin.

 Steep

Out-and-Back Picnic Option

The family-friendly, out-and-back option to the base of the falls involves 500 feet of elevation gain and takes a little over an hour round-trip. Figure on at least an extra half hour for a picnic and short climb to the top of the falls.

About 600 yards up the trail, there's a nice overlook ►7 near the top of the falls. The route continues climbing up through a regenerating lodgepole burn area to the Fairy Creek/Little Firehole Meadows Trail junction. ►8

Turn right, crest the ridge atop the Madison Plateau, and descend to the Biscuit Basin Overlook ►9 for an impressive overview of the aftermath of **Viewpoint** 🔭 the 1988 fires and the entire Upper Geyser Basin. With decent binoculars, you can enjoy a good bird's-eye view of several major active geysers, including Old Faithful.

From the overlook, the trail descends via switchbacks more than 500 feet over 0.9 mile to rejoin the Mystic Falls Trail. ►10 Fork left at the now-familiar junction and retrace your steps back through Biscuit Basin to the parking area. ►11

🚶 MILESTONES

►1	0.0 Start at Biscuit Basin trailhead parking lot
►2	0.2 Left at boardwalk loop junction
►3	0.3 Left at unsigned Mystic Falls Trail junction
►4	0.6 Left at Mystic Falls Trail loop junction
►5	0.65 Right at Summit Lake/Little Firehole Meadows Trail junction
►6	1.2 Mystic Falls
►7	1.5 Mystic Falls Overlook
►8	1.7 Right at Fairy Creek/Little Firehole Meadows Trail junction
►9	2.5 Biscuit Basin Overlook
►10	3.4 Mystic Falls Trail junction
►11	4.0 Return to parking area

Old Faithful and Observation Point

For most folks, Old Faithful is a must-see. If you haven't seen the most famous geyser in the world's most active geyser basin, can you really say that you've been to Yellowstone?

Best Time

Any time of day or night is a wonderful time to see her majesty in action. The boardwalks are accessible year-round (weather permitting), while the loop trail is typically hikable May–October. Make sure to time your visit with an eruption (the average interval hovers around 90 minutes) by checking the predicted schedule with rangers at the visitor center. Or check the Web cam at tinyurl.com/oldfaithfulcam.

Finding the Trail

From the north, go south from Madison Junction on Grand Loop Road 15.5 miles to the Old Faithful exit. From the east, go 17 miles west from West Thumb on Grand Loop Road over Craig Pass (8,262 feet). After exiting from either direction, follow signs from the overpass for about a mile to the visitor center and Old Faithful geyser parking areas.

Logistics

The Old Faithful Visitor Center posts eruption prediction schedules for five major geysers (Castle, Daisy, Grand, Old Faithful, and Riverside) in the Upper Geyser Basin. Predictions are also made for

TRAIL USE
Hike

LENGTH
2.4 miles, 1.5 hours

VERTICAL FEET
±250

DIFFICULTY
– 1 **2** 3 4 5 +

TRAIL TYPE
Loop

SURFACE TYPE
Dirt

FEATURES
Child Friendly
Handicap Accessible
Steep
Great Views
Photo Opportunity
Geothermal
Moonlight Hiking

FACILITIES
Visitor Center
Restrooms
Picnic Tables
Phone
Water

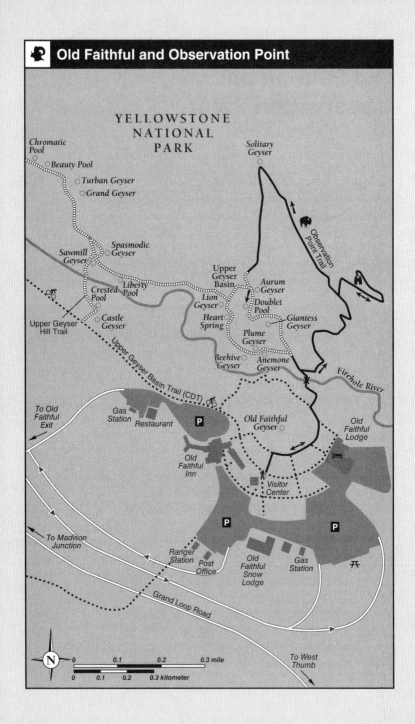

Old Faithful and Observation Point

YELLOWSTONE
NATIONAL
PARK

Chromatic Pool
Beauty Pool
Turban Geyser
Grand Geyser
Solitary Geyser
Spasmodic Geyser
Sawmill Geyser
Liberty Pool
Crested Pool
Upper Geyser Hill Trail
Castle Geyser
Upper Geyser Basin
Lion Geyser
Aurum Geyser
Doublet Pool
Heart Spring
Giantess Geyser
Plume Geyser
Beehive Geyser
Anemone Geyser
Observation Point Trail
Firehole River

Upper Geyser Basin Trail (CDT)

To Old Faithful Exit

Gas Station
Restaurant
P
Old Faithful Geyser
Old Faithful Lodge

Old Faithful Inn

Visitor Center

To Madison Junction

P
Ranger Station
Post Office
Old Faithful Snow Lodge
Gas Station
P

Grand Loop Road

N
0   0.1   0.2   0.3 mile
0   0.1   0.2   0.3 kilometer

To West Thumb

Great Fountain, 8 miles north of Old Faithful off Firehole Lake Drive, in the Lower Geyser Basin. These predictions are also posted at Old Faithful's lodgings and at the Madison Information Station, or call 307-344-2751 for recorded details.

All predictions are estimates; Old Faithful's performance intervals, for example, have varied historically from 45 to 120 minutes, with the current average time frame running 65–95 minutes.

If the next eruption is predicted (not scheduled!) for less than 30 minutes after you arrive, start the hike to Observation Point straightaway. Otherwise, grab a snack or drink, and check out the lobby of the inn or the visitor center's displays and short films. In any case, allow at least 20–30 minutes for the short but aerobic climb to the overlook.

> Though probably Yellowstone's most famous, Old Faithful is neither the largest nor the most regular geyser in the park. The largest active geyser in the world is Steamboat Geyser in the Norris Geyser Basin, erupting up to 400 feet in height (see Trail 19).

Trail Description

From the northwest side of the parking lot, ▶1 follow signs to the visitor center ▶2 and check the

NOTES

Urban Legend

A group of bored seasonal employees once received a severe reprimand from the National Park Service after they engaged in a clever bit of street theater. A few minutes before Old Faithful was predicted to erupt, they rolled out a large red wagon wheel and pretended that they were cranking open the geyser's subterranean plumbing so that the crucial H20 would appear, mocking visitors' expectations of timeliness.

On Demand?

In the height of summer, it's not uncommon to witness impatient crowds of spectators clapping in unison to urge the geyser on while complaining that their bus might leave if the darn thing doesn't perform as "scheduled."

Tours and Secrets of the Old Faithful Inn

The free guided tours of the inn are highly recommended, especially if you're an architecture or history buff. The inn is exactly one-eighth of a mile from the geyser, the legal limit. Construction began in 1904 with a $140,000 loan from railroad magnates.

Architect Robert Reamer's vision was to craft something that looked as if it had grown out of the surrounding landscape. Today, you'll find a fire in the main lobby fireplace most mornings and evenings. Tuesday–Saturday evenings, longtime pianist George tickles the ivories on the mezzanine. Around the central fireplace, look for the massive blacksmithed popcorn poppers, which have been retired due to damage.

Notice how the lobby windows are staggered to simulate natural light streaming through a forest. The entire theme, in fact, is asymmetrical; Reamer abhorred symmetry. You can distinguish the original construction from newer additions by the pitch of the roof: the Old House has a steeply pitched roof, while the newer ones are much flatter. Five second-story rooms overlooking the main portico are favorites with large families because they are large (reserve well in advance) and offer nice geyser-basin views. Only 10 rooms in the original Old House have private bathrooms.

Today, bellhops are the only people who get to live in the inn full-time. Most live in the wing known as Bat's Alley, where they have private bathrooms and enjoy the rooftop "pebble beach." Even-numbered rooms in the Old House, 46–54, face Old Faithful, but increasingly lodgepole saplings are encroaching on the geyser views, and by law they are not allowed to be trimmed. A shared bathtub and showers are upstairs. Rooms 134 and 145 have private bathrooms. The smallest rooms, all with queen beds, still have original log walls. Construction of the east wing blocked views of Old Faithful that used to be enjoyed from the inn's main dining room.

If you have a reservation at the inn, ask a bellhop if you can come along for the early-morning flag-raising ritual on the rooftop "widow's walk" or in the evening when the flags are retrieved. Only two guests are allowed to join the bellhop for each shift. It's a great photo op and includes a private tour of the historic inn's otherwise off-limits Crow's Nest.

predicted eruption times so you can plan the best hiking strategy.

From the visitor center, find the plastic-lumber boardwalk ►3 circling Old Faithful, and follow it counterclockwise (right) for a few hundred yards. Branch right to leave the boardwalk at the signed

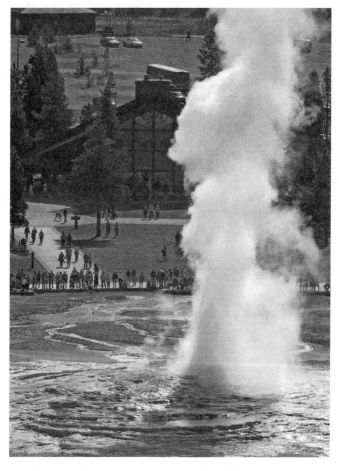

Old Faithful *erupts dramatically.*

What to Do Before an Eruption?

If you have time to burn before the next anticipated eruption, there are several intriguing options. The visitor center shows a film that gives a general introduction to the park, starting 30 minutes before an eruption is predicted. Another film about the inner workings of Old Faithful screens 15 minutes after each flare-up.

Or grab a drink from the bar or espresso cart on the mezzanine level of the Old Faithful Inn and—if you can stand the diesel fumes from the idling buses—sit out on the deck and watch the geyser warm up. In the captivating lobby, pick up a self-guiding brochure from the front desk and check out the massive central fireplace and interior stylings of "parkitecture" pioneer Robert C. Reamer. Stairs in the rustic rafters shown above climb to the now off-limits "Crow's Nest."

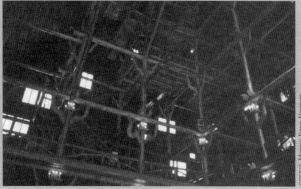

CREDIT: Morgan Konn Nystrom

turnoff for the Observation Point Trail, ►4 which soon crosses the Firehole River on a wooden footbridge. ►5

Soon after the bridge, head uphill to your right on the dirt path ►6 where the left fork leads to the Geyser Hill boardwalk loop. A bit of hard breathing and 0.5 mile later, take the signed right fork of the Observation Point loop trail ►7 up to the overlook ►8 for an expansive panorama of the Upper Geyser Basin. Catch your breath, check your watch, and

Viewpoint

find a comfortable spot with an unobstructed view of the activity below.

Heading back downhill, complete the Observation Point loop and turn right at the bottom of the hill. ▶9 Next, traverse 0.3 mile of mixed open forest—such good bear habitat that the trail is sometimes closed—to reach Solitary Geyser. ▶10 Solitary began its life as a hot spring but morphed into a gusher after its water was diverted for use in a swimming pool in the 1940s. Today, the ex-spring spouts up to 15 feet every four to eight minutes.

Head 0.3 mile downhill to the Geyser Hill boardwalk ▶11 junction. The level, wheelchair-accessible boardwalk winds past named and unnamed active geysers, including several near-perpetual spouters. Interpretive signs and self-guided trail brochures explain some of the intriguing hydrothermal phenomena.

When you're ready to conclude your hike, head back on the boardwalk toward Old Faithful. Where the Geyser Hill boardwalk ends, continue straight ahead on the paved walkway to return to the Firehole River footbridge. ▶12 Retrace your steps clockwise on the boardwalk ▶13 around Old Faithful—it may well be poised to erupt again—back to the visitor center ▶14 and parking lot. ▶15

Named for its predictability by the Washburn Expedition in 1870, Old Faithful's average interval between eruptions has lengthened due to earthquakes and vandalism, but it remains as predictable as it was more than a century ago. Its outbursts last anywhere from 90 seconds to 5 minutes, reach heights of 106–184 feet, and expel 3,700–8,400 gallons of boiling water.

Geysers Galore

Unrepentant geyser-gazers who can't get enough have plenty of exciting options for extending the hike from Old Faithful. It's possible to follow a network of boardwalks and paved bike paths—part of the Continental Divide National Scenic Trail—northwest 2 miles, beyond Geyser Hill past the predictable Grand and Riverside Geysers (90 minutes–2 hours round-trip, including time for gazing), to the much-ogled Morning Glory Pool.

The word *geyser* comes from the Icelandic verb meaning "to gush."

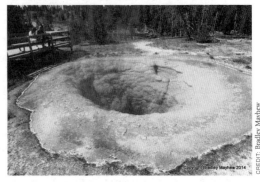

Morning Glory Pool *is a crowd favorite and a worthwhile detour from the Upper Geyser Basin Trail.*

🚶 MILESTONES

- ►1 0.0 Start at Old Faithful parking lot
- ►2 0.1 Visitor center and restrooms
- ►3 0.2 Counterclockwise (right) around Old Faithful boardwalk
- ►4 0.3 Right onto Observation Point Trail
- ►5 0.35 Firehole River Bridge
- ►6 0.4 Right at Geyser Hill Trail boardwalk junction
- ►7 0.9 Right onto Observation Point loop trail
- ►8 1.0 Observation Point overlook
- ►9 1.1 Right at Observation Point Trail junction
- ►10 1.4 Left (downhill) from Solitary Geyser
- ►11 1.7 Left at Geyser Hill boardwalk junction
- ►12 1.9 Straight at end of boardwalk to Firehole River footbridge
- ►13 2.0 Left (clockwise) around Old Faithful boardwalk
- ►14 2.3 Visitor center
- ►15 2.4 Return to parking lot

Shoshone Lake and Shoshone Geyser Basin

With no road access, forest-lined Shoshone Lake is the largest backcountry lake in the Lower 48. An amazing geyser basin, good fishing, boat-in camping, and the possibility of extended backpacking and kayaking trips add to the allure. Nearly a third of all the park's backcountry use is concentrated around the lake.

Best Time

Lewis and Shoshone Lakes are usually ice-free by the second or third week in June. Grant's Pass (8,000 feet), between Lone Star Geyser and the west end of Shoshone Lake, typically isn't free of snow until late June or early July. Early-season flooding is common at some lakefront campsites, so many sites aren't available for reservation before July 1 or July 15. Contact a backcountry office for current conditions and for early-season walk-up permits. If you're planning a late-season trip, say for October, monitor the weather carefully.

Finding the Trail

From the north, head 2.5 miles south on Grand Loop Road from the Old Faithful overpass, and turn right into the Lone Star Geyser parking lot on the south side of the road. From the southeast, go 14.5 miles west from West Thumb Junction over Craig Pass (8,262 feet), and turn left into the parking lot. The trailhead parking area is just south of the Kepler Cascades turnout, which is a parking alternative if the Lone Star lot is full.

TRAIL USE
Hike, Backpack

LENGTH
17.0 miles, 2–5 days

VERTICAL FEET
±600

DIFFICULTY
– 1 2 3 4 **5** +

TRAIL TYPE
Out-and-back

SURFACE TYPE
Dirt

FEATURES
Backcountry Permit
Lake
Stream
Autumn Colors
Wildflowers
Birds
Wildlife
Great Views
Photo Opportunity
Camping
Geothermal

FACILITIES
Patrol Cabin
Boat Launch

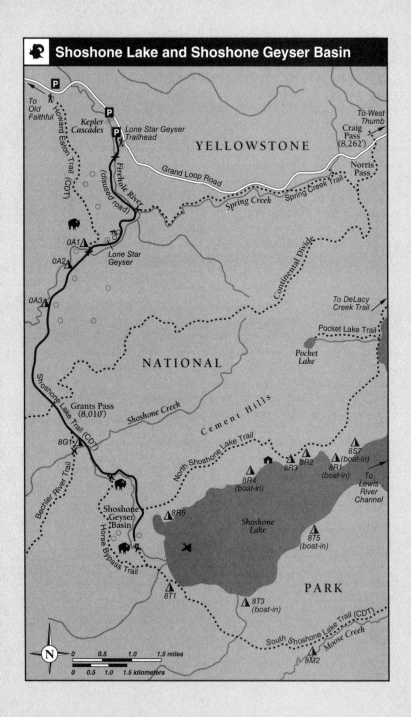

Shoshone Lake and Shoshone Geyser Basin

To Old Faithful

To West Thumb

P

Kepler Cascades

P Lone Star Geyser Trailhead

Craig Pass (8,262')

YELLOWSTONE

Norris Pass

Howard Eaton Trail (CDT)

Grand Loop Road

Firehole River

(disused road)

Spring Creek

Spring Creek Trail

0A1

Lone Star Geyser

Continental Divide

0A2

To DeLacy Creek Trail

0A3

Pocket Lake Trail

Pocket Lake

NATIONAL

Shoshone Lake Trail (CDT)

Grants Pass (8,010')

Shoshone Creek

Cement Hills

North Shoshone Lake Trail

8G1

8S7 (boat-in)

8R3 8R2

8R1 (boat-in)

Bechler River Trail

8R4 (boat-in)

To Lewis River Channel

8R5

Shoshone Geyser Basin

Shoshone Lake

Horse Bypass Trail

8T5 (boat-in)

PARK

8T1

8T3 (boat-in)

South Shoshone Lake Trail (CDT)

Moose Creek

N

0   0.5   1.0   1.5 miles

0   0.5   1.0   1.5 kilometers

8M2

Logistics

Shoshone Lake has more boat-in campsites than hike-in sites. Wood fires are banned along the entire lakeshore; only campsite 8M2, well away from the lake, allows fires. All campsites have primitive toilets and a party limit of eight people, except 8T1, which is limited to one tent and four people.

Boat access is via the boat dock at Lewis Lake Campground and the 3.5-mile Lewis River Channel, which enters Shoshone Lake at its southeast corner. Mandatory boating permits ($5–$20) are available from the South Entrance, Grant Village Backcountry Office, and Bridge Bay Ranger Station. Grand Teton National Park boat permits are honored in Yellowstone. See the Appendix (page 348) for the locations of and contact details for all Yellowstone backcountry offices.

The Shoshone Lake Trail is part of the Continental Divide Trail system, which links 3,100 miles of America's wildest and most dramatic backcountry. Beyond Shoshone Lake, it continues southeast to Heart Lake, the Snake River headwaters, and the Teton Wilderness.

Trail Description

From the Lone Star trailhead, ▶1 an abandoned service road heads south along the upper Firehole River. After passing the remains of an old waterworks, the paved road traces the east bank of the river as it heads upstream.

After passing the Spring Creek Trail junction ▶2 at 1.6 miles, you may hear Lone Star Geyser ▶3 before you see it. For a detailed description of the geyser and environs, see Trail 29, page 233. You can get a jump on the hike by cycling this first 2.5 miles.

 Geothermal

A few hundred yards beyond the geyser basin, turn left after 2.7 miles at the well-signed Shoshone Lake Trail junction, ▶4 where bison are often spotted wallowing around thermal areas in view of the trail. If you are planning an extended trip, there are three decent first-night trailside campsites in the next 1.5 miles.

 Wildlife

First up, the wide-open campsite OA1 ▶5 is the only one that allows stock parties. Four hundred yards down-trail, across the Upper Firehole River, campsite OA2 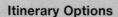6 is the best choice. Almost a mile farther upstream, at 4.1 miles, campsite OA3 ►7 is near Firehole Springs. Beyond here, the trail leaves the river and starts to climb up through unburned forest to the Continental Divide, reaching unsigned Grants Pass (8,010 feet) at the 6-mile mark. ►8

OPTIONS

Itinerary Options

The return hike to Shoshone Geyser Basin is just about doable as a very long day hike, especially if you shave 5 miles off the hike by cycling the section from the trailhead to Lone Star Geyser and back. Much better is to make this an overnight trip, camping en route at site 8G1, 8R5, or 8T1. Better still, turn this into a three-day shuttle hike by continuing along the North Shoshone Lake Trail, spending the second night on the lakeshore at site 8R3, 8R2, 8S3, or 8S2 before hiking out to DeLacy Creek Trailhead for a 21-mile walk.

For the full loop of Shoshone Lake and return to Lone Star Geyser, you are looking at a four- or five-day trip from the Lone Star trailhead.

There are a total of three trail-accessible, five boat-in, and two mixed hiking–boating campsites along Shoshone Lake's north shore. The south shore has eight boat-in sites, one tent-only site, and one two-party, hiking–boating site at the head of the Lewis River Channel. The remaining two trail-accessible sites (8M1 and 8M2) are well removed from the south shore and are shared with stock parties. Wood fires are prohibited at all Shoshone Lake sites.

Alternate Trailheads

For the quickest route to Shoshone Lake, the DeLacy Creek trailhead, about halfway between Old Faithful and West Thumb Junction, is the place. The hike to the north lakeshore is 4–5 hours and 6 miles round-trip, with 200 feet of elevation loss on the way down.

Soon after the anticlimactic pass, you drop down along an upper fork of Shoshone Creek to the signed Bechler River Trail junction. ▶9 The hiker- and llama-only campsite 8G1 ▶10 (no wood fires) is a hundred yards off-trail to the right, in Shoshone Meadows, 6.5 miles from the trailhead.

Watch for moose as you descend along and cross over Shoshone Creek on a footbridge. A mile downhill from the junction, keep to the main trail; don't take the signed horse bypass trail that forks off across a footbridge to the right (it loops 2.2 miles around to the south side of Shoshone Geyser Basin). ▶11

 Wildlife

Continue down the pretty drainage for another mile to the North Shoshone Lake Trail junction, ▶12 8.3 miles from the trailhead. The left fork contours above the lake's north shore past the splendid hiker- only campsite 8R5 fronting Basin Point Bay, offering an excellent overnight option. This section of trail is officially called the North Shoshone Lake Trail but is known more casually as the North Shore Trail.

Following instead the right fork of the main Shoshone Lake Trail, you pass through a marshy area and soon arrive at the extraordinary and very volatile Shoshone Geyser Basin. ▶13 Unlike heavily visited frontcountry geyser basins, there's a notable absence of boardwalks, railings, and signage here. Please tread lightly through the fragile thermal areas; help keep the basin pristine by using common sense and keeping your wits about you as you explore the captivating thermal features rarely found so near the trail.

 Geothermal

Shoshone Geyser Basin is Yellowstone's most active backcountry hydrothermal area, with around 70 geysers in active phases at any given time.

Besides the aforementioned campsite 8R5, trail- side, hiker-only campsite 8T1 (one tent and four- person limit) is the closest to the basin, a few hundred yards south of the junction of the horse bypass trail and the trail along the south shore. If you can't secure a reservation at one of these two

Boating Safety on Shoshone Lake

Frequent high winds and extremely cold water (which is often 40°–50°F and rarely warms above 60°F) pose serious challenges for canoeists and kayakers on the 8,000-acre lake. Suitable bailing and personal flotation devices are required at all times. For maximum safety, avoid open-water crossings, and travel close to the shore and in the early morning and late afternoon, when winds are calmer.

It's not possible to paddle upstream for the northernmost mile of the Lewis River channel. Instead, you must wade through up to 3–4 feet of cold water and drag your boat through the rocky-bottomed stream. Motors are allowed for crossing Lewis Lake but must be left at the south end of the channel. Finally, the National Park Service suggests that boat-in campers select a site on the southern lakeshore for the first night of any trip.

popular sites, it's another 3 miles in either direction to the next options.

Our trail description ends here, but, depending on how many days you have to experience this fascinating area, your explorations should be just beginning. Once you've finished relaxing, fishing, watching the myriad wildlife and waterfowl, and enjoying the lake, retrace your steps northwest on the Shoshone Lake Trail, back to the Lone Star trailhead. ▶14

Lake 〰

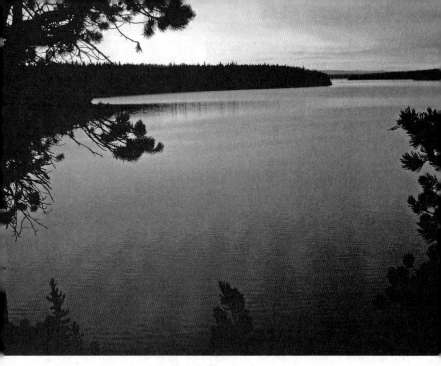

An overnight *backpacking trip rewards with sunset views over Shoshone Lake.*

CREDIT: Bradley Mayhew

👤	**MILESTONES**
▶1	0.0 Start at Kepler Cascades turnout/Lone Star trailhead parking lots
▶2	1.6 Right at Spring Creek Trail junction
▶3	2.5 Lone Star Geyser
▶4	2.7 Left at Shoshone Lake Trail junction
▶5	2.9 Campsite OA1
▶6	3.3 Campsite OA2
▶7	4.1 Campsite OA3
▶8	6.0 Grants Pass
▶9	6.4 Left at Bechler River/Shoshone Lake Trail junction
▶10	6.5 Campsite 8G1
▶11	7.4 Stay on main trail at Horse Bypass Trail junction
▶12	8.3 Right at North Shoshone Lake (North Shore) Trail
▶13	8.5 Shoshone Geyser Basin
▶14	17.0 Return to Lone Star trailhead parking lots

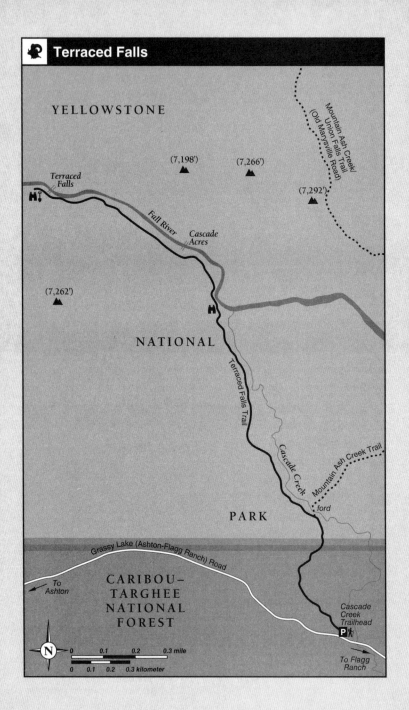

Terraced Falls

YELLOWSTONE

Terraced Falls

(7,198')

(7,266')

Mountain Ash Creek/
Union Falls Trail
(Old Marysville Road)

(7,292')

Fall River

Cascade
Acres

(7,262')

NATIONAL

Terraced Falls Trail

Cascade Creek

Mountain Ash Creek Trail

PARK

ford

Grassy Lake (Ashton-Flagg Ranch) Road

To
Ashton

CARIBOU–
TARGHEE
NATIONAL
FOREST

Cascade
Creek
Trailhead

To Flagg
Ranch

N

0   0.1   0.2   0.3 mile

0   0.1   0.2   0.3 kilometer

Terraced Falls

This remote riverside trail is difficult to access, but once you're there, it's a level, short hike and offers an up-close look at one of the Cascade Corner's bigger multitier waterfalls, set in a dramatic, volcano-forged canyon. If you're already in the area, it's a great late-season option and combines nicely with an overnight trip to Union Falls.

TRAIL USE
Hike
LENGTH
3.6 miles, 1–2 hours
VERTICAL FEET
±250
DIFFICULTY
– 1 **2** 3 4 5 +
TRAIL TYPE
Out-and-back
SURFACE TYPE
Dirt

FEATURES
Child Friendly
Canyon
Stream
Waterfall
Autumn Colors
Cool & Shady
Great Views
Photo Opportunity
Secluded
Geologic Interest

FACILITIES
None

Best Time

There are no fords, so theoretically the trail can be hiked from about mid-June through October. In reality, the Grassy Lake access road is often rough going during late spring and early summer, and like the rest of the Bechler region, it can be quite buggy until August. Grassy Lake Road closes for the winter as soon as snow levels make keeping the road open impractical. It's most enjoyable when fall colors peak, around the autumnal equinox.

Finding the Trail

From Yellowstone's South Entrance, go 2.5 miles south and turn right at Flagg Ranch. Follow the signs for Grassy Lake Road (called Ashton–Flagg Ranch Road, Reclamation Road, or USFS Road 261 on older maps). Drive west through the John D. Rockefeller Jr. Memorial Parkway area (administered by Grand Teton National Park) along a bumpy gravel road, past eight free, primitive campgrounds (with toilets and picnic benches but no water). After 9 miles, without much fanfare, the road enters the Caribou-Targhee National Forest. This section of

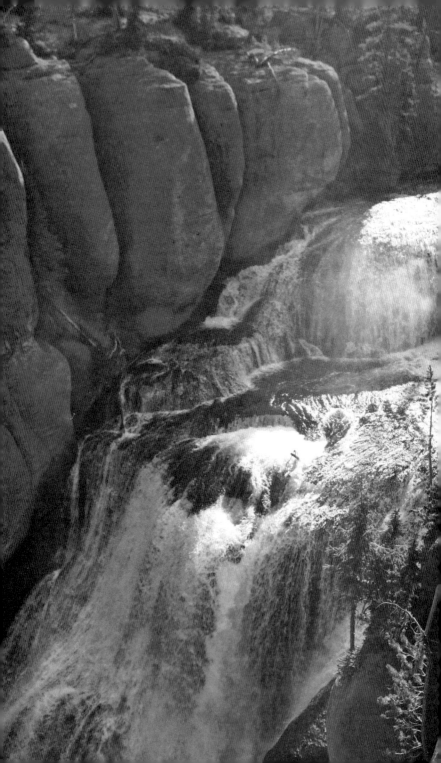

road near the reservoir has a terrible reputation, but it's not that bad, especially in later summer. This is one hike where the drive there is more taxing than the hiking trail.

Fortunately, the Cascade Creek trailhead is only 1.5 miles beyond the dam, on the northwest end of Grassy Lake Reservoir, on the right (north) side. If the small trailhead parking area is full (not likely), there's a large parking area directly across the road, with free dispersed camping among the lodgepole pines.

From the west in Ashton, Idaho, it's an even rougher 36-mile scramble over gravel Forest Service roads. Part of the route follows an old wagon trail, and often it feels that way, though to be fair the road has improved greatly in recent years.

The Terraced Falls overlook sits atop the geographic limit of Yellowstone's Cascade Corner. It straddles the edge of lava flows that ended here approximately 70,000 years ago.

Trail Description

From the National Park Service–signed Cascade Creek (9K5) trailhead ►1 in the Caribou-Targhee National Forest, the little-used but well-maintained trail descends gently through lodgepole pine forest 0.3 mile to the southern Yellowstone National Park boundary. ►2 The boundary is indicated both by posted signs and a notice board that posts National Park Service regulations. Soon the route meets a cutoff trail to the Pitchstone Plateau, ►3 next to an easy ford of Cascade Creek.

Take the left branch just before the ford for the Terraced Falls Trail. The path winds through mixed lodgepole pine stands as it traces the west bank of Cascade Creek. After 0.6 mile the creek joins the Fall River at a lovely confluence. ►4 En route, stop to admire the long set of rapids known as Cascade Acres.

 Viewpoint

Terraced Falls, *with its graceful lines, is one of Bechler's most accessible waterfalls.*
CREDIT: Bradley Mayhew

Waterfall 🏞️

Although the Fall River isn't always in view for the final 0.7 mile to the picture-perfect Terraced Falls overlook, ▶5 it's almost always within earshot.

The maintained trail dead-ends at the overlook of the falls. The river continues flowing downstream through a rugged canyon to plunge over inaccessible Rainbow Falls and eventually meet the Bechler River just upstream from Cave Falls, near the Bechler Ranger Station.

After you've finished picnicking and exploring around the falls, retrace your steps to return to the trailhead parking area. ▶6

🚶 MILESTONES

▶1 0.0 Start at Cascade Creek trailhead
▶2 0.3 Straight at Yellowstone National Park boundary
▶3 0.5 Left on Terraced Falls Trail just before Cascade Creek ford
▶4 1.1 Cascade Creek/Fall River confluence
▶5 1.8 Terraced Falls overlook
▶6 3.6 Return to trailhead parking area

Union Falls and Mountain Ash Creek

The most impressive backcountry waterfall in Greater Yellowstone and a sublime swimming hole await at the end of this hearty daylong hike. A couple of campsites near Union Falls allow for an easy overnight trip.

Best Time

Like most of the Cascade Corner, it's buggy and wet here until early August. Things dry out by late summer, but the falls are most impressive during the first half of July. The 9U group of campsites, all within 5 miles of the falls, don't dry out until early July. The heaviest trail usage happens before Labor Day, when scouting troops and day-trippers on horseback are out in force. Depending on the weather, October can be a wonderful time to hike here.

Finding the Trail

Getting to the trailhead is half the fun: From Yellowstone's South Entrance, go 2.5 miles south and turn right at Flagg Ranch. Follow the signs for Grassy Lake Road (called Ashton–Flagg Ranch Road, Reclamation Road, or USFS Road 261 on older maps).

Continue 9 miles west through the John D. Rockefeller Jr. Memorial Parkway area (administered by Grand Teton National Park) along the decent, graded gravel road past eight free primitive campgrounds. At 9 miles, without much fanfare, the road enters the Caribou-Targhee National Forest and begins to rapidly deteriorate. Depending on the

TRAIL USE
Hike, Backpack, Horse

LENGTH
15.8 miles, 8–10 hours

VERTICAL FEET
±1,800

DIFFICULTY
– 1 2 3 4 **5** +

TRAIL TYPE
Out-and-back

SURFACE TYPE
Dirt

FEATURES
Backcountry Permit
Canyon
Stream
Waterfall
Autumn Colors
Photo Opportunity
Camping
Swimming
Secluded
Geologic Interest

FACILITIES
Horse Staging

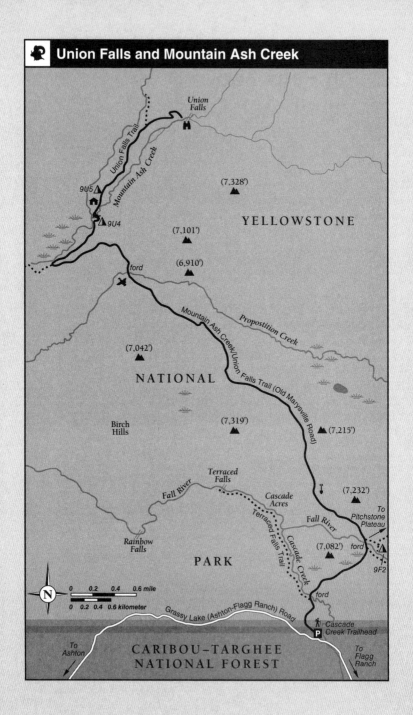

Union Falls and Mountain Ash Creek

Union Falls

(7,328')

YELLOWSTONE

Union Falls Trail

9U5

Mountain Ash Creek

9U4

(7,101')

ford

(6,910')

Propostition Creek

Mountain Ash Creek/Union Falls Trail (Old Marysville Road)

(7,042')

NATIONAL

(7,215')

Birch Hills

(7,319')

Terraced Falls

Cascade Acres

(7,232')

To Pitchstone Plateau

Fall River

Terraced Falls Trail

Fall River

ford

9F2

Rainbow Falls

PARK

Cascade Creek

(7,082')

0   0.2   0.4   0.6 mile

0   0.2 0.4 0.6 kilometer

N

Grassy Lake (Ashton–Flagg Ranch) Road

ford

Cascade Creek Trailhead

P

To Ashton

CARIBOU–TARGHEE
NATIONAL FOREST

To Flagg Ranch

season, the stretch around the reservoir can be easy going or a spine-jarring washboard riddled with huge, tire-eating potholes.

Fortunately, the Cascade Creek trailhead is only 1.5 miles beyond the dam, on the northwest end of Grassy Lake Reservoir, on the right (north) side. If the small trailhead parking area is full (not likely), there's a large parking area directly across the road, with free dispersed camping among the lodgepole pines.

From the west in Ashton, Idaho, it's an even rougher 36-mile scramble over gravel Forest Service roads. The road follows an old wagon route, and often it feels that way.

Trail Description

Beyond the Cascade Creek trailhead ▶1, the first 0.3 mile of trail descends gradually through the Caribou-Targhee National Forest to a sign for the south boundary of Yellowstone National Park ▶2.

A few hundred yards beyond a notice board—which posts National Park Service regulations, our trail meets the Terraced Falls Trail, ▶3 (see Trail 33, page 258). If you are overnighting at Union Falls, it's worth adding on the 2.6-mile detour to see Terraced Falls, either now or on the way back. The Cascade Creek ford here is short and shallow, if ice-cold, but you can generally find a dry route

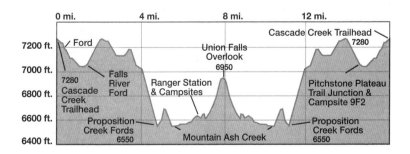

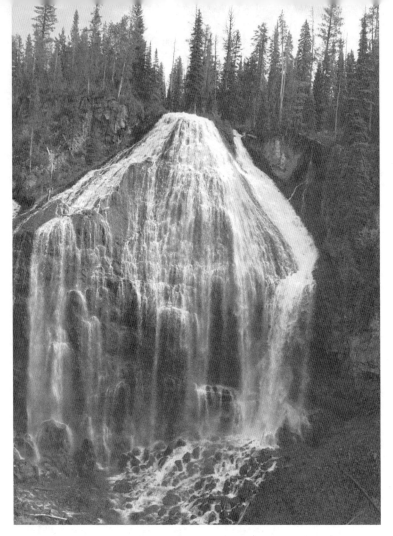

Union Falls *is one of Yellowstone's tallest plunges and one of the most beautiful falls in the backcountry.*

across the logjam. Beyond the ford, the trail crests a short, forested ridge and then drops back down through willow-choked marshland to a junction with the Mountain Ash Creek Trail, above the Fall River ford. ▶4 This ford, at 1.2 miles, is 50 feet wide, and the thigh-high current can be quite swift through July. Later in the season, it's an easy, if slippery, less-than-knee-high crossing; bring wading shoes and a stick or trekking pole. By mid-September, it's barely calf-high.

Camping

The Pitchstone Plateau Trail junction, ▶5 also the turnoff for campsite 9F2, is immediately beyond the ford. Forking left toward Union Falls, it's a steady climb several hundred feet away from the river onto a forested plateau. As the sounds of the river fade, the trail levels off in a mature stand of mixed conifers.

Geologic Interest

As a valley opens up to the left, watch for shiny, black volcanic rock to start showing up underfoot. It's a rocky descent down an open slope, along an 1880s wagon road route, to Proposition Creek, ▶6 at 4.9 miles from the trailhead. Blue jays flit about the fir–spruce forest around the two easy fords here. Don't be surprised by the chipmunks trawling the dense underbrush for mushrooms alongside the trail in the fall. After 0.8 mile, you arrive at another junction overlooking Mountain Ash Creek, ▶7 where the trail doubles back and makes a hard right upstream along the creek.

Alternate Trailheads

OPTIONS

From the Bechler Ranger Station trailhead, it's 12.5 scenic, nearly flat miles one-way to Union Falls.

From the Fish Lake trailhead—0.5 mile down a very rough, high-clearance four-wheel-drive track off Grassy Lake Road—it's 7.8 level miles one-way to the falls, including a couple of significant river fords. The unmaintained track down to Fish Lake trailhead is mostly used by stock parties. The Fish Lake Trail itself passes by several pretty lakes and through a small but beautiful slice of the U.S. Forest Service–administered Winegar Hole Wilderness before entering Yellowstone National Park.

A couple of miles east of the Cascade Creek trailhead near Grassy Lake Reservoir, the Grassy Lake trailhead is a slightly longer and less scenic approach to the Union Falls Trail, which it joins at the Pitchstone Plateau Trail junction.

Camping After 0.5 mile along the south bank, look for a footbridge across the creek just before the signpost for the pleasant, hiker-only campsite 9U4 ►8 (wood fires allowed, two-night limit). The seasonal Union Falls Patrol Cabin ►9 is a few hundred yards beyond the bridge on the left side, 6.4 miles from the trailhead. A spur trail heads several hundred yards off to the left to the equally pleasant campsite 9U5 ►10 (no wood fires, two-night limit), which is popular with stock parties. This site enjoys easy access to a shallow northern fork of Mountain Ash Creek that's warm enough for dipping in, and there's a large meadow out the front door; it's well worth the extra trek a few hundred yards off the trail.

Beyond the Ranger Station, it's a bit slow going on the sandy, horse-worn trail for the next mile. Fortunately, only foot travel is allowed beyond the final unsigned fork ►11, where there's a horse-hitching area.

Swimming The left fork, which deceptively appeared to be the main fork during my last visit, dead-ends after 0.3 mile at an unnamed waterfall and sublime, luke-warm swimming hole known as Ouzel Pool (also called Scout Pool for the heavy use it receives by Boy Scout troops in midsummer). Carefully dog-paddle your way into a natural seat at the base of the falls to experience an indescribable natural whirlpool pummeling.

Waterfall The unsigned right fork—which may still appear to be a mere runoff gully—winds around uphill 0.5 mile to the Union Falls ►12 overlook, 7.9 miles from the trailhead.

Photo Opportunity No doubt about it, the multifaceted, 250-foot plunge is a real gusher. Just follow your ears toward the oceanlike sound: you'll hear it well before the falls come into view. Depending on the season, the precipitous, unmaintained path down to the base

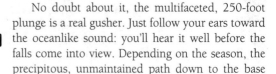

of the falls can be slick and treacherous, thanks to heavy mist from the falls.

If you can pull yourself away (it's getting late, no?), retrace your steps back to the Cascade Creek trailhead parking area. ▶13

🚶 MILESTONES

▶1	0.0 Cascade Creek trailhead
▶2	0.3 Yellowstone National Park boundary
▶3	0.4 Ford Cascade Creek at Terraced Falls Trail junction
▶4	1.2 Fall River ford
▶5	1.3 Left at Pitchstone Plateau junction; campsite 9F2 turnoff
▶6	4.9 Proposition Creek fords
▶7	5.7 Right at Mountain Ash Creek Trail junction
▶8	6.2 Campsite 9U4
▶9	6.4 Union Falls Patrol Cabin
▶10	6.6 Campsite 9U5 spur trail
▶11	7.4 Right at unsigned horse-hitch junction
▶12	7.9 Union Falls
▶13	15.8 Return to Cascade Creek trailhead

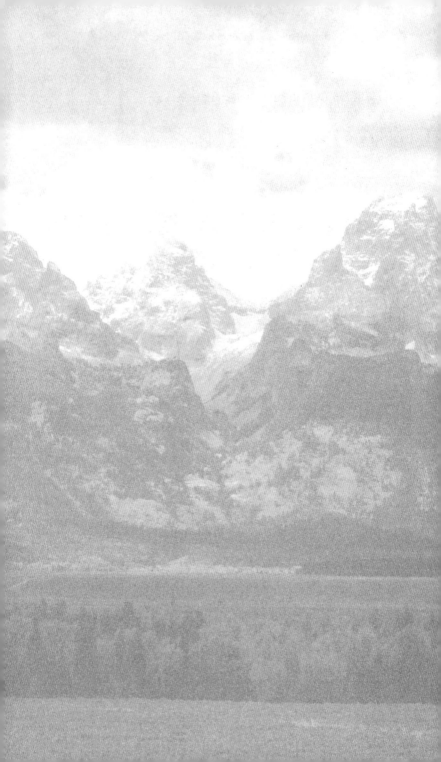

Grand Teton National Park

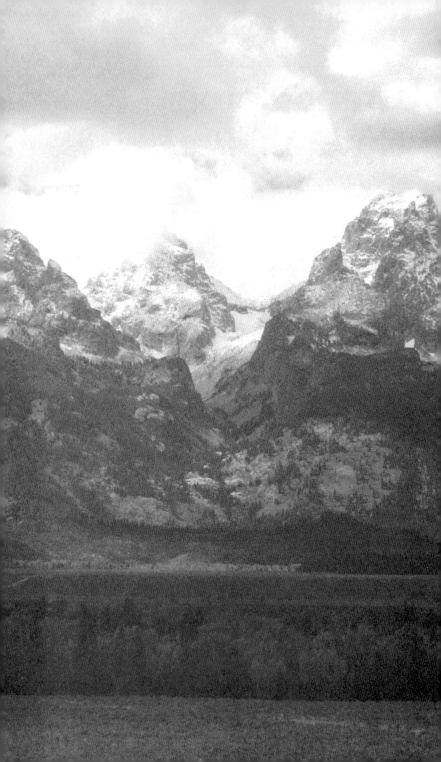

Grand Teton National Park

I t's often said that the Teton Range is what mountains are supposed to look like. Indeed, the range is a textbook example of alpine topography and one of the world's most iconic concentrations of rock and ice, with its jagged peaks rising abruptly several thousand feet from Jackson Hole and the broad Snake River Plain.

As you traverse the sagebrush flats that dominate the Jackson Hole valley floor, the *trois* Tetons appear to follow your eyes, like the *Mona Lisa*—a mesmerizing experience, no matter how many times you have laid eyes on them. In fact, the peaks' allure seems to grow with each new glimpse, as local climbers can attest.

If Yellowstone is primarily about natural spectacle (Old Faithful, bison photo ops, dazzling thermal areas, charismatic megafauna, and so on), then the Teton experience is more active and participatory: in summer, it's all about hiking, climbing, fishing, floating, paddling, and mountaineering. In Yellowstone, it's easiest to observe wildlife along the roads, but in the Tetons your best bet is often to beeline for the high country. One distinct advantage is that the Tetons are blissfully bug-free year-round, while Yellowstone can be quite the opposite in the early summer until August.

While the granitic peaks are the obsession of an international coterie of climbers, it's the lovely piedmont lakes and glacial canyons that attract legions of day hikers and backpackers to the park's 250 miles of trails. The hiking season runs roughly May–October, depending on elevation and weather conditions. Snowfields usually disappear from valley trails by sometime in June but linger on canyon trails and at higher elevations through the end of July. Many summers' worth of world-class alpine and subalpine hiking and climbing await.

Since more folks get out of their cars and hit the trails here than in Yellowstone, it pays to plan ahead, especially if you prefer to camp. During

Overleaf and opposite: *Panorama of the Teton Range, looking west across Jackson Hole*

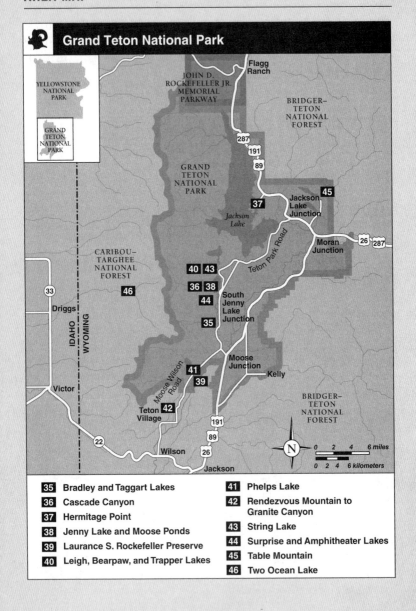

Grand Teton National Park

YELLOWSTONE NATIONAL PARK

GRAND TETON NATIONAL PARK

JOHN D. ROCKEFELLER JR. MEMORIAL PARKWAY

Flagg Ranch

BRIDGER–TETON NATIONAL FOREST

287
191
89

GRAND TETON NATIONAL PARK

Jackson Lake

37

Jackson Lake Junction

45

Moran Junction

26 287

CARIBOU–TARGHEE NATIONAL FOREST

Teton Park Road

40 43

36 38

44

35

South Jenny Lake Junction

33

Driggs

46

IDAHO
WYOMING

Moose Junction

Moose Wilson Road

41

39

Kelly

Victor

Teton Village

42

BRIDGER–TETON NATIONAL FOREST

191

89

22

Wilson

26

0   2   4   6 miles

0   2   4   6 kilometers

N

Jackson

35	Bradley and Taggart Lakes	**41**	Phelps Lake
36	Cascade Canyon	**42**	Rendezvous Mountain to Granite Canyon
37	Hermitage Point	**43**	String Lake
38	Jenny Lake and Moose Ponds	**44**	Surprise and Amphitheater Lakes
39	Laurance S. Rockefeller Preserve	**45**	Table Mountain
40	Leigh, Bearpaw, and Trapper Lakes	**46**	Two Ocean Lake

Grand Teton National Park

TRAIL	DIFFICULTY	LENGTH	TYPE	USES & ACCESS	TERRAIN	FLORA & FAUNA	EXPOSURE	OTHER
35	3	5.8	Loop	Day Hiking, Horses, Child-Friendly	Lake	Autumn Colors, Wildflowers, Birds, Wildlife	Great Views	Geologic Interest
36	4	9.1	Out-and-back	Day Hiking, Horses, Backpacking	Canyon, Lake, Stream, Waterfall	Autumn Colors, Wildflowers, Wildlife	Cool & Shady, Great Views	Camping, Geologic Interest, Steep
37	4	9.4	Loop	Day Hiking, Horses, Backpacking, Child-Friendly	Lake	Wildflowers, Birds, Wildlife	Cool & Shady, Great Views, Photo Opportunity	Camping
38	3	7.0	Loop	Day Hiking, Horses, Child-Friendly, Wheelchair Access	Lake, Waterfall	Autumn Colors, Birds, Wildlife	Cool & Shady, Great Views, Photo Opportunity	Geologic Interest
39	2	3.0	Loop	Day Hiking, Child-Friendly	Lake, Stream	Autumn Colors, Wildflowers, Birds, Wildlife	Cool & Shady, Great Views, Photo Opportunity	Swimming
40	2/3	2.2/8.4	Out-and-back	Day Hiking, Horses, Backpacking, Child-Friendly	Lake	Autumn Colors, Wildflowers, Birds, Wildlife	Cool & Shady, Great Views, Photo Opportunity	Camping, Swimming
41	2	4.0	Out-and-back	Day Hiking, Horses, Backpacking, Child-Friendly	Lake, Stream	Autumn Colors, Wildflowers, Birds, Wildlife	Cool & Shady, Great Views, Photo Opportunity	Camping, Swimming, Geologic Interest
42	4	12.4	Loop	Day Hiking, Horses, Backpacking	Canyon, Mountain, Summit, Stream	Autumn Colors, Wildflowers, Birds, Wildlife	Great Views, Photo Opportunity	Camping, Geologic Interest, Steep
43	2	3.4	Loop	Day Hiking, Horses, Child-Friendly, Wheelchair Access	Lake, Stream	Autumn Colors, Wildflowers, Wildlife	Cool & Shady, Great Views, Photo Opportunity	Swimming, Geologic Interest
44	5	9.6	Out-and-back	Day Hiking, Backpacking	Canyon, Mountain, Lake	Autumn Colors, Wildflowers, Birds, Wildlife	Great Views, Photo Opportunity	Camping, Geologic Interest, Steep
45	4	14.0	Out-and-back	Day Hiking	Mountain, Summit, Stream	Wildflowers	Great Views	Steep
46	3	6.4	Loop	Day Hiking, Horses	Summit, Lake	Autumn Colors, Wildflowers, Birds, Wildlife	Great Views, Photo Opportunity	Swimming, Geologic Interest

USES & ACCESS	TYPE	TERRAIN	FLORA & FAUNA	OTHER
Day Hiking	Loop	Canyon	Autumn Colors	Camping
Bicycling	Out-and-back	Mountain	Wildflowers	Swimming
Horses	Point-to-point	Summit	Birds	Historic/Secluded
Backpacking		Lake	Wildlife	Geologic Interest
Child-Friendly	DIFFICULTY -12345+ less more	Stream	EXPOSURE	Geothermal
Wheelchair Access		Waterfall	Cool & Shady	Moonlight
Permit			Great Views	Steep
			Photo Opportunity	

July and August, trailhead parking areas fill early, especially at South Jenny Lake, String Lake, Lupine Meadows, Death Canyon, and Granite Canyon. Get an early start and obey posted regulations to avoid parking tickets. Most trailheads don't have water or restrooms.

The holy grail for gung-ho backpackers is the sky-high Teton Crest Trail, which traverses 40 exhilarating miles while straddling the range's rugged spine. The most popular stretch runs from Rendezvous Mountain (10,450 feet) in the south to Paintbrush Divide (10,720 feet) and String

Lake (6,875 feet) in the north. Due to the high elevation, the Crest Trail's short season runs roughly mid-July–mid-September, with the first month or so being the best for wildflowers. Most people opt to do the hike in three to four nights, from south to north to take advantage of the high-altitude start and leave the most challenging sections for last. Even with a net 3,575-foot elevation loss hiking south to north, there's still plenty of roller-coaster terrain along the way. For an even longer trip, it's possible to begin south of the park, on the eastern side of Teton Pass at the Ski Lake trailhead (7,800 feet), in the Bridger-Teton National Forest.

The park's five developed, first-come, first-served frontcountry campgrounds ($24–$25 per night, $10–$11 per hiker/bicyclist site) are run by concessionaires Grand Teton Lodge Company and Signal Mountain Lodge. Most campgrounds fill up by noon during the summer, and Jenny Lake fills before 9 a.m. Advance reservations are available (and advised) only for group campsites and RV sites.

From most to least popular, frontcountry campgrounds include the tent-only Jenny Lake (49 sites, open early May–mid-September), popular with climbers; Signal Mountain (81 sites, open early May–mid-October), with an RV dump station and good Jackson Lake views; chaotic Colter Bay (350 sites, open late May–late September), near services at Colter Village, with a separate RV park; secluded Lizard Creek (60 sites, open early June–early September), popular with boaters; and inconveniently located Gros Ventre (300 sites, open early May–mid-October), which has a dump station and is always the last to fill. The maximum stay in the park is 30 nights per year and 14 nights at each campground, except Jenny Lake, where it's 7 nights.

Just outside the park, the Bridger-Teton National Forest has some popular (but unreservable) camping options as well. These include free, primitive, dispersed sites north of the quaint settlement of Kelly on Shadow Mountain (two-night limit); $12 sites in scenic Curtis Canyon, up a rough road 8 miles east of the National Elk Refuge; $5 primitive sites at Sheffield Creek just south of Flagg Ranch; and eight free, minimally developed sites spread out along the first 9 miles of the unpaved Grassy Lake Road, west of Flagg Ranch.

RVs can get sites with hookups at Signal Mountain Campground ($47–$59), Gros Ventre ($51), Colter Bay RV Park ($58–$68), Colter Bay Campground ($51), and Headwaters at Flagg Ranch ($71). Reservations are available at Colter Bay RV Park at 307-543-3100 and Headwaters at 307-543-2861.

The best deal inside the park is the dorm bunks ($25 per nonmember, $16 per member) at the American Alpine Club's Grand Teton Climbers' Ranch, 3 miles south of Jenny Lake off Teton Park Road. Call 307-733-7271 or visit americanalpineclub.org/gtcr; open early June–mid-September. Advance reservations are available online, and walk-ins are welcome if space is available (call ahead).

See the Appendix (page 349) for a summary of in-park lodging options (all nonsmoking and without phones or TVs), most of which are open between May and October, weather permitting.

Permits and Maps

None of this chapter's day hikes requires permits. All overnight trips require a backcountry camping permit ($25 per permit). One-third of the backcountry campsites are reservable in advance (applications accepted at recreation.gov or in person January 1–May 15, for a nonrefundable service fee of $35), while the rest are filled on a first-come, first-served basis starting the first week of June at park permit offices. Download the park's Backcountry Camping brochure at tinyurl.com/gtnpbackcountrybrochure, or contact the Backcountry Permits Office for details. Call 307-739-3309 or 307-739-3397.

The park headquarters are across the road from the year-round Craig Thomas Discovery & Visitor Center, where there's a 3-D relief map of the park and exhibits on history, natural history, climbing, and Indian arts, and where you can arrange permits, watch videos about the park, and buy an extensive range of books and maps. Free Wi-Fi is available here. Call 307-739-3399 or visit nps.gov/grte. Open 8 a.m.–7 p.m. in summer, 8 or 9 a.m.–5 p.m. the rest of the year.

The Jenny Lake Ranger Station also issues permits and is the best place to get updates on backcountry hiking and climbing conditions, though it's not the best place to get backcountry permits for other parts of the park, such as Jackson Lake. Call 307-739-3343; open daily, 8 a.m.–7 p.m., in summer, with reduced spring and fall hours.

Nearby, the summer-only and recently renovated Jenny Lake Visitor Center has a bookstore, helpful staff, a 3-D map of Jackson Hole, and good interpretive geological displays. Call 307-739-3392; open daily, 8 a.m.– 7 p.m., late June–August (until 4:30 p.m. in early and late season).

On the northeast side of Jackson Lake, 25 miles north of Moose, the Colter Bay Visitor Center has a good bookstore, videos, free Wi-Fi, and the most helpful rangers for issuing permits around Jackson Lake. Call 307-739-3594; open daily, 8 a.m.–7 p.m., from June–August, with reduced hours in May and September–October.

Grand Teton National Park

Laurance S. Rockefeller Preserve . . 305

Explore the latest addition to Grand Teton National Park, a former dude ranch and Rockefeller family summer retreat, via 8 miles of minimally signed trails that weave through a diverse range of sagelands, forests, and wetlands and alongside tumbling creeks. A gem of a picnic spot awaits on the southern shore of Phelps Lake.

TRAIL 39

Hike, Horse
3.0 miles, Loop
Difficulty: 1 **2** 3 4 5

Leigh, Bearpaw, and
Trapper Lakes 311

This family-friendly outing is easily extended into a stress-free overnighter. All three lakes are far enough away from the road to make you feel like you are in the backcountry. At midsummer, Leigh Lake is a favorite swimming hole and popular horseback-riding destination.

TRAIL 40

Hike, Backpack, Horse
2.2 or 8.4 miles, Out-and-back
Difficulty: 1 **2** 3 4 5

Phelps Lake. 316

This popular, low-elevation outing climbs gently through shady, mature forest to a scenic overlook of a charming glacial lake. Fish and wildflowers are abundant, and the three lakefront campsites feel miles from the trailhead. Reserve ahead for an easy, family-friendly overnighter.

TRAIL 41

Hike, Backpack, Horse
4.0 miles, Out-and-back
Difficulty: 1 **2** 3 4 5

Rendezvous Mountain to
Granite Canyon 320

This route is spectacular—and 95% downhill—so it sees traffic whenever the weather is decent and the tram is in service. Lower Granite Canyon is a riot of vegetation and wildlife. With so many critters flitting about, it can feel busy even when no other hikers are around.

TRAIL 42

Hike, Backpack, Horse
12.4 miles, Loop
Difficulty: 1 2 3 **4** 5

TRAIL 43

Hike, Horse

3.4 miles, Loop

Difficulty: 1 **2** 3 4 5

String Lake 328

One of the park's most rewarding easy hikes traces the shoreline of a tranquil lake at the foot of the awe-inspiring Teton Range. Swimming and boating options add to the alluring mix.

TRAIL 44

Hike, Backpack

9.6 miles, Out-and-back

Difficulty: 1 2 3 4 **5**

Surprise and Amphitheater Lakes . . 332

Don't try this challenging route on your first day at altitude. The supersteep hike is one of the park's most popular for good reason: it provides quick access to a couple of the most scenic alpine lakes in North America.

TRAIL 45

Hike

14 miles, Out-and-back

Difficulty: 1 2 3 **4** 5

Table Mountain 338

For some of the best views of the Tetons, you have to leave the park and drive into neighboring Idaho. You'll feel eyeball to eyeball with the epic range on this popular classic.

TRAIL 46

Hike, Horse

6.4 miles, Loop

Difficulty: 1 2 **3** 4 5

Two Ocean Lake 343

This easy hike around a serene lake in the park's sparsely visited northeast corner is the antithesis of what most visitors expect from their Teton experience. What the route lacks in breathtaking switchbacks and alpine vistas it more than makes up for in lovely flora, abundant wildlife, and fine panoramas of the Teton Range. If you're up for great views and a more ambitious climb, continue on to Grand View Point.

Bradley and Taggart Lakes

Escape the crowds at Jenny Lake with this scenic, leisurely wander through meadows and regenerating forest to a pair of lovely glacial lakes. The untouched forests around Bradley Lake provide a vivid contrast to the Taggart Lake burn area. Both lakes are lined with secluded beaches and teem with fish, but sorry, there's no swimming allowed.

Best Time

Almost any time between May and October is a good time to visit these low-elevation lakes. As elsewhere, you'll be the most comfortable and spot the most wildlife outside of the midday hours, as shade is in short supply in the burn areas. Rangers lead guided hikes to Taggart Lake June–August, daily at 9 a.m.

Finding the Trail

From the south, head north out of Jackson 8 miles on US 26/89/191 past the park's southern boundary, and turn left at Moose Junction. Continue 1 mile past the visitor center to the Moose Entrance Station. Go 2.3 miles north and turn left into the ample Taggart Lake trailhead parking area, on the west side of Teton Park Road. From the north, starting at Jackson Lake Junction, go 17.5 miles south on Teton Park Road, past the Jenny Lake Visitor Center, and turn right into the parking area. Pick up a field guide and map at the trailhead ($1 donation or return it when finished).

TRAIL USE
Hike, Horse

LENGTH
5.8 miles, 3–4 hours

VERTICAL FEET
±550

DIFFICULTY
− 1 2 **3** 4 5 +

TRAIL TYPE
Loop

SURFACE TYPE
Dirt

FEATURES
Child Friendly
Lake
Autumn Colors
Wildflowers
Birds
Wildlife
Great Views
Geologic Interest

FACILITIES
Restrooms
Picnic Tables

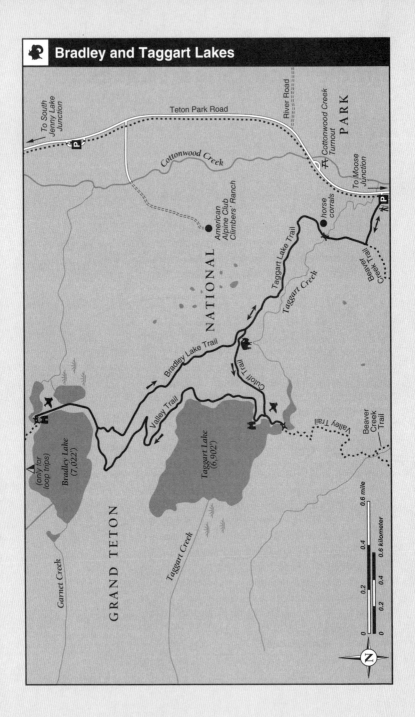

Bradley and Taggart Lakes

To South Jenny Lake Junction

Teton Park Road

River Road

Cottonwood Creek Turnout

PARK

To Moose Junction

Cottonwood Creek

American Alpine Club Climbers' Ranch

horse corrals

NATIONAL

Taggart Lake Trail

Taggart Creek

Beaver Creek Trail

Bradley Lake Trail

Cutoff Trail

Valley Trail

Bradley Lake (7,022')

(only for loop trips)

Taggart Lake (6,902')

Valley Trail

Beaver Creek Trail

GRAND TETON

Garnet Creek

Taggart Creek

0.6 mile

0.6 kilometer

0.4

0.2

0

N

Trail Description

From the parking area, ▶1 the wide trail heads west across a rolling sagebrush flat dotted with wildflowers. At the foot of the glacial moraine, the trail splits at a T-junction ▶2 signed for the Beaver Creek Trail.

The right fork, the Taggart Lake Trail, heads north, branching off the road-size trail onto the main hiking trail, which crosses Taggart Creek on a wooden footbridge. After tracing the creek and passing horse corrals, the trail swings left and skirts the flank of the burned moraine. The Tetons appear and, if you're lucky, the delights of postfire regeneration—busy birds, active wildlife, and blooming wildflowers—are very much in evidence.

About 30 minutes into the hike, you meet the junction of trails to Taggart and Bradley Lakes ▶3 at 1.3 miles. Take the left fork for Taggart Lake, tracing the ridge of the glacial moraine, then descending through stands of quaking baby aspens and open sagebrush. After 1.6 miles you reach Taggart Lake, where you can take a short detour left (south) at the Taggart Lake/Valley Trail junction ▶4 along the south shore to the outlet of Taggart Lake (6,902 feet). On a clear day, from the bridge over the outlet stream, you'll find unobstructed views of the remarkable Grand Teton (13,770 feet). If you are short on time, you could turn back here for a 3.2-mile hike.

Retrace your steps north along the lakeshore back to the junction, ▶5 and then continue north on the Taggart Lake/Valley Trail, which switchbacks steeply for 20 minutes over the moraine dividing Taggart and Bradley Lakes. The Valley Trail passes a junction for the Bradley Lake Trail, headed back to the trailhead, just before it hits the well-forested southeast shore of Bradley Lake (7,022 feet). The lake was originally formed by the glacial ice that once poured out of Garnet Canyon.

The timbered ridges that confine both lakes, known as lateral moraines, are composed of glacial debris; they give some idea of how thick the glaciers once were.

 Wildflowers

 Viewpoint

 Lake

Early-Season Access

Early in the season—say, mid-May—the Beaver Creek Trail is a good alternative to reach Taggart Lake via the Valley Trail (4.2 miles round-trip), when the more northerly Bradley Lake route remains covered by snow. Either lake can be visited by itself as a loop hike, and any of these routes can be done in either direction without an increase in difficulty.

Grand Teton Pathway

The paved, multiuse Grand Teton Pathway offers a rare chance for some wonderful, safe cycling in the shadow of stunning Teton views. The 20-mile path runs from Jackson to Moose and then parallels Teton Park Road past the Taggart Lake trailhead en route to Jenny Lake. It's a great family ride from either Jenny Lake or Moose, and you can use the trail to get to the Taggart Lake trailhead and make the Taggart and Bradley Lakes hike before cycling back. It's a 5-mile ride to the trailhead from Jenny Lake or 3 miles from Moose. From Moose to Jenny Lake is 7.5 miles. The nonmotorized trail is open to in-line skaters, walkers, and runners (no pets) and is wheelchair accessible. If you don't have your own bike, you can rent one at Dornans (dornans.com) in Moose or at Hoback Sports (hobacksports.com) or Teton Mountain Bike Tours (tetonmtbike .com) in Jackson. Figure on $40 for a day's hire.

Viewpoint 🔭

Before turning tail for home, take time to explore the placid lakeshore. It's worth making the detour ▶6 0.3 mile left (north) along the lakeshore to the bridge spanning the lake's narrow neck for more stunning, up-close Teton views. The bridge was out of service in 2016 but should have been replaced by 2017. Retrace your steps back to the Bradley Lake Trail ▶7 for the final, 2.2-mile home stretch of the loop, climbing over the moraine with fine views of Taggart Lake, descending through aspen for excellent Teton views, and continuing past the turnoff to Taggart Lake. ▶8 Return to the now-familiar junction for the Taggart Lake trailhead ▶9 and the parking area. ▶10

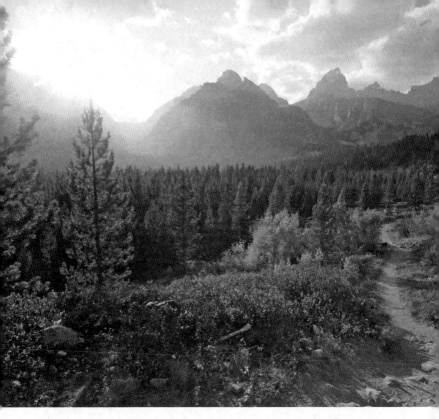

Lovely afternoon light *on the Bradley Lake Trail, with the Tetons in the distance*

CREDIT: Bradley Mayhew

🚶	MILESTONES

- ▶1   0.0 Start at Taggart Lake trailhead parking area
- ▶2   0.2 Right on Taggart Lake Trail at Beaver Creek Trail junction
- ▶3   1.3 Left on Valley Trail
- ▶4   1.6 Left along shore for optional detour to Taggart Lake outlet
- ▶5   1.9 North (straight ahead) on Valley Trail at Taggart Lake Trail junction
- ▶6   3.0 Left along shore at Bradley Lake Trail (optional detour)
- ▶7   3.6 Left on Bradley Lake Trail
- ▶8   4.5 Straight (southeast) at Cutoff Trail junction
- ▶9   5.6 Left at junction for Taggart Lake trailhead
- ▶10   5.8 Return to parking area

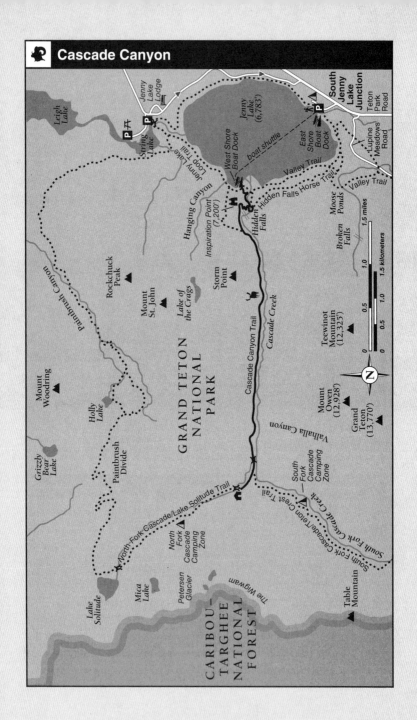

Cascade Canyon

String Lake

Leigh Lake

Jenny Lake Lodge

P

String Lake

P

Jenny Lake Loop Trail

West Shore Boat Dock

Jenny Lake (6,783')

boat shuttle

East Shore Boat Dock

P

South Jenny Lake Junction

Teton Park Road

Lupine Meadows Road

Valley Trail

Valley Trail

Hanging Canyon

Inspiration Point (7,200')

Hidden Falls

Hidden Falls Horse Trail

Moose Ponds

Broken Falls

Rockchuck Peak

Mount St. John

Lake of the Crags

Storm Point

Paintbrush Canyon

Cascade Creek

Cascade Canyon Trail

Teewinot Mountain (12,325')

Mount Woodring

Holly Lake

Grizzly Bear Lake

Paintbrush Divide

GRAND TETON NATIONAL PARK

Valhalla Canyon

Mount Owen (12,928')

Grand Teton (13,770')

N

1.5 miles

1.5 kilometers

1.0

1.0

0.5

0.5

0

0

South Fork Cascade Camping Zone

South Fork Cascade/Teton Crest Trail

North Fork Cascade/Lake Solitude Trail

North Fork Cascade Camping Zone

Lake Solitude

Mica Lake

Petersen Glacier

The Wigwam

South Fork Cascade Creek

Table Mountain

CARIBOU–TARGHEE NATIONAL FOREST

Cascade Canyon

This challenging extension of the popular Jenny Lake and Moose Ponds loop (see Trail 38, page 298) is the park's most popular and crowded canyon trail. In summer, it's a bottleneck of sorts, at the confluence of several major climbing and backpacking trails. Thanks to the scenic boat shuttle, it's also one of the most beautiful and direct routes into the wild heart of the Tetons.

Best Time

Snow can linger in the upper reaches of the canyon until early July. Because they are at relatively low elevation, the lower stretches of the canyon are accessible June–October. Hidden Falls is at its most spectacular early in the season. Afternoon thundershowers, which appear with little warning, are common in the canyon.

Finding the Trail

From the south, follow US 26/89/191 north out of Jackson 8 miles past the park's southern boundary and turn left at Moose Junction. Continue 1 mile past the visitor center to the Moose Entrance Station. Go 7 miles north on Teton Park Road and turn left at the South Jenny Lake Junction. Follow the signs for the East Shore Boat Dock another 0.5 mile (making a couple of right turns) through the developed area around the visitor center/ranger station to arrive at the trailhead parking area. From the north, starting at Jackson Lake Junction, take Teton Park Road 12.5 miles south (past North Jenny Lake

TRAIL USE
Hike, Backpack, Horse
LENGTH
9.1 miles, 5–6 hours
VERTICAL FEET
±1,100
DIFFICULTY
– 1 2 3 **4** 5 +
TRAIL TYPE
Out-and-back
SURFACE TYPE
Dirt

FEATURES
Canyon
Lake
Stream
Waterfall
Autumn Colors
Wildflowers
Wildlife
Cool & Shady
Great Views
Camping
Geologic Interest

FACILITIES
Visitor Center
Ranger Station
Restrooms
Phone
Water
Horse Staging

Teewinot comes from the Shoshone word meaning "many pinnacles." The name is thought to have once applied to the entire Teton range.

Junction) and turn right into the South Jenny Lake parking area.

Logistics

Jenny Lake's parking lots often fill to capacity in midsummer. Arrive as early as possible to find a space. The area around the Jenny Lake Visitor Center was rebuilt in 2016 and 2017, with new lakeshore viewing areas ("viewing nodes") and updated facilities.

Lake

Taking a seasonal shuttle boat across Jenny Lake cuts out the first 2 miles of hiking in each direction. Catch the first boat to beat the crowds to the falls. Jenny Lake Boating shuttles depart Jenny Lake's East Shore Boat Dock for the Cascade Canyon trailhead dock every 15 minutes daily, weather permitting, between May 15 and early September. From June to early September, hours of operation are 7 a.m.–7 p.m., with service reduced to 10 a.m.–4 p.m. during May. Fares are $9 one-way or $15 round-trip for passengers ages 11 and older, and $6 one-way or $8 round-trip for children ages 2–11. Starting in June, you can also rent canoes and kayaks ($20 per hour

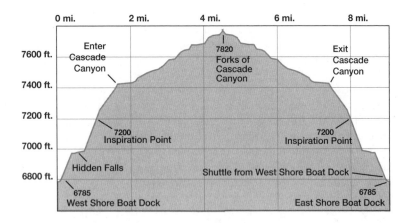

or $75 per day). A one-hour lake cruise costs $19 for adults and $11 for children and runs a couple of times a day. Call 307-734-9227 or see jennylake boating.com for schedules.

Rangers lead guided hikes to Inspiration Point via the boat shuttle daily at 8:30 a.m. A maximum of 25 hikers are accepted, so arrive early at the Jenny Lake Visitor Center to sign up.

Trail Description

From the parking area near the visitor center, ►1 follow signs to the East Shore Boat Dock, on the southeast end of the lake. ►2 During the high season, you can catch a shuttle boat for the scenic, 12-minute ride across the lake to the West Shore Boat Dock, ►3 where there are no visitor services.

Once on the opposite side of the lake, follow signs to your left (south) for a couple hundred yards along the well-beaten paths to the signed Jenny Lake Loop Trail junction. ►4 Turn right (west) on the middle trail at the four-way intersection to follow a path that parallels the north side of Cascade Creek before crossing over it on a footbridge. Follow signs to the viewpoint of the 200-foot Hidden Falls, ►5 tucked away in a spruce–fir forest behind a split-rail fence. This section of trail was under reconstruction in 2016 but should have reopened by 2017.

Heading back toward the lake and away from the falls, turn left and follow signs across a bridge over Cascade Creek. Soon you start the 0.4-mile climb (also signed for Cascade Canyon) to Inspiration Point (7,200 feet) ►6 for sweeping views east across the Snake River Valley to the Gros Ventre Range and back west to the Cathedral Group: Teewinot Mountain (12,325 feet); the Grand Teton (13,770 feet); and Mount Owen (12,928 feet), the second-highest peak in the Teton Range. This

In summer, rangers lead interpretive hikes from the Jenny Lake Visitor Center to Hidden Falls and Inspiration Point, which can cause some crowding on the main trails. Little-used horse trails provide less-crowded alternatives.

 Viewpoint

 Waterfall

 Viewpoint

OPTIONS

North and South Forks of Cascade Canyon

You can extend this hike into an overnight trip by getting a backcountry permit for either the North Fork or South Fork Cascade Canyon camping zones, which start just beyond the trail fork near the head of the canyon.

The South Fork, usually snow-free by mid-July, gains 2,600 feet over 5.1 scenic miles en route to Hurricane Pass (10,372 feet) on the park's western boundary.

The North Fork climbs a gentler 1,200 feet in 2.7 miles to the eastern shore of 50-acre Lake Solitude (9,035 feet), a misnomer for this striking and extremely popular destination. If you plan on camping, you can take the two-day Cascade Canyon–Paintbrush Divide and Canyon route—the park's most popular high-country loop—which gains 3,850 feet over 19.2 miles.

Skipping the Shuttle Boat

If the boats aren't running or you'd rather skip the shuttle, it's a straightforward, flat, and well-signed 2-mile walk around the southern and western lakeshore via the Valley Trail or Hidden Falls Horse Trail to reach Hidden Falls (see Trail 38, page 298).

In summer, rangers lead interpretive hikes from the Jenny Lake Visitor Center to Hidden Falls, which can cause some crowding on the main trails. An infrequently used horse trail that starts north of the West Shore Boat Dock skips the crowded area around Hidden Falls and intersects with the Cascade Canyon Trail a few hundred yards above Inspiration Point.

section of trail was rebuilt in 2016 with rock helicoptered in from Idaho.

Most casual visitors do not make it beyond Inspiration Point, so the farther you go up the canyon, the more peaceful things should become. Begin the gradual, gentle 0.6-mile climb—past the horse bypass trail intersection—to the mouth of the U-shaped Cascade Canyon, ▶7 where the majesty of the mile-high, glacially sculpted walls really begins to sink in.

Canyon

Several large talus slopes—home to many vocal marmots, as well as pikas—intersect the trail from the right as it follows the north side of Cascade Creek and traverses prime wild-berry habitat. (Look for raspberries, huckleberries, thimbleberries, and grouse whortleberries.) If you can properly identify them, you are welcome to pick small quantities for personal use, but leave some for the critters that frequent the area, too.

Moose migrate up the canyon during the summer and are often spotted browsing around the marshier stretches of Cascade Creek.

Thanks to the sheer canyon walls, you'll enjoy great views beyond the Douglas-fir canopy all the way up the canyon. Just before the Forks of Cascade Canyon ►8 junction (look for the huge limber pine specimen), the trail crosses over Cascade Creek on a footbridge and starts to climb more noticeably again. (See Options for a short description of the North and South Fork Trails.)

About 0.3 mile up the North Fork Trail, the Cascade Patrol Cabin makes a nice picnic spot before you do a U-turn and retrace your steps down the canyon to the shuttle boat ►9 to the East Shore Boat Dock ►10 and the South Jenny Lake trailhead parking area. ►11

☰ MILESTONES

- ►1   0.0 Start at South Jenny Lake parking area
- ►2   0.1 Visitor center and East Shore Boat Dock
- ►3   0.1 Shuttle boat to West Shore Boat Dock
- ►4   0.3 Jenny Lake Loop Trail junction
- ►5   0.6 Hidden Falls
- ►6   1.0 Inspiration Point
- ►7   1.6 Enter Cascade Canyon
- ►8   4.5 Forks of Cascade Canyon
- ►9   9.0 Back at West Shore Boat Dock
- ►10   9.0 Shuttle boat to East Shore Boat Dock
- ►11   9.1 Return to South Jenny Lake parking area

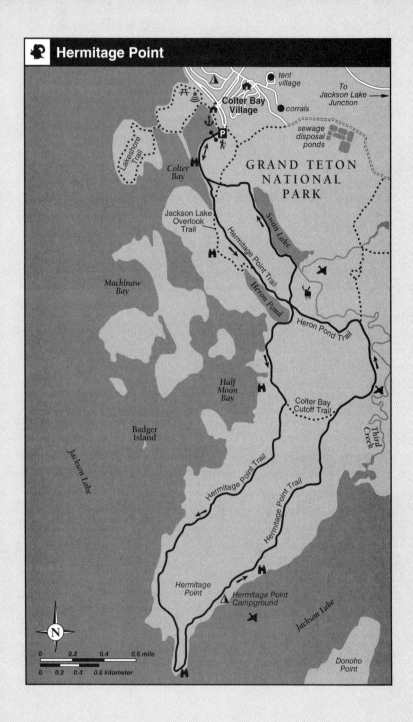

Hermitage Point

tent village

To Jackson Lake Junction

Colter Bay Village

corrals

Lakeshore Trail

sewage disposal ponds

Colter Bay

GRAND TETON NATIONAL PARK

Jackson Lake Overlook Trail

Swan Lake

Hermitage Point Trail

Mackinaw Bay

Heron Pond

Heron Pond Trail

Half Moon Bay

Colter Bay Cutoff Trail

Badger Island

Third Creek

Jackson Lake

Hermitage Point Trail

Hermitage Point Trail

Hermitage Point

Hermitage Point Campground

Jackson Lake

N

0   0.2   0.4   0.6 mile

0   0.2   0.4   0.6 kilometer

Donoho Point

Hermitage Point

This easygoing but rewarding shoreline jaunt leaves the crowds at Colter Bay behind. The forested habitat is ever-changing, and the views across Jackson Lake are amazing. It's a flexible route, too: add an overnight at one of the park's best low-elevation campgrounds for the perfect first-time backcountry adventure.

Best Time

The trail is hikable mid-May–October. In the hottest months of the summer, it's most enjoyable in the early morning or late afternoon. Dawn and dusk are the best times for spotting wildlife. Sunset behind the Tetons is magical from Colter Bay.

Finding the Trail

From the south, head north out of Jackson on US 26/89/191 for 26 miles past the park's southern boundary. At Moran Junction, turn left onto US 26/287, go 4 miles past the park entrance station, and bear right at Jackson Lake Junction. Turn left into Colter Bay Village, 5.2 miles beyond Jackson Lake Junction. Follow the signs 1 mile to the Colter Bay Visitor Center. The visitor center is just to the right of the final T-junction; the marina and trailhead are to your left.

Park near the boat ramp at the marina. The trailhead is in the southeast corner of the large parking area, between the boat ramp and the nondescript brown pump house.

TRAIL USE
Hike, Backpack, Horse

LENGTH
9.4 miles, 4–6 hours

VERTICAL FEET
±150

DIFFICULTY
– 1 2 3 **4** 5 +

TRAIL TYPE
Loop

SURFACE TYPE
Mixed

FEATURES
Child Friendly
Lake
Wildflowers
Birds
Wildlife
Cool & Shady
Great Views
Photo Opportunity
Camping

FACILITIES
Visitor Center
Restrooms
Picnic Tables
Phone
Water
Boat Launch
Horse Staging

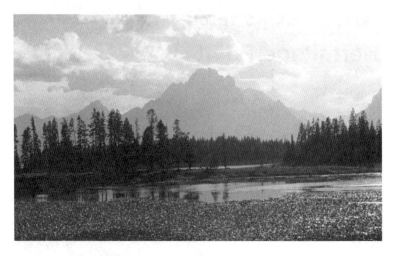

Beavers *are busy at Heron Pond; Mount Moran looms in the background.*

Logistics

All the trail junctions described here are signed; ignore the numerous unmarked junctions with horse trails and unofficial trails. There are public restrooms near the trailhead at the visitor center and marina. Pick up a free trail map from the box at the service-road entrance gate.

Trail Description

From the trailhead, ►1 follow the wide gravel service road past the gate and along the shore overlooking the marina while soaking up the views across Colter Bay to Mount Moran (12,605 feet). At the end of the service road, stay right at the first trail junction. ►2 The route turns into a singletrack trail and enters a mixed lodgepole pine and fir forest.

Viewpoint 🔭

A few hundred yards farther along, your next option is to turn right on the Jackson Lake Overlook Trail ►3 or forge ahead on the flat route. If you're in the mood and have the gumption, it's well worth the short, gentle ascent and the slightly longer loop to take in the breezy views from the sagebrush meadow

atop the knoll. Jackson Lake is actually obscured
by pines, but there's a nice panorama of the Teton
Range. The overlook route rejoins the lower trail
after 0.5 mile, just before the north end of lily-laden,
yellow-green Heron Pond. ►4

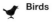 Lake

After skirting the edge of the pond and passing several unmarked spurs leading down toward
the shoreline, make a hard right 1.4 miles beyond
the trailhead at the four-way trail junction. ►5 The
trail hugs the pond's southern shore, bringing you
close enough to see beavers working on their lodges
and to hear the ducks, pelicans, and Canada geese
splashing about. Dense lodgepole stands obscure
the lake from view until you reach the Colter Bay
cutoff trail junction at 2.2 miles, ►6 beyond which
most of the horses and crowds disappear.

 Birds

At the junction, follow the right fork along the
peninsula, and watch for tantalizing glimpses of the
Teton Range across the lake to your right. A small
grove of majestic, towering aspens appears on the
left just before the views really open up. After what
seems like much longer than a mile, the dense, dog-
hair forest finally gives way to sagebrush meadows
and, on clear days, truly grand views.

 Viewpoint

Kid-Friendly Shortcuts

OPTIONS

If you have little ones in tow or want to opt out of the longer
loop midway, there are three opportunities to cut the hike
short, using signed cutoff trails to return to Colter Bay. You
can loop back around at the north end of Heron Pond (2 miles
round-trip via the Jackson Lake Overlook) or the south end of
Heron Pond (2.6 miles round-trip), or make a longer loop about
0.8 mile beyond Heron Pond by taking the Colter Bay cutoff
trail (5.4 miles round-trip).

The mercifully undeveloped Hermitage Point ►7 is breezy, but when it's sunny it can be a wonderful place for a picnic amidst the fragrant sagebrush. Many unofficial trails lead to all manner of photo opportunities around the point.

 Camping

Afterward, proceed 0.5 mile from the sign on the far side of the point, past a short spur trail to the Hermitage Point campground, ►8 one of the park's nicest low-elevation backcountry campsites. It's perfectly perched above the shoreline 4.9 miles from the trailhead, though a bit exposed; this gives it stunning, 180-degree views. The site fronts a placid bay that harbors tons of birdlife—bring your binoculars.

Immediately beyond the campground, the trail climbs away from the lake, straight up a moraine wall to an overlook, then drops through mixed-fir forest and more sagebrush meadow to the east end of the previously seen Colter Bay cutoff trail. ►9

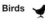 **Wildlife**

At this juncture, the cutoff saves no distance, so forge ahead on the main trail alongside Third Creek. Watch for moose lurking in the willows and raptors soaring against the backdrop of the Teton Wilderness to the east.

Just below the southeast arm of Swan Lake, turn left at the signed junction for the Heron Pond Trail. ►10 Crest a small, forested rise, and then drop down past a glimpse of Swan Lake to a now-familiar four-way junction at Heron Pond. ►11

Take a hard right (not the path you followed previously along the shore of the pond), and head north over a gentle rise and 0.3 mile down to the west shore of Swan Lake. The lake is named after a pair of rare and endangered trumpeter swans who have abided here for two decades. The couple have yet to produce any offspring but have been observed defending their nesting patch from other swans. Other creatures that share the lake's resources include beavers, moose, elk, deer, herons, cranes, and less-showy birds.

Birds

 Wildlife

After you travel north along the lakeshore for almost a mile and take in the lake and its gregarious inhabitants, make a soft left toward Colter Bay at yet another well-signed four-way junction. ►12 Merge right onto the service road ►13 to finish the loop at the Colter Bay/Hermitage Point trailhead parking area. ►14

⊼ MILESTONES

►1   0.0 Start at Hermitage Point trailhead

►2   0.2 Right at first junction

►3   0.4 Right at Jackson Lake Overlook Trail (optional)

►4   1.0 Right at north end of Heron Pond to rejoin main trail

►5   1.4 Hard right at four-way trail junction

►6   2.2 Right at Colter Bay cutoff trail junction

►7   4.4 Left around Hermitage Point

►8   4.9 Straight past Hermitage Point campground

►9   6.6 Right past cutoff trail junction

►10   7.3 Left on Heron Pond Trail at Swan Lake junction

►11   7.8 Right at Heron Pond four-way junction to Swan Lake

►12   8.7 Soft left at four-way junction to Colter Bay

►13   Right on service road to Colter Bay/Hermitage Point trailhead

►14   9.4 Return to parking area

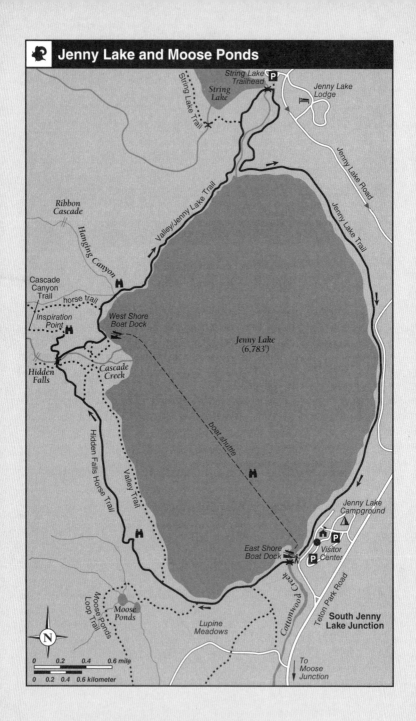

Jenny Lake and Moose Ponds

String Lake Trailhead
Jenny Lake Lodge
String Lake
String Lake Trail
Jenny Lake Road
Valley/Jenny Lake Trail
Ribbon Cascade
Hanging Canyon
Jenny Lake Trail
Cascade Canyon Trail
horse trail
Inspiration Point
West Shore Boat Dock
Jenny Lake (6,783')
Hidden Falls
Cascade Creek
boat shuttle
Hidden Falls Horse Trail
Valley Trail
Jenny Lake Campground
East Shore Boat Dock
Visitor Center
Moose Ponds Loop Trail
Moose Ponds
Lupine Meadows
Cottonwood Creek
Teton Park Road
South Jenny Lake Junction

N

| 0 | 0.2 | 0.4 | 0.6 mile |
| 0 | 0.2 | 0.4 | 0.6 kilometer |

To Moose Junction

Jenny Lake and Moose Ponds

Grand Teton's most popular day hike deserves all the accolades heaped upon it, but the route also suffers from the overcrowding the attention brings. The wide, well-maintained trail skirts the shoreline of the park's second-largest lake and is almost completely flat. An optional shuttle boat (one-way or round-trip) goes most of the way to the photogenic focal point, Hidden Falls.

Best Time

It can be impossible to find parking around noon in summer, so aim to arrive early, or consider a late-afternoon start. When the shuttle boats are running, the trail is much less crowded, and your chances of seeing wildlife increase exponentially. The loop around the lake is hikable May–October and is a good, snow-free early- or late-season option.

Finding the Trail

From the south, take US 26/89/191 north out of Jackson 8 miles past the park's southern boundary and turn left at Moose Junction. Continue 1 mile past the visitor center to the Moose Entrance Station. Go 7 miles north and turn left at the South Jenny Lake Junction. Follow the signs for the East Shore Boat Dock another 0.5 mile (making a couple of right turns) through the developed area around the visitor center and ranger station to arrive at the trailhead parking area. From the north, starting at Jackson Lake Junction, take Teton Park Road 12.5 miles south (past North Jenny Lake Junction) and turn right at the South Jenny Lake junction.

TRAIL USE
Hike, Horse

LENGTH
7.0 miles, 3–4 hours

VERTICAL FEET
±525

DIFFICULTY
– 1 2 **3** 4 5 +

TRAIL TYPE
Loop

SURFACE TYPE
Paved, Dirt

FEATURES
Child Friendly
Handicap Accessible
Lake
Waterfall
Autumn Colors
Birds
Wildlife
Cool & Shady
Great Views
Photo Opportunity
Geologic Interest

FACILITIES
Visitor Center
Restrooms
Picnic Tables
Phone
Water
Horse Staging

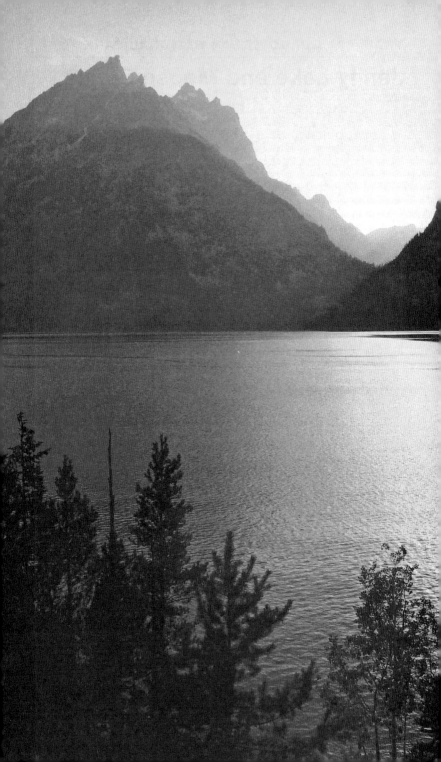

Logistics

Seasonal shuttle boats depart Jenny Lake's East Shore Boat Dock for the Cascade Canyon trailhead dock every 15 minutes daily, weather permitting, between May 15 and early September. From June 1 to September 15, hours of operation are 7 a.m.– 7 p.m., with service reduced to 10 a.m.–4 p.m. in May and the second half of September.

Fares are $9 one-way or $15 round-trip for passengers ages 11 and older, and $6 one-way or $8 round-trip for children ages 2–11. Call 307-734-9227 or visit jennylakeboating.com for more information.

Alternatively, you can set up a car shuttle by leaving a vehicle at the String Lake trailhead to avoid the final 2.9-mile stretch that parallels the road.

> The terminal moraine around Jenny Lake was deposited by a glacier flowing out of Cascade Canyon during the Pinedale Glaciation period, which ended around 10,000 years ago.

Trail Description

From the East Shore Boat Dock ►1 near the visitor center, head out toward the Tetons around the southwest side of Jenny Lake (6,783 feet). You'll cross Cottonwood Creek on a footbridge soon after passing the boat-launch area. The wide trail here may feel more like a highway, especially if the shuttle boat is not running.

Just beyond the Moose Ponds Loop Trail junction ►2, the trail forks at an unsigned junction. Take the high route, ►3 an unsigned horse trail, for better views and to avoid the crowds. As the trail winds up above the lakeshore, there are several scenic viewpoints looking back out to the east across the lake to Jackson Hole. The lower, more crowded Valley Trail follows the lakeshore.

Jenny Lake *and Cascade Canyon*

CREDIT: Bradley Mayhew

Waterfall

Viewpoint

After 1.3 mile the trail's forks reunite near the spur trails leading to the West Shore Boat Dock. ▶4 If you wish to cut your hike short for some reason here, you can catch the shuttle boat back across the lake to the visitor center. Otherwise, follow the signs a few hundred yards to the base of 200-foot Hidden Falls, ▶5 which is really a cascade (a series of small falls) instead of one free-falling torrent of water. Semantics aside, it still exerts that romantic, mesmerizing effect unique to pristine falling water.

The area below the falls is a well-signed maze of well-beaten paths. Follow the signs for Cascade Canyon to avoid ending up at the boat dock.

Heading back toward the lake from the base of the falls, the well-marked trail crosses over Cascade Creek on a bridge at the mouth of the U-shaped canyon and ascends along the north side of the creek. It's well worth a bit of exertion to climb the 0.4 mile beyond the falls to Inspiration Point (7,200 feet). ▶6

Note: If crowds look like they might pose a problem along the narrow trail to Inspiration Point, you can head a couple hundred yards north (right) from the boat dock and look for a horse trail that heads directly for the Cascade Canyon Trail. When it rejoins the main footpath, backtrack down the canyon (to the left) a few hundred yards to reach Inspiration Point.

After retracing your steps down from Inspiration Point back toward the boat dock, the Jenny Lake Trail (also known as the Valley Trail) hugs the lakeshore through a severe burn area, the aftermath of the lightning-sparked Alder Fire that consumed more than 300 acres in 1999. A few hundred yards beyond a scenic viewpoint, pause where a stream called Ribbon Cascade tumbles off the hillside to look up Hanging Canyon.

Look back up Cascade Canyon, to your left, for a glimpse of the Cathedral Group—from left to right: Teewinot Mountain (12,325 feet), the Grand Teton

Shuttle Boat

You can shortcut the first 2 miles of the hike by catching a
shuttle boat across the lake to the West Shore Boat Dock.
If you ride the boat in both directions, the round-trip hike to
Hidden Falls and Inspiration Point is only 2 miles total. If you
only want to take the shuttle boat one way, try starting at the
String Lake trailhead near Jenny Lake Lodge and looping
southwest around the less-trodden west shore, which cuts out
the two most crowded miles.

Moose Ponds Loop

Done by itself from the East Shore Boat Dock, the 3-mile
Moose Ponds Loop is a very pleasant, lightly traveled
90-minute outing. Four-tenths of a mile beyond the trailhead,
drop down a moraine to your left from the overview point to
the Moose Ponds. These three ponds and adjacent marshes
at the base of Teewinot Mountain offer a good chance to spot
some waterfowl and wildlife, especially in the early morning or
late evening. Willows, aspens, and wildflowers abound as you
first approach the ponds. On the far (south) side of the ponds,
the trail passes through a mature mixed subalpine fir and
Engelmann spruce forest. Either retrace your steps or follow
the trail as it loops around the last pond, through the sagebrush flats in Lupine Meadows, to end up back near the South
Jenny Lake parking area.

Cascade Canyon

Intrepid adventurers will want to continue upstream from
Hidden Falls and Inspiration Point to the Forks of Cascade
Canyon (an extra 9 miles round-trip, 3–4 hours, and 1,000 feet
of elevation gain), a strenuous climb to views of the Cathedral
Group. See Trail 36 (page 286) for a full description.

(13,770 feet), and Mount Owen (12,928 feet). In Hanging Canyon, a steep, unofficial (unmarked and unmaintained) climbers' trail gains 2,700 feet in less than 3 miles as it picks its way through boulder fields and climbs up the glacier-carved canyon past Ramshead Lake to Lake of the Crags, an imposing cirque.

You shouldn't encounter many hikers again until the String Lake trailhead junction ▶7. Soon after the junction, the trail cuts away from the lakeshore and crosses a footbridge over the rapids between String Lake and Jenny Lake ▶8 near the String Lake parking lot.

Along the final 2.9-mile stretch, the Teton views are impressive, but the traffic noise on the adjacent one-way scenic drive drowns out any illusion that you are in a pristine natural area. The trail hugs the eastern shore of Jenny Lake as it weaves in and out of lodgepole pine forest before ending up back at the South Jenny Lake parking area. ▶9

🚶 MILESTONES

▶1 0.0 Start at visitor center and East Shore Boat Dock
▶2 0.4 Right at Moose Ponds Trail junction
▶3 0.7 Fork left onto unsigned Hidden Falls Horse Trail
▶4 2.0 Left at West Shore Boat Dock cutoff
▶5 2.2 Hidden Falls
▶6 2.6 Inspiration Point
▶7 3.8 Right at the trail junction
▶8 4.1 Right after bridge over Jenny Lake inlet
▶9 7.0 Return to South Jenny Lake parking area

Laurance S. Rockefeller Preserve

This charming new addition to the park encourages visitors to explore one of the most wildlife-rich and scenic low-elevation areas of the Tetons. It's a lovely introduction to the full spectrum of Tetons ecosystems. The trails gently climb across ecotones, from sageland to woodlands and wetlands, before arriving at stunningly serene, 525-acre Phelps Lake.

Best Time

The preserve's trails are shaded enough to make the hiking pleasant any time of day, although early morning and late afternoon are the most serene times. As with other relatively low-elevation areas around Jackson Hole, snow can linger into June. Wildflowers pop up soon after the snowmelt, and birdlife is most diverse in early summer. Autumn colors peak in late August and early September.

Finding the Trail

From south of the park in the town of Jackson, head 1 mile southwest through town on US 26/89/191 to the WY 22 junction. Turn right and go west 4.5 miles to WY 390 (Moose Wilson Road). Turn right and go 7 miles north, past Teton Village and Jackson Hole Mountain Resort. Continue north through the park's Granite Canyon Entrance Station, where the road turns to dirt and is rough in patches; proceed 4.5 miles north, 1.75 miles past the Granite Canyon trailhead, and turn right down a gravel road, passing through a well-signed, ranch-style entrance gate for the Laurance S. Rockefeller (LSR) Preserve.

TRAIL USE
Hike

LENGTH
3.0 miles, 1.5–2 hours

VERTICAL FEET
±250

DIFFICULTY
– 1 **2** 3 4 5 +

TRAIL TYPE
Loop

SURFACE TYPE
Dirt

FEATURES
Child Friendly
Lake
Stream
Autumn Colors
Wildflowers
Birds
Wildlife
Cool & Shady
Great Views
Photo Opportunity
Secluded

FACILITIES
Visitor Center
Restrooms
Picnic Tables

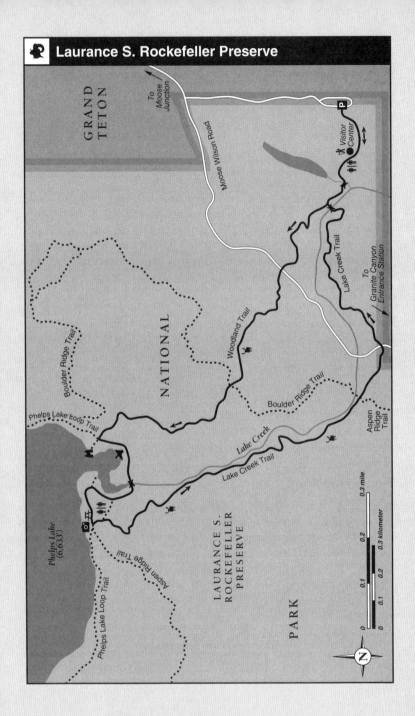

Laurance S. Rockefeller Preserve

GRAND TETON

To Moose Junction

Moose Wilson Road

P

Visitor Center

Lake Creek Trail

To Granite Canyon Entrance Station

Woodland Trail

NATIONAL

Boulder Ridge Trail

Phelps Lake Loop Trail

Boulder Ridge Trail

Aspen Ridge Trail

Lake Creek

Lake Creek Trail

Lake Creek Trail

Phelps Lake (6,633')

Aspen Ridge Trail

LAURANCE S. ROCKEFELLER PRESERVE

Phelps Lake Loop Trail

PARK

0.3 mile

0.1   0.2

0.3 kilometer

0   0.1   0.2

N

From the north, look for the junction with Teton Park Road across from the visitor center in Moose. Drive south 3.5 miles on a narrow, winding, paved but scenic stretch of Moose Wilson Road and turn left at the signed preserve turnoff. RVs, trailers, and vehicles more than 23 feet long are not allowed on Moose Wilson Road.

Logistics

Get to the preserve before 10 a.m. to ensure a parking spot, as cars are strictly limited to 50. Pick up a preserve trail map on arrival. Rangers lead free guided hikes to Phelps Lake daily at 9:30 a.m.; make a reservation by calling 307-739-3654. If the weather turns foul, you could do worse than to curl up with a book in the lodgelike reading room of the LEED-certified (Platinum-rated) visitor center; open June–September, daily, 8 a.m.–5 p.m. Kids ages 6–12 can pick up a Native Explorers backpack full of activities at the visitor center. There is also a daily talk on Laurance Rockefeller at 10 a.m.

Early or late in the season, inquire about trail conditions at the Craig Thomas Discovery & Visitor Center in Moose.

Trail Description

From the preserve visitor center, ▶1 head west through a sagebrush meadow across a seasonal stream on a footbridge, passing the park's only wheelchair-accessible waterfall. After 0.1 mile, fork right at the signed Lake Creek–Woodland Trail junction, ▶2 just beyond a bridged crossing of Lake Creek. Dads can enjoy teaching their kids about the signposted "rock snot" here.

Just uphill, pass through a split-rail fence and watch for traffic as you cross Moose Wilson Road ▶3 (no parking allowed), where the mixed spruce, fir,

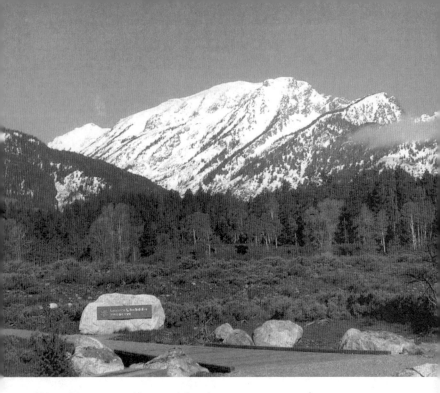

Teton vistas *contrast with a crystal-clear sky.*

Wildlife

Birds

Lake

Viewpoint

and lodgepole pine forest starts to take over as you climb gently. Watch carefully here for owls, moose, elk, deer, and even signs of bears. Sharp eyes may notice the faint traces of the decommissioned JY Ranch road, which the trail crisscrosses and roughly parallels.

Colorful stands of aspen, cottonwood, and Rocky Mountain maple and huckleberry fill out the mixed forest's lush understory and provide good bird-watching opportunities. After passing the signed Boulder Ridge Trail junction, the trail flattens out a bit before a final, gentle ascent to a four-way junction, near the southern shore of Phelps Lake (6,633 feet). ►4 Turn left and wind along the lakeshore, crossing the lake's cascading outlet on finely crafted bridges, and then seek out a rough-cut log bench or scenic picnic spot around the LEED-certified restrooms tucked away just off the lakeshore.

Detour: If you're not ready to head home, the Phelps Lake Trail continues west, meandering along the lakeshore 0.7 mile to secluded Huckleberry Point, with metal boardwalks spanning seasonal marsh wetlands en route.

To return to the trailhead, turn left away from the lakeshore on Lake Creek Trail, at a three-way junction ►5 to begin the gradual descent past the former JY Ranch site—watch for a large, open meadow on your right as the trail begins to closely parallel Lake Creek. A trail sign at the southern end of this meadow marks the start of the final, scenic 1.1-mile stretch back to the visitor center, once again crossing Moose Wilson Road. ►6

NOTES

The Rockefeller Conservation Legacy

Valued at $160 million, the 1,106-acre Laurance S. Rockefeller (LSR) Preserve was donated to the National Park Service (NPS) in 2001 but was opened to the public only in late 2007. The property was the final parcel of the 3,100-acre Rockefeller summer family retreat, purchased by John D. Rockefeller in 1932, and was originally home to the pioneering JY Ranch, Jackson Hole's first dude ranch (circa 1907). Between 2004 and 2007, 30 buildings, as well as roads, utilities, and other outbuildings were removed in an effort to remove all traces of human presence, and developed areas were reclaimed to blend with the natural landscape. Several of the structures, including the oldest cabins and dining and recreation buildings, were relocated to another Rockefeller property outside the park. The remaining structures were donated to the NPS for housing and service facilities within the park. Other ongoing restoration projects within the preserve include wildlife habitat enhancement, nonnative vegetation eradication, and reconnection of fragmented wetlands. The idea behind the preserve is to focus on the contemplative, spiritual side of the landscape, reflecting Rockefeller's own belief in the restorative power of nature.

►1   0.0 Start at the LSR Preserve visitor center trailhead

►2   0.1 Fork right at Lake Creek–Woodland Trail junction

►3   0.2 Cross Moose Wilson Road (no parking)

►4   0.9 Left at junction near southern shore of Phelps Lake

►5   1.3 Left at Lake Creek Trail junction

►6   3.0 Return to LSR Preserve visitor center

Route Options

OPTIONS

The longer Aspen Ridge and Boulder Ridge loops, which fork off the main Woodland and Lake Creek Trails, trace glacial ridges and include more strenuous terrain. Neither sees a great deal of traffic. The scenic Phelps Lake loop, which connects via the Valley Trail with the Phelps Lake Trail (page 316), is 7 miles long and takes about four hours.

Leigh, Bearpaw, and Trapper Lakes

The easy outing to Leigh Lake is a favorite of families and those looking for a stress-free overnight option. The lake is big enough and just far enough away from the road to feel like it's in the backcountry, but close enough to attract parents with small children. It's also a favorite summer swimming hole and popular horseback-riding destination. Campsites around the much smaller and forested Bearpaw and Trapper Lakes provide an extra measure of seclusion but lack the sandy beaches and mountain views.

Best Time

The hike is very pleasant at any time. The snow is usually gone by mid-May, and the trail is passable through October. Swimming is best in July and August. Beware of hypothermia-inducing temperatures in Leigh Lake before the end of June. Early morning is particularly charming here, when the lake is calm, light on the mountains is at its best, and crowds are at their lightest.

Finding the Trail

From the south, take US 26/89/191 north out of Jackson; proceed 8 miles past the park's southern boundary and turn left at Moose Junction. Continue 1 mile past the visitor center to the Moose Entrance Station. Go 11 miles north and turn left at the North Jenny Lake Junction. Continue 1.5 miles and turn right near Jenny Lake Lodge, just before the road becomes one-way. Follow the signs a few hundred yards to the String Lake Picnic Area parking lot.

TRAIL USE
Hike, Backpack, Horse

LENGTH
2.2 miles to Leigh Lake, 8.4 miles to Trapper Lake; 2–3 hours

VERTICAL FEET
Negligible

DIFFICULTY
– 1 **2 3** 4 5 +

TRAIL TYPE
Out-and-back

SURFACE TYPE
Dirt

FEATURES
Child Friendly
Lake
Autumn Colors
Wildflowers
Birds
Wildlife
Cool & Shady
Great Views
Photo Opportunity
Camping
Swimming

FACILITIES
Restrooms
Picnic Tables
Horse Staging

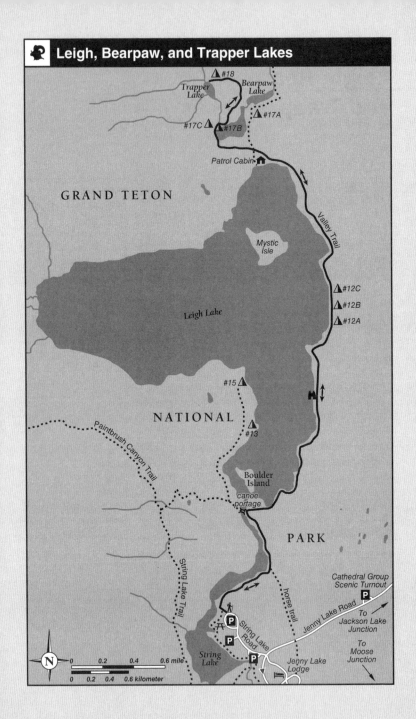

Leigh, Bearpaw, and Trapper Lakes

Trapper Lake

▲ #18

Bearpaw Lake

▲ #17A

#17C ▲   ▲ #17B

Patrol Cabin 🏠

GRAND TETON

Valley Trail

Mystic Isle

▲ #12C

▲ #12B

▲ #12A

Leigh Lake

#15 ▲

NATIONAL

▲ #13

Paintbrush Canyon Trail

Boulder Island

canoe portage

PARK

String Lake Trail

horse trail

Cathedral Group Scenic Turnout

🅿

To Jackson Lake Junction

To Moose Junction

Jenny Lake Road

🅿 String Lake Road

🅿

🅿

String Lake

Jenny Lake Lodge

N

0   0.2   0.4   0.6 mile

0   0.2   0.4   0.6 kilometer

From the north, starting at Jackson Lake Junction, go 9 miles south on Teton Park Road and turn right at North Jenny Lake Junction. Continue 1.5 miles and turn right into the picnic-area parking lot.

Trail Description

Start from the trailhead (6,875 feet) near the northwest corner of the String Lake Picnic Area parking lot. ▶1 The wide, packed-sand trail sees lots of horse traffic as it starts out through lodgepole pine forest. After a horse trail from Jenny Lake Lodge joins in on the right side, the trail meets the signed canoe portage ▶2 for Leigh Lake, 0.9 mile beyond the trailhead.

From the canoe portage junction, follow the right fork and continue 1.1 miles north along the south shore of Leigh Lake (6,877 feet). ▶3 This is also a good area to forage for berries.

Starting after 1.1 miles, you'll pass a series of wonderful, white-sand swimming beaches, ▶4 where the views of Mount Moran reflected in the lake are fit for the cover of a box of chocolates.

Less than a mile farther along the lakeshore, you'll pass the first of three East Shore campsites (12A, 12B, and 12C), ▶5 all fabulous spots to spend the night and only 3 miles from the trailhead. The first site is for groups only but gets released to nongroups after 3 p.m. They are also very popular with boating families. Each is about a minute's walk from the other. If you do spend the night here, take proper bear precautions; pitch your tent on a pad, if provided; build fires only in grates; put your food and toiletries in the provided bear boxes or on the poles; and beware of the waves (yes, waves) caused by wind on the lake.

Beyond the head of the lake, past a burn area and opposite a turnoff for the Leigh Lake Patrol Cabin, the trail forks to the right for tree-lined and marshy Bearpaw Lake ▶6 and backcountry campsite

Just below Mount Moran, Falling Ice Glacier often calves frozen blocks into the lake and contributes to Leigh Lake's unique blue-green tint.

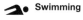 Swimming

The glaciers hugging the sides of Mount Moran are up to 100 feet thick.

 Camping

Backcountry Campsites

Lake lovers and anglers will want to continue on to Bearpaw
and Trapper Lakes and possibly even bushwhack a bit to reach
remote Bearpaw Bay or Little Grassy Island campsites on the
south shore of Jackson Lake. Be particularly aware of grizzlies if you tackle this off-trail section. It's also possible to hike
to campsites 13 and 15 on an unmaintained trail just after the
bridge crossing at the String Lake inlet, near the portage sign.
Note that the Leigh Lake backcountry campsites are among the
park's most popular, so try to reserve these before May 15.

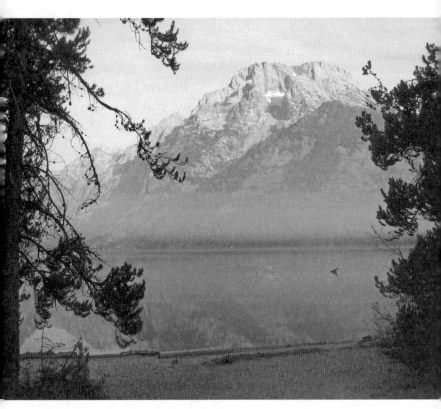

Leigh Lake *is lined with private beaches and lovely backcountry campsites.*

CREDIT: Bradley Mayhew

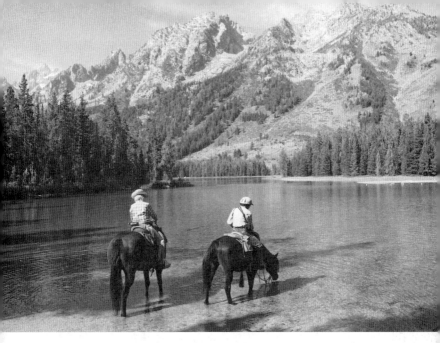

Thirsty horses *drink from crystal-clear Leigh Lake.*

CREDIT: Bradley Mayhew

17B. Straight on takes you to lakeshore campsite 17A and nearby 17C. About 0.6 mile farther is Trapper Lake, ►7 with some views of Mount Moran and one private campsite (18).

If you can pull yourself away, retrace your steps to the String Lake parking area. ►8

🚶	**MILESTONES**

►1	0.0 Start at String Lake Picnic Area parking lot
►2	0.9 Right at Leigh Lake Trail junction (canoe portage)
►3	1.1 Leigh Lake
►4	2.2 Sandy beach
►5	3.0 East Shore (12-series) campsites
►6	3.7 Right at Bearpaw Lake junction (3.9 to Bearpaw Lake)
►7	4.2 Trapper Lake
►8	8.4 Return to String Lake parking lot

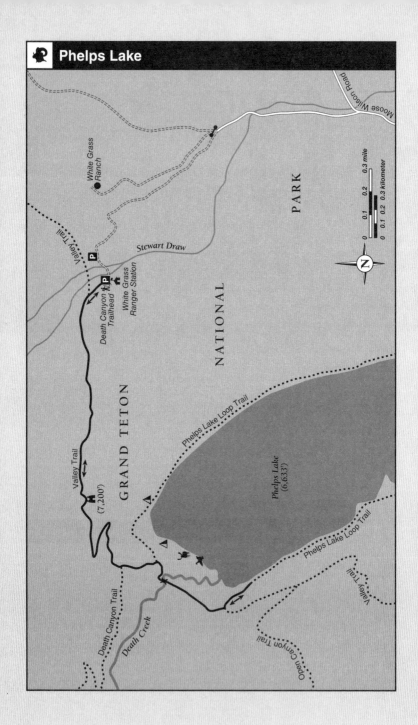

Phelps Lake

White Grass Ranch

Moose Wilson Road

PARK

NATIONAL

GRAND TETON

Valley Trail

Stewart Draw

White Grass
Ranger Station

Death Canyon
Trailhead

Valley Trail

(7,200')

Death Canyon Trail

Death Creek

Phelps Lake Loop Trail

Phelps Lake
(6,633')

Phelps Lake Loop Trail

Open Canyon Trail

Valley Trail

0   0.1   0.2   0.3 mile
0 0.1 0.2 0.3 kilometer

Phelps Lake

Beyond the scenic overlook of the park's fourth-largest lake, this rewarding route provides access to a group of three charming lakefront campsites that feel miles from the trailhead. Wildflowers, trout, moose, and black bears are abundant. Reserve campsites as far ahead as possible for this popular, family-friendly overnighter.

Best Time

Snow usually disappears from the trail by mid-June. Wildflowers appear soon after the snowmelt, and bird-watching is most diverse in early summer. Autumn colors peak in late August and early September. There's enough shade to make the trail pleasant any time of day.

Finding the Trail

From south of the park in the town of Jackson, head 1 mile southwest through town on US 26/89/191 to the WY 22 junction. Turn right and go west 4.5 miles to WY 390 (Moose Wilson Road). Turn right and go 7 miles north, past Teton Village and Jackson Hole Mountain Resort. Continue north through the park's Granite Canyon Entrance Station, where the road turns to dirt; proceed 5 miles north, past the Granite Canyon trailhead, and turn left on a paved road signed for Death Canyon. Bear left after 0.3 mile: the pavement ends after 0.5 mile, and the rough, one-lane dirt road (no trailers or mobile homes allowed) gets worse for the next mile until it passes a larger parking area (best for low-clearance vehicles). There

TRAIL USE
Hike, Backpack, Horse
LENGTH
4.0 miles, 2–3 hours
VERTICAL FEET
±420 to overlook, ±850 to lake
DIFFICULTY
– 1 **2** 3 4 5 +
TRAIL TYPE
Out-and-back
SURFACE TYPE
Dirt

FEATURES
Child Friendly
Lake
Stream
Autumn Colors
Wildflowers
Birds
Wildlife
Cool & Shady
Great Views
Photo Opportunity
Camping
Swimming
Geologic Interest

FACILITIES
Restrooms
Horse Staging

317

Granite Canyon Car Shuttle

If you have two cars, you can extend the hike into a 6.1-mile point-to-point outing by leaving a vehicle at the signed Granite Canyon trailhead (6,356 feet), on the west side of Moose Wilson Road, just north of the Granite Canyon Entrance Station.

Long-Distance Backpacking Routes

Popular overnight backpacking options that use the Death Canyon trailhead en route to the Teton Crest Trail include the 19.3-mile loop from Granite Canyon via Open Canyon; a 24.8-mile (one or two nights) route to Jenny Lake via Static Peak Divide; a more challenging 29.5-mile (two or three nights) route to the String Lake Picnic Area; a 25.7-mile (two nights) loop to Granite Canyon trailhead; and the demanding 36-mile (four nights) trip to String Lake via Paintbrush Canyon. Download or pick up a Backcountry Planning brochure (tinyurl.com/gtnp backcountrybrochure) for details.

are parking spots all along the road until it dead-ends soon after at the crowded trailhead parking area near the White Grass Ranger Station.

From the north, look for the junction with Teton Park Road across from the Moose Visitor Center. Drive south 3 miles on a narrow, winding, paved but scenic stretch of Moose Wilson Road and turn right at the signed Death Canyon Trailhead Road junction.

Trail Description

From the Death Canyon trailhead (6,780 feet) near the seasonal White Grass Ranger Station, ▶1 keep left at the signed Valley Trail T-junction, ▶2 0.1 mile beyond the parking area.

For the next 0.8 mile, the well-beaten path—once a popular horseback-riding route for dudes staying at the White Grass Ranch—rises gradually through meadows, mixed-conifer forest, and colorful groves of aspens, crossing a couple of streams flush with thimbleberries. Ignore all the unmarked horse trails that intersect the trail as it climbs to the overlook.

Once atop the lateral moraine—deposited more than 15,000 years ago by a mass of ice pouring out of Death Canyon—there are nice picnic spots tucked among the boulders to the left, and good views over the lake to the Jackson Hole valley from the Phelps Lake Overlook (7,200 feet). ▶3

 Geologic Interest

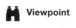 Viewpoint

For an easy, hourlong outing, some folks prefer to turn back here and return to the trailhead. To experience the variety of habitats around the lakeshore and for a better look up the glacial, U-shaped canyon, follow the switchbacks down the steeper, southern face of the moraine 0.7 mile to the Death Canyon Trail junction. ▶4

The spur trail for the three lovely campsites perched above the lake's northern shore branches off to the left from the Phelps Lake Trail just beyond the Death Canyon Trail junction. For fishing access and some good bird-watching, continue south along the western lakeshore after crossing Death Creek on a footbridge, and follow a side trail down to the shore and inlet of Phelps Lake. ▶5 Retrace your steps back to the trailhead parking area. ▶6

 Camping

 Birds

🚶 MILESTONES

▶1   0.0 Start at Death Canyon (White Grass) trailhead
▶2   0.1 Left at Valley Trail T-junction
▶3   0.9 Phelps Lake Overlook
▶4   1.6 Left at Death Canyon Trail junction
▶5   2.0 Phelps Lake
▶6   4.0 Return to trailhead parking area

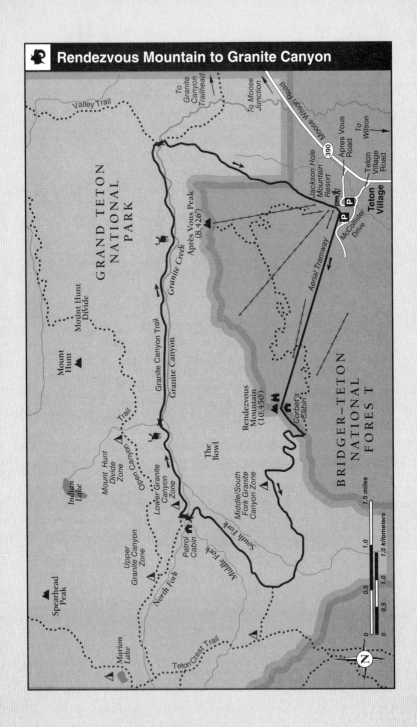

Rendezvous Mountain to Granite Canyon

Rendezvous Mountain to Granite Canyon

Where else in the United States can you fill your lungs with such rarefied alpine air without breaking a sweat? This route is spectacular—and 95% downhill—so it gets traffic whenever the weather is decent and the tram is in service. No other trail gives you a taste of Teton's upper canyons while only demanding a downhill stroll in return.

Best Time

The tram operates Memorial Day–late September, but inclement weather can halt operations, and snow can linger around Rendezvous Peak through July. Catch the first tram so you can enjoy a picnic lunch along the way and have plenty of time to hang out along the creek in the canyon. Better yet, reserve a backcountry campsite and make it an overnight trip. Fall colors peak around the autumnal equinox (September 21).

Finding the Trail

From Jackson, head 1 mile south on US 26/89/191 to the WY 22 junction. Turn right and go west 4.5 miles to WY 390 (Moose Wilson Road). Turn right and head north 7 miles to Teton Village and Jackson Hole Mountain Resort. Turn left into the parking area and follow the signs to the aerial tram ticket booth. From the Moose Visitor Center, drive south 8 miles on Moose Wilson Road, past the Granite Canyon trailhead and Granite Canyon Entrance Station to Teton Village.

TRAIL USE
Hike, Backpack, Horse

LENGTH
12.4 miles, 6–8 hours

VERTICAL FEET
+400/–4,100

DIFFICULTY
– 1 2 3 **4** 5 +

TRAIL TYPE
Loop

SURFACE TYPE
Dirt

FEATURES
Canyon
Mountain
Summit
Steep
Stream
Autumn Colors
Wildflowers
Birds
Wildlife
Great Views
Photo Opportunity
Camping
Geologic Interest

FACILITIES
Visitor Center
Restrooms
Phone
Water

Logistics

Horses are not allowed between the tram and the Middle Fork Cut-Off Trail junction, a one-hour to 90-minute hike down. Enjoy the singing mountain songbirds and woodpeckers drumming away.

This hike starts outside the park, high above Teton Village (locally known simply as "the Village") from Jackson Hole Mountain Resort. For details, see jacksonhole.com.

The resort's aerial tram (round-trip tickets are $42 for adults, $25 for children ages 6–17; free for descent only) runs in summer Memorial Day–late September. Hours of operation vary seasonally: from 9 a.m.–5 p.m. in the low season, and from 9 a.m.–6 p.m. in the high season. The tram runs every half hour and takes 12 minutes to climb more than 4,000 feet to the top of Rendezvous Mountain; see tram-formation.com for details. Pick up a free copy of the Jackson Hole Daily newspaper to score a $5 coupon off the cost of the tram.

High winds and inclement weather can disrupt tram service; contact the resort's Guest Service Center for updates on current conditions. Call 307-739-2753. If you miss the last tram down from the summit at 6:30 p.m., it's a long, 7.2-mile walk back down along the service road. Note that weather conditions at the summit are always much cooler and windier than at the base.

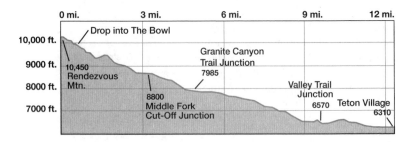

Trail Description

Enjoy the expansive views from the aerial tram ▶1 during the ride up Rendezvous Mountain. Upon exiting the tram platform, above treeline at the summit (10,450 feet), ▶2 you can take care of any last-minute needs at Corbet's Cabin, where there are restrooms, fresh waffles, and hot drinks. Soak up the endless views, check out the Grand Teton in the telescope, and then head left (south) along the ridge down the Summit Trail/service road.

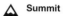 Summit

 Viewpoint

Tread lightly in this fragile alpine zone: several varieties of delicate alpine wildflowers, lichens, and stunted krummholz Engelmann spruce and whitebark pine flourish in revegetation zones near the trail. Continue straight ahead (not left) at the first signed junction, after 0.4 mile, ▶3 your only chance to bail out and return to Teton Village. Soon after, at the second signed junction, enter Grand Teton National Park by turning right and following the signs for Granite Canyon. ▶4

 Wildflowers

Detour: A minor trail continues straight at the junction, scrambling up a minor peak to the west, offering a short side trip. The same trail continues southwest to a larger peak, but you don't really have the time to tackle this summit if you are headed for Granite Canyon.

The main trail quickly drops into a big cirque aptly called The Bowl. The stunted spruce forest here marks timberline. After a short climb, you enter the Middle/South Fork Granite Canyon camping zone, where the trail crosses several small stream culverts and bisects a wildflower meadow before crossing the South Fork of Granite Creek.

 Wildflowers

After 3.5 miles, beyond the Middle Fork Cut-Off junction, ▶5 follow the ridgeline between the Middle and South Forks of Granite Creek through open meadows down to a spruce–fir forest. A sign announces the end of the Middle Fork camping zone, and then the trail crosses two babbling creek

Loop and Overnight Options

If you're looking for a scenic workout, you can hike 7.2 miles (4,100 vertical feet) up the service road and ride the aerial tram back down to the base area for free. If the weather looks dodgy up top, you might opt for one of several shorter, well-signed loops around the summit. Or you can extend the trip by adding an overnight at Marion Lake (9,240 feet, 15.9 miles total) or in one of the three designated camping zones along the Granite Canyon Trail.

You can avoid the final dull Valley Trail stretch of the full loop by setting up a car shuttle at the Granite Canyon trail-head, just inside the park along Moose Wilson Road, 2 miles north of Teton Village.

The Uphill Option

You can save some cash by making this hike in reverse, starting at Teton Village, hiking up Granite Canyon, and taking the tram down for free. The catch: You have to ascend 4,100 feet the hard way. Be sure also to check the weather and make sure you catch the last tram down. The initial trail can be tricky to find from the tram in Teton Village, so pick up a resort map to get yourself oriented. Make your way to the Bridger Center and Teewinot lift; then follow the uphill path to the right, crossing a dirt road and the high ropes course, passing a trail-board map en route. Cross a second dirt road at the Après Vous lift, and follow the green signs for the Valley Trail to the signposted border of Grand Teton National Park.

Canyon

forks on sturdy wooden footbridges. Just beyond the second bridge, look for the Granite Canyon Patrol Cabin off-trail to your left at 5.2 miles (there's an emergency toilet here). It's located just before the trail junction for Open Canyon, Marion Lake, and the Teton Crest Trail. ▶6 Turn right (east) here to start the gradual, 4.7-mile descent on the Granite Canyon Trail to the mouth of the canyon.

Almost immediately after this junction, the trail enters fragrant forest and the Lower Granite Canyon camping zone, where you'll pass 10 signposted sites over the next 90 minutes of walking. Several viewpoints high above Granite Creek afford views down to meadows and the canyon mouth. Before the trail eventually drops down alongside the creek, watch for moose and mule deer browsing in meadows—you may even see them foraging side by side.

Another sign indicates a group campsite, shortly before the trail passes below a small waterfall on the left and a stock bridge over the resulting stream. The trail drops through sagebrush meadows, past areas signed as closed for regrowth, before leveling off alongside a charming stretch of Granite Creek.

The cool, breezy lower half of the canyon is often choked with luxuriant vegetation. Ripe, rosy mountain-ash fruits are the most conspicuous eye-catchers. There are a couple of nice riverfront campsites, just before the canyon's right wall closes in to its narrowest point, opposite a large talus field riddled with raspberry bushes. From here, the trail levels off before a final abrupt descent, which begins where the trail trends away from the creek to exit the canyon.

 Wildlife

Snack alert: In early summer, keep an eye out for the ripe, wild, red raspberries on bushes that poke out of rocky slopes and talus fields.

 Camping

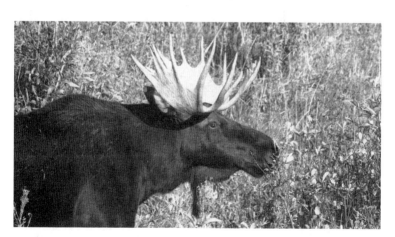

Yield to moose: *In Lower Granite Canyon, I had a surprise encounter with a skittish cow moose and her very peeved bull (and his huge rack), who stared me down where the trail passes through their favorite willow thicket. I was unnerved enough to start singing to myself.*

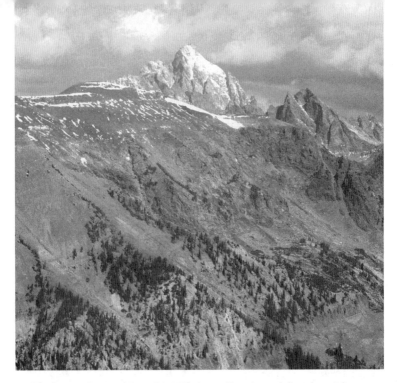

On clear days, *the Grand Teton (13,770 feet) is visible to the north from the aerial tram platform atop Rendezvous Mountain.*

Don't be startled by the well-camouflaged grouse that like to jump out of the woods just after the trail drops below treeline.

Viewpoint 👀

The impact of heavy horse use becomes more apparent near the canyon mouth as the trail approaches the Valley Trail ►7 junction after 9.9 miles. The trail forks again 0.1 mile after crossing Granite Creek for the final time on a stock bridge. Beyond this junction, follow signs for the Valley Trail and/or Teton Village, ignoring all unsigned horse trails that join in from the left.

The final 2.4 miles of the Valley Trail is the least appealing section of the entire route. It can be very dusty due to heavy equestrian use, with several mild ups and downs. It's an anticlimactic ending to an invigorating hike, but it does have some nice panoramas across Jackson Hole, fine displays of fall color, and deer and quail lying in wait alongside the trail.

A sign at the park boundary points the way (right) uphill to Teton Village. The trail passes briefly through a maintenance yard, then winds through an aspen grove before reaching a resort service road. Ignore all bike-route signs and turn left on the gravel service road, following the signs past the Après Vous ski lift. Continue down past a number of ski-in trophy houses and the Four Seasons lodge to arrive at the base of the tram in the Village. ▶8

🚶 MILESTONES

▶1   0.0 Start at Teton Village–Jackson Hole Mountain Resort parking area; buy tickets and board aerial tram

▶2   0.0 Exit tram platform and walk left on Rendezvous Mountain Trail

▶3   0.4 Straight (not left) at junction for Teton Village parking area

▶4   0.5 Right at Grand Teton National Park boundary

▶5   3.5 Right at Middle Fork Cut-Off junction

▶6   5.2 Right at Granite Canyon Patrol Cabin

▶7   9.9 Right at Valley Trail junction

▶8   12.4 Return to Teton Village

NOTES

Peak Après-Hike Experiences

When you return to civilization, why not stop for a drink? If you're feeling very civilized, drop in at the stylish yet informal Ascent Lounge at the Four Seasons, conveniently located next to the trail as it descends to the resort's base area.

For a less refined atmosphere, pop into the Mangy Moose Restaurant and Saloon, near the bottom of the tram in Teton Village, for some live music, a free-range buffalo burger, or, best of all, a frosty pint of Moose Drool. Call 307-733-9779 or see mangymoose.com to check the live music schedule.

If you are here on a Sunday in July or August, time your hike with one of the free weekly music concerts that take place next to the tram. See concertsoncommons.com for the current lineup.

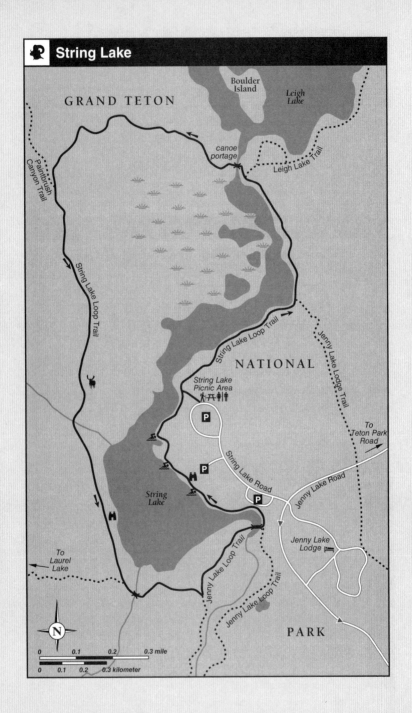

String Lake

GRAND TETON

Boulder Island

Leigh Lake

Paintbrush Canyon Trail

canoe portage

Leigh Lake Trail

String Lake Loop Trail

String Lake Loop Trail

NATIONAL

Jenny Lake Lodge Trail

String Lake Picnic Area

To Teton Park Road

String Lake Road

String Lake

Jenny Lake Road

Jenny Lake Loop Trail

Jenny Lake Lodge

To Laurel Lake

Jenny Lake Loop Trail

PARK

N

| 0 | 0.1 | 0.2 | 0.3 mile |
| 0 | 0.1 | 0.2 | 0.3 kilometer |

String Lake

This is one of the most relaxing and easygoing—and thus very popular—hikes in the park. The nearly flat trail winds through a variety of habitats and traces the shoreline of the smallest in a string of tranquil piedmont lakes, all at the foot of the awe-inspiring Teton Range. Lots of opportunities for swimming and boating make this a great family and warm-weather option.

Best Time

Whenever you can get in and out of the park, this hike is a good choice. There are a couple of short, sunny sections, but most of the route remains cool and shady all day long. Swimming is most enjoyable in July and August, after the lake has warmed up a bit.

Finding the Trail

From the south, take US 26/89/191 north out of Jackson; proceed 8 miles past the park's southern boundary and turn left at Moose Junction. Continue 1 mile past the visitor center to the Moose Entrance Station. Drive 11 miles north and turn left at North Jenny Lake Junction. Continue 1.5 miles and turn right just before the road becomes one-way. Pass the busy String Lake trailhead parking lot and continue a couple hundred yards to the much larger String Lake Picnic Area parking. From the north, starting at Jackson Lake Junction, go 9 miles south on Teton Park Road and turn right at North Jenny Lake Junction. Continue 1.5 miles and turn right into the trailhead parking lot.

TRAIL USE
Hike, Horse

LENGTH
3.4 miles, 1–2 hours

VERTICAL FEET
±270

DIFFICULTY
− 1 **2** 3 4 5 +

TRAIL TYPE
Loop

SURFACE TYPE
Dirt, Paved

FEATURES
Child Friendly
Handicap Accessible
Lake
Stream
Autumn Colors
Wildflowers
Wildlife
Cool & Shady
Great Views
Photo Opportunity
Swimming
Geologic Interest

FACILITIES
Restrooms
Picnic Tables
Boat Launch
Horse Staging

Leigh and Jenny Lake Detours

We describe the loop counterclockwise, but you can do it in either direction without increasing the difficulty.

To extend the hike, add an out-and-back detour to the south shore of Leigh Lake (0.4 mile round-trip) or an extension to the north shore of Jenny Lake (0.4 mile round-trip). The backcountry campsites around Leigh Lake are wonderful spots for overnight canoe trips and first-time family wilderness outings. For details, see Trail 40 (page 311).

Logistics

The String Lake Picnic Area parking has toilets, water, picnic benches, and an area for launching kayaks and canoes. If you plan to use a kayak, canoe, or stand-up paddleboard (SUP) you will need to purchase a $10 permit in advance at a backcountry office. If you are bringing in your watercraft from out of state, you will also need a Wyoming Aquatic Invasive Species decal, which costs $5 for Wyoming residents or $15 for nonresidents. No permits are needed for inflatable tubes.

Trail Description

From the String Lake picnic area, ▶1 the trail quickly turns to packed sand and starts to see horse traffic as it passes through lodgepole pine forest. After a horse trail from Jenny Lake Lodge joins in from the right, the trail meets the canoe portage to Leigh Lake, at 0.8 mile from the trailhead. ▶2

Lake

Cross the babbling brook that links Leigh Lake and String Lake via a long, sturdy footbridge. ▶3 Once across the bridge, you can't help but notice the large glacial erratic boulders. The well-worn footpaths around the rocks aren't beaten by climbers looking to practice boulder-scaling but by savvy huckleberry seekers who flock here in early summer, trying to beat the bears to their treasure. A tempting seat offers a convenient place to take a break if you need it.

Geologic
Interest

Beyond the berry patches, the trail ducks once again into mature mixed-conifer forest and starts a steady climb up to the String Lake Trail junction, ▶4 where the right fork leads steeply up into Paintbrush Canyon. Take the left branch toward Jenny Lake.

The trail opens up and traverses a few aspen-dotted meadows below Rockchuck Peak (11,144 feet) and nearby Mount Saint John as it heads south above the west shore of String Lake, offering fine views. Moose can sometimes be found in the willows here in the early morning hours. Shortly after the trail drops down to the shoreline, it passes through a small burn area. At this point, explorers can make a short side trip to a scenic picnic spot at Laurel Lake (7,625 feet). Before the trail crosses a footbridge over a feeder stream, follow an unmarked but well-worn path to the right, which climbs uphill about 0.5 mile to the tiny lake.

After returning to the main trail, at the Jenny Lake–Valley Trail junction, ▶5 bear left to cross the bridge over String Lake's outlet stream, and continue to the String Lake trailhead parking lot, ▶6 where a paved, wheelchair-accessible path winds around the peaceful lakeshore. There are great views of the towering Cathedral Group (Teewinot Mountain, Mount Owen, and the Grand Teton) and sandy beaches offering a cooling dip in the lovely, clear lake. Bring a towel, tube, and cooler and end the hike in style. ▶7

 Wildlife

 Viewpoint

 Stream

 Viewpoint

 Swimming

🚶 **MILESTONES**

▶1	0.0 Start at String Lake picnic area parking lot
▶2	0.8 Left at Leigh Lake Trail junction
▶3	0.9 Bridge across Leigh Lake outlet
▶4	1.5 Left at String Lake Trail junction
▶5	2.8 Left across bridge at Jenny Lake–Valley Trail junction
▶6	3.1 String Lake trailhead parking lot
▶7	3.4 Return to String Lake picnic area

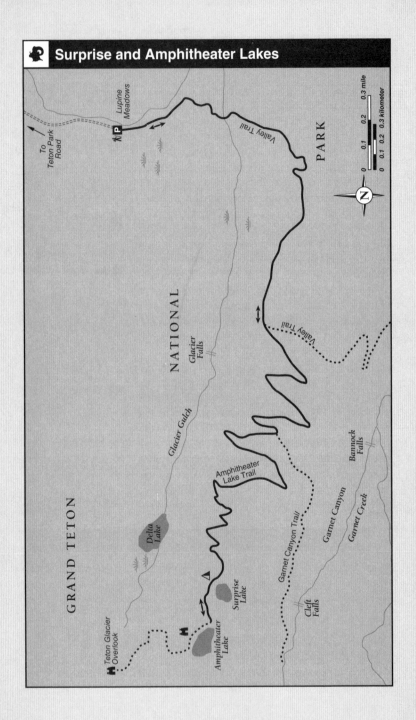

Surprise and Amphitheater Lakes

Surprise and Amphitheater Lakes

Welcome to the Tetons. Don't try this aerobic hike on your first day at altitude. It climbs nearly a thousand feet per mile—but the views are worth every last gasp of breath. The route is one of the park's most popular for good reason: it provides quick access to some of the most scenic alpine lakes in North America. Overachievers often add an extension to the stunning Teton Glacier Overlook.

Best Time

Snow often persists on higher portions of the route until as late as late June or early July, and it can start reappearing by mid-September. The lakes are ice-free for only a few months a year. The exposed switchbacks can be quite hot in the midday summer sun. Set out early to beat the crowds and to allow maximum time for enjoyment, recovery, and lakeside relaxation up top.

Finding the Trail

From the south, take US 26/89/191 north out of Jackson; proceed 8 miles past the park's southern boundary and turn left at Moose Junction. Go past the Moose Visitor Center through the Moose Entrance Station. Continue north on Teton Park Road 6.6 miles. Turn left at the signed Lupine Meadows junction. Follow the gravel road across the new Cottonwood Creek bridge 1.5 miles to the ample Lupine Meadows parking area and trailhead. From the north, starting at Jackson Lake Junction, go 13.3 miles south on Teton Park Road and turn right at the Lupine Meadows junction.

TRAIL USE
Hike, Backpack

LENGTH
9.6 miles, 5–6 hours

VERTICAL FEET
±3,000

DIFFICULTY
– 1 2 3 4 **5** +

TRAIL TYPE
Out-and-back

SURFACE TYPE
Dirt

FEATURES
Canyon
Mountain
Steep
Lake
Autumn Colors
Wildflowers
Birds
Wildlife
Great Views
Photo Opportunity
Camping
Geologic Interest

FACILITIES
Restrooms

Logistics

Amenities and last-minute supplies can be found near the Jenny Lake Visitor Center, a mile north of the Lupine Meadows junction. Bring plenty of water, as there's little between the trailhead and the tarns.

Trail Description

Geologic Interest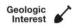

The Lupine Meadows trailhead parking area ▶1 (6,732 feet) is named after the colorful members of the pea family that dominate the surrounding sagebrush flats with luxuriant, blooming pastel displays every summer.

In sharp contrast to the open outwash plain deposited by glaciers around the parking area, the trail, a popular climbers' access route, quickly enters the cover of a mature mixed-conifer forest as it heads south on disintegrating asphalt.

After 1.7 miles, at the first junction with the Valley Trail, which leads down to Bradley Lake, ▶2 the Amphitheater Lake Trail forks off the Valley Trail and starts to switchback up an exposed ridge (known as a lateral moraine) between Burned Wagon and Glacier Gulches, with views over the lake to Jackson Hole. Above here, ruffed grouse calmly sit along the trail, and wildflowers are often abundant on the sunny slopes.

Wildflowers

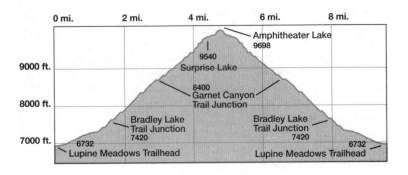

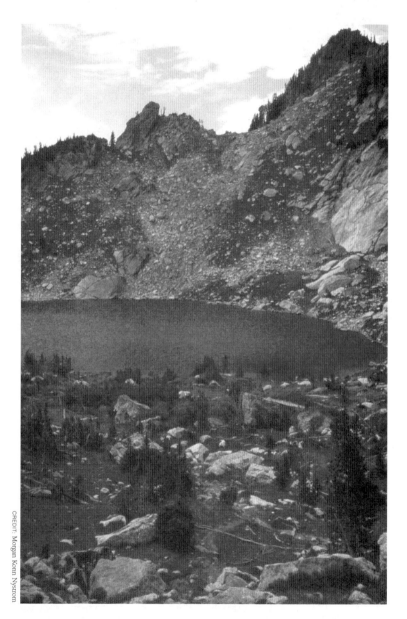

CREDIT: Morgan Konn Nystrom

Amphitheater Lake *occupies a stunning cirque at the foot of Disappointment Peak.*

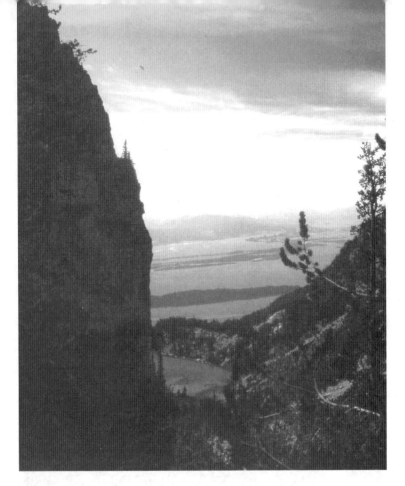

Teton Glacier Overlook *offers views of Delta Lake and Jackson Hole.*

Steep

Lake

Beyond the Garnet Canyon Trail junction ▶3 (8,400 feet), at 3 miles, the straight-ahead switch-back climb will knock the velvet off all but the most fit antlers. Pack an extra cache of chocolate (or other quick-energy food).

Stay on designated trails to preserve the beautiful, fragile subalpine habitat surrounding the perfectly circular Surprise Lake ▶4 (9,540 feet). A single backcountry campsite offers an opportunity for overnights, though the site is sometimes closed in late summer as bears arrive to eat whitebark pine

Teton Glacier Overlook and Garnet Canyon

From Amphitheater Lake, you can continue 0.3 mile one-way around the northeast shore to the highly recommended Teton Glacier Overlook. It offers impressive views into the next valley and back over aquamarine Delta Lake to Jackson Hole.

You could also extend the hike by adding a 2.2-mile, two-hour detour up Garnet Canyon to get to a large boulder field, spectacular views of the Middle Teton (12,804 feet), and a popular climbing base at the Meadows camping area.

nuts. Just a few hundred yards above and beyond, Amphitheater Lake ▶5 (9,698 feet) occupies a stunning cirque at the foot of Disappointment Peak (11,618 feet).

After you have finished picnicking and exploring around the lakes, retrace your steps downhill to return to the trailhead parking area. ▶6

🚶 MILESTONES

▶1   0.0 Start at Lupine Meadows parking area
▶2   1.7 Right at Valley Trail junction (signed for Bradley Lake)
▶3   3.0 Right at Garnet Canyon Trail junction
▶4   4.6 Right at Surprise Lake
▶5   4.8 Amphitheater Lake
▶6   9.6 Return to Lupine Meadows parking area

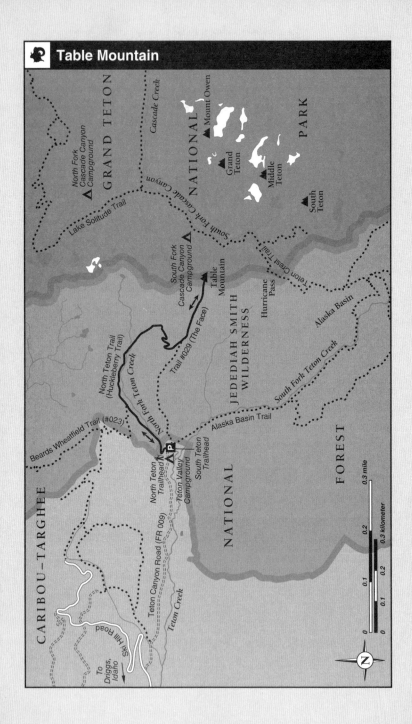

Table Mountain

North Fork
Cascade Canyon
Campground

GRAND TETON

Cascade Creek

Mount Owen

Grand
Teton

Middle
Teton

NATIONAL

PARK

South
Teton

Lake Solitude Trail

South Fork
Cascade Canyon
Campground

South Fork Cascade Canyon

Table
Mountain

North Teton Trail
(Huckleberry Trail)

Trail #029 (The Face)

North Fork Teton Creek

Hurricane
Pass

Alaska Basin

JEDEDIAH SMITH
WILDERNESS

Teton Crest Trail

South Fork Teton Creek

Beards Wheatfield Trail (#023)

Alaska Basin Trail

North Teton
Trailhead

South Teton
Trailhead

Teton Valley
Campground

NATIONAL

FOREST

CARIBOU–TARGHEE

Teton Canyon Road (FR 009)

Ski Hill Road

Teton Creek

To
Driggs, Idaho

0.1   0.2   0.3 mile

0.1   0.2   0.3 kilometer

N

Table Mountain

This popular uphill hike is the best Grand Teton hike that is not actually in the park. The rewards for the drive out of the park are fabulous views of Teton peaks and an alternative view of the range from the Idaho side.

Best Time

The trail is accessible mid-July–September; before and after this you should be prepared for snow. It's a good idea to get an early start as afternoon storms can obscure views and create hazardous conditions in summer.

Finding the Trail

From downtown Driggs, Idaho, take East Little Avenue and then Ski Hill Road east through the tiny settlement of Alta 5 miles toward Grand Targhee Resort. Take the turnoff right onto unpaved Teton Canyon Road (Forest Road 009) and go 4.7 miles to Teton Valley Campground. Just beyond the campground is the North Teton trailhead, the first of two trailheads here (the second South Teton trailhead, a couple hundred yards farther, has a toilet and water). You can hike straight from the Teton Valley Campground if staying there. The region is most easily visited if you are doing a loop of Grand Teton and Yellowstone National Parks, while driving to or from West Yellowstone.

TRAIL USE
Hike

LENGTH
14 miles, 7–9 hours

VERTICAL FEET
±4,120

DIFFICULTY
– 1 2 3 **4** 5 +

TRAIL TYPE
Out-and-back

SURFACE TYPE
Dirt

FEATURES
Mountain
Summit
Stream
Wildflowers
Great Views
Steep

FACILITIES
Restrooms
Water

Grand Targhee

If you have a free day in your itinerary, head to nearby Grand Targhee Resort for mountain biking, downhill rides (bikes can be hired), horseback riding, a ropes course, a zip line, bungee jumping, and a climbing wall. Music lovers can time their hike with the well-regarded bluegrass music festival in mid-August, but make sure you reserve accommodations in advance. See grandtarghee .com or call 800-TARGHEE (800-827-4433) for details.

Table Mountain was the very spot chosen by photographer William Jackson to immortalize the Tetons in his iconic 1872 photographs.

Logistics

To get an early start, overnight at the Caribou-Targhee National Forest Teton Valley Campground ($12 per site, open mid-May–mid-September). Sites are reservable for a $9 fee at recreation.gov or by calling 877-444-6777. Nearby Reunion Flat is mostly a group campground. There are several primitive camping spots along Teton Canyon Road en route to the trailhead. The trail is outside Grand Teton National Park in Idaho's Caribou-Targhee National Forest. Pack a warm jacket for the windy summit.

Trail Description

The trailhead sign at the parking lot ►1 points the way on North Teton Trail 24, also called the Huckleberry Trail. After five minutes, a horse trail joins from a separate trailhead parking area, as the trail climbs through groves of aspen. A sign indicates that you are entering the Jedediah Smith Wilderness, named after a 19th-century trapper, explorer, and mountain man. The initially steep climb eases as you follow the North Fork of Teton Creek. Look for moose during this section of trail.

Wildlife

After the junction with the Beards Wheatfield Trail (23), ►2 continue through open meadows bursting with wildflowers in July. The trail gets rockier as you get closer to the river, winding around giant slabs of rock. Cross the creek on log

Wildflowers

bridges twice in 10 minutes (fill up on water here) and you'll soon see the upper bowl ahead of you. Passing more meadows, the trail swings to the right and starts to switchback up the grassy ridge, looping to the right to traverse the ridge and reveal views of the mesalike butte of Table Mountain, with Grand Teton towering behind.

Viewpoint

A rock cairn marks the otherwise unsigned junction with Trail 29, ▶3 an alternative but much steeper route called The Face that climbs directly from South Teton Trailhead. Most people who come up this route decide to go down the other

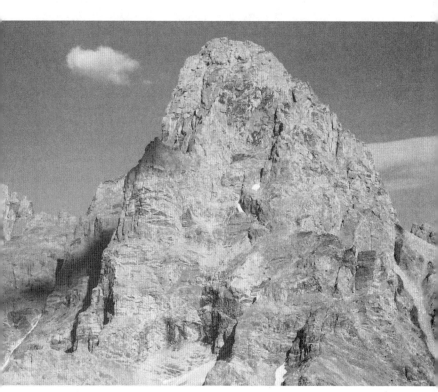

Grand Teton *from Table Mountain*

CREDIT: Bradley Mayhew

The Face

A shorter but steeper trail nicknamed The Face (29) climbs from near the South Teton Trailhead straight up the mountainside to join the main trail to Table Mountain near the summit, though be warned: it's a very steep trail. It's therefore possible to hike up The Face to Table Mountain and then descend the main Huckleberry Trail for a loop hike. The trailhead for The Face is a little tricky to find, leading off from next to the vault toilet at the South Teton Trailhead. Don't confuse this minor path with the main Alaska Basin Trail.

way (it's particularly slippery downhill). Continue up the ridge toward Table Mountain, past the last whitebark pines and following cairns through a rock field. The long, grassy alpine ridge gets increasingly

Steep steep as you make the final steep scramble up to the 11,106-foot summit of Table Mountain. ▶4 Figure on 3.5 hours from the trailhead to the windy summit, also called Table Rock. The epic views center on 13,770-foot Grand Teton, but you can also see Middle Teton, South Teton, and Mount Owen, with

Summit the South Fork of Cascade Canyon far below you, and Hurricane Pass and Alaska Basin to the right.

For slightly closer views of the South Fork of Cascade Canyon, it's possible to descend to the right (south) of Table Mountain and continue for 10 minutes along the rocky plateau behind Table

Viewpoint Mountain.

Figure on about three hours to return via the same route to the North Teton Trailhead. ▶5

🚶 MILESTONES

▶1	0.0 North Teton Trailhead
▶2	1.5 Junction with Beards Wheatfield Trail
▶3	6.2 Junction with Trail 29 (The Face)
▶4	7.0 Table Mountain summit
▶5	14.0 Back at North Teton Trailhead

Two Ocean Lake

This level loop hike around a mountain lake is a perfect early- or late-season altitude-acclimatization route. It also offers a nice escape from the crowds that flock to trails on the park's popular western side. Arrive early or stay late for the best chance at spotting deer, elk, or moose. Whenever you arrive, definitely allow time to ascend Grand View Point for some amazing views.

Best Time

Since it is at a lower elevation than most of the park, Two Ocean Lake is typically accessible (depending on snow level and road conditions) late May–early October. For spotting birds and wildlife, the early morning or late afternoon is best. On warm days, it's best to visit the sunnier, more exposed north shore in the morning to avoid the heat. The shady south shore is fine any time. Thanks to its length and relative inaccessibility, the trail is often crowd-free, even on perfectly sunny summer days.

Finding the Trail

From Moran Junction in the park's northeast sector, head 1 mile north on US 89/191/287 past the Moran Entrance Station. Turn right on paved Pacific Creek Road and go 2 miles; at the fork, bear left onto the graded dirt road signed for Two Ocean Lake and continue 2.3 miles to the signed parking area. Springtime downpours can cause the temporary closure of this road—if there's been recent heavy rain, double-check the road's status at a ranger station or visitor center;

TRAIL USE
Hike, Horse
LENGTH
6.4 miles, 3–4 hours
VERTICAL FEET
±150
DIFFICULTY
– 1 2 **3** 4 5 +
TRAIL TYPE
Loop
SURFACE TYPE
Dirt

FEATURES
Summit
Lake
Autumn Colors
Wildflowers
Birds
Wildlife
Great Views
Photo Opportunity
Secluded
Geologic Interest

FACILITIES
Restrooms
Picnic Tables
Boat Launch
Horse Staging

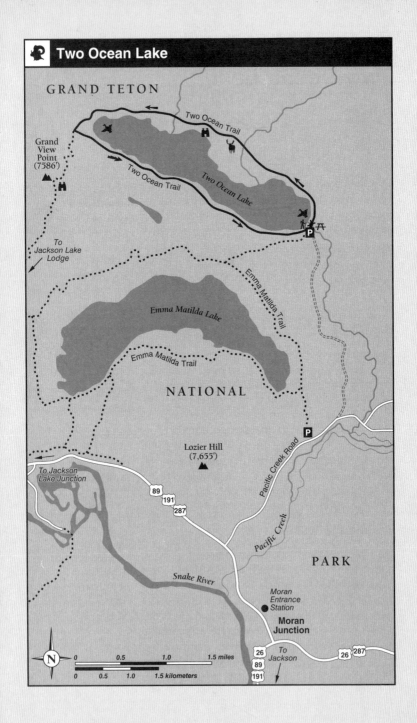

Two Ocean Lake

GRAND TETON

Two Ocean Trail

Grand
View
Point
(7586')

Two Ocean Trail

Two Ocean Trail

Two Ocean Lake

To
Jackson Lake
Lodge

P

Emma Matilda Trail

Emma Matilda Lake

Emma Matilda Trail

NATIONAL

To Jackson
Lake Junction

P

Lozier Hill
(7,655')

Pacific Creek Road

89
191
287

Pacific Creek

PARK

Snake River

Moran
Entrance
Station

Moran
Junction

N

0   0.5   1.0   1.5 miles

0   0.5   1.0   1.5 kilometers

26
89
191

To
Jackson

26   287

you may have to choose another trail. At other times, all vehicles should be able to navigate the unpaved section. To start on the north shore, look for the trailhead near the picnic area. For the south shore, look for the trailhead past the restrooms.

Logistics

The loop around Two Ocean Lake can be done in either direction with no change in elevation gain. You can start on the north or south shore, depending on whether you want to tackle the more difficult part first or leave it for last.

Trail Description

Find the north shore trailhead, ▶1 just past the picnic benches, where a sign points the way 4.3 miles to Grand View Point. Cross a small bridge over the outlet stream of Two Ocean Lake ▶2 (6,896 feet), which meanders along Two Ocean Road for a couple of miles before its confluence with Pacific Creek. Waterfowl are abundant around the lake, and grizzlies have been seen gorging themselves on berries, so remain bear-aware.

After contouring along the open lakeshore 0.5 mile, the singletrack trail trends northwest, away from the shore, and enters a shady, mixed aspen and conifer forest. Ignore the horse trails that head down into the boggy meadows, and monitor the lakefront willow thickets for browsing moose. Even the main routes can get muddy in low-lying areas during early summer.

The trail continues above the north shore, losing views of the lake and crossing several seasonal creeks that water meadows of sagebrush and prolific wildflowers. After about 45 minutes of walking, look for a forested knoll at the northwest end of the lake, which offers a fine picnic spot just off the main trail. ▶3

Two Ocean Lake's name refers to an early assumption that because it is close to the Continental Divide, its waters must drain into both the Atlantic and Pacific Oceans. They don't, but the nearby Two Ocean Plateau, in Yellowstone's bottom-right corner, is bisected by the Continental Divide, and its waters do drain to both oceans.

 Birds

 Wildlife

 Wildflowers

Grand View Point Side Trip

The uphill, out-and-back detour from Two Ocean Lake up the north flank of Grand View Point (7,586 feet) adds at least an hour and 700 feet of elevation gain. On clear days, two volcanic outcroppings atop the well-named vista point make scenic picnic spots and offer amazing near-360-degree panoramas, including eye-level views of Mount Moran and the central Tetons and east to some of the remotest territory in the Lower 48. The second, balder clearing has the best views. This detour adds 2 miles to the hike. If you can arrange a car shuttle, you could follow trails downhill all the way to Jackson Lake Lodge (2.9 miles), finishing the hike with a beer on the fabulous deck of the lodge's Blue Heron Lounge.

Birds

Three miles from the trailhead, a sign announces the head of Two Ocean Lake, ▶4 at its western end. A small, unmarked trail leads down to the lakeshore, where ducks, swans, and other waterfowl are often found basking in the bay.

Back on the main trail and across a small bridge, a signed junction marks the route's most important decision point: ▶5 continuing straight ahead 1.3 miles takes you up the steep north side of Grand View Point (see Options) via a series of switchbacks, a recommended extension to this hike.

Viewpoint

Back on the main trail after the detour, the views from the lake's shady south shore are obscured by morainal ridges, so the final 3.1 miles are less spectacular than the first half of the hike, with no mountain views.

From the junction for Grand View Point, the trail descends through pine forest to cross a couple of streams before gently climbing more than 100 feet above Two Ocean Lake's southern shoreline. The landscape on the home stretch of the trail varies: you'll encounter lodgepole pine and old-growth spruce–fir forests, clearings, bridged stream crossings, bogs, and wildflower meadows—offering a look at a selection of flora not seen on the sunnier north shore.

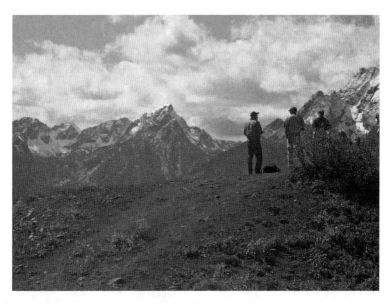

Taking in a phenomenal vista of **Grand View Point** *(see Options, opposite)*

After a final bridged crossing of a small bog, the trail crests a gentle rise at the Two Ocean parking and picnic area, ▶6 on your left shortly after the signed junction for the trail to Emma Matilda Lake.

🚶 MILESTONES

▶1	0.0	Start at Two Ocean Lake parking area
▶2	0.1	Cross stock bridge
▶3	1.5	Find a shady picnic spot with Grand Teton views
▶4	3.0	Western end of Two Ocean Lake
▶5	3.3	Straight to Grand View Point or left to return to trailhead
▶6	6.4	Return to parking area

Appendixes

Major Public Agencies

National Park Service (NPS) nps.gov

Phone numbers for specific divisions are listed below. See tinyurl.com /national-parks-pass for details on buying a National Parks and Federal Recreation Lands Annual Pass ($80).

National Park Foundation

888-467-2757, 202-354-6460, nationalparks.org

Yellowstone National Park nps.gov/yell

General visitor information: 307-344-7381, TTY 307-344-2386

Albright Visitor Center: 307-344-2263

Bechler Ranger Station: 406-581-7074

Canyon Visitor Center: 307-344-2550

Fishing Bridge Visitor Center: 307-344-2450

Grant Village Visitor Center: 307-344-2650

Madison Information and Junior Ranger Station: 307-344-2821

Norris Information Station: 307-344-2812

Old Faithful Visitor Center: 307-344-2751

West Yellowstone Multiagency Visitor Center: 307-344-2876

Central Backcountry Office: 307-344-2160, YELL_Backcountry_Office@nps.gov

Recorded camping and lodging report: 307-344-2114

Beartooth Highway road conditions: 888-285-4636

Yellowstone National Park road conditions: 307-344-2117

Lake Hospital: 307-242-7241

Mammoth Medical Clinic: 307-344-7965

Old Faithful Medical Clinic: 307-545-7325

Park lost and found: 307-344-2109; lodging lost and found: 307-344-5387

Grand Teton National Park

nps.gov/grte, facebook.com/grandtetonnps

P.O. Drawer 170, Moose, WY 83012-0170

General visitor information: 307-739-3300 or 307-739-3600,
TDD 307-739-3400

Colter Bay Visitor Center: 307-739-3594

Craig Thomas Discovery & Visitor Center: 307-739-3399

Flagg Ranch Information Center: 307-543-2372

Jenny Lake Ranger Station: 307-739-3343

Jenny Lake Visitor Center: 307-739-3392

Backcountry Permits Office: 307-739-3602 or 307-739-3309,
fax 307-739-3438

Camping and lodging information: 307-739-3603

Climbing information and permits: 307-739-3604

Grand Teton Medical Clinic: 307-543-2514, 307-733-8002 after hours

Lost and found: 307-739-3450

Park emergency dispatch: 307-739-3301

Report a bear in campground: 307-739-3301

River-flow information: 800-658-5771

Road conditions: 307-739-3614, 307-739-3682 in winter

Weather report: 307-739-3611

Lodging

In Yellowstone National Park

Xanterra (pronounced zan-TAIR-uh) **Parks and Resorts:** Yellowstone's only
in-park accommodations concessionaire runs four campgrounds, nine
lodgings, and an RV park. See the regional introductions for details on
specific lodges and campgrounds and visit yellowstonenationalpark
lodges.com. Note: all rates are per night.

General information and same-day reservations: 307-344-7901

Camping, lodging, and dining reservations: 866-439-7375 or 307-344-
7311, TDD 307-344-5395, fax 307-344-7456

In Grand Teton National Park

American Alpine Club's Grand Teton Climbers' Ranch: Open early June–mid-September, the reservable four- to eight-bed dorm bunks ($16 for members, $25 for nonmembers) are the best budget-lodging deal inside the park. No pets are allowed. 307-733-7271, americanalpineclub.org/grand-teton-climbers-ranch.

Dornans: Runs the recommended Spur Ranch Cabins at Moose Junction in summer (May 16–October 15) for $225–$350 for one or two bedrooms and in the winter/shoulder season (October 16–May 15) for $125–$175. Open year-round. Hearty meals are served alfresco at picnic tables or around a fire inside tepees. 307-733-2522, dornans.com.

Grand Teton Lodge Company: Manages a wide variety of accommodations, most open late May–early October. Colter Bay Village offers basic canvas tent cabins with wood-burning stoves ($69) and better-value cabins (shared bathroom, $90; private bathroom, $165–$210). The well-situated Jackson Lake Lodge has standard hotel-style rooms (doubles $309–$419; suites $729–$809) and opens earlier than most other park accommodations. The chic Jenny Lake Lodge has finely appointed log cabins ($485) and exclusive suites ($669). Package rates at the lodge include breakfast, horseback riding, and a five-course dinner. 307-543-3100, 800-628-9988, gtlc.com.

Headwaters Lodge: Situated 6 miles north of Grand Teton National Park's northern boundary and 2 miles south of Yellowstone National Park's South Entrance at Flagg Ranch. Open mid-May–mid-September; call for winter availability, which varies from year to year depending on snowmobiling regulations. Camper cabin $74; doubles $220–$310; reservable tent site for one or two people $35; RV site $72. 307-543-2861, 800-443-2311, flaggranch.com.

Jackson Hole Mountain Resort: This year-round resort 12 miles northwest of Jackson is home to world-class skiing and myriad summer activities. There are 2,500 acres of in-bounds terrain and a vertical drop of 4,139 feet—the greatest continuous plunge in the United States. Half the runs traverse expert terrain, and the open backcountry gate system accesses more than 3,000 out-of-bounds acres. Accommodation options range from private, budget-sparing rooms at the family-friendly Hostel ($49–$129; 307-733-3415, thehostel.us) to studio condos and fully furnished, ski-in luxury chalets. 307-733-2292, jacksonhole.com.

Jackson Hole Central Reservations: 307-733-4005, 888-838-6606; jacksonholewy.com

Jackson Hole Resort Lodging: 800-443-8613, jhrl.com

Signal Mountain Lodge: Two miles southwest of Jackson Lake Junction on Teton Park Road. Open early May–mid-October. Options include log cabins (one or two rooms, $192–$217), motel rooms ($243–$353), kitchenette bungalows ($243–$394), lakefront suites ($353–$394), and one three-room cabin ($413). 307-543-2831, signalmtnlodge.com.

Other Grand Teton–Area Resources

Bridger-Teton National Forest

Grand Teton visitors often camp, hike, boat, or fish in this National Forest, which borders the park on three sides. All campsites except group sites are first come, first served. 307-739-5500, www.fs.usda.gov/btnf.

Caribou-Targhee National Forest

This national forest, which borders the park on its west side, is home to the Jedediah Smith and Winegar Hole Wilderness areas. 208-524-7500, www.fs.usda.gov/ctnf.

Jackson Hole and Greater Yellowstone Visitor Center

Jackson's helpful interagency center is loaded with detailed information and has extensive wildlife-related videos and exhibits. The bookstore is well stocked, and there are public phones for making free calls for local lodging reservations. Sells all passes and permits. 307-733-3316; 532 N. Cache Drive, Jackson, WY. Open 8 a.m.–7 p.m. in summer, 8 a.m.–5 p.m. in winter; closed Thanksgiving and Christmas. tinyurl.com/jhgyvisitorcenter.

Upwards of 5,000 elk and 1,000 bison overwinter October–May at the U.S. Fish & Wildlife Service's 25,000-acre National Elk Refuge, between Grand Teton National Park and Jackson. Other inhabitants include 47 types of mammals and 175 bird species. 307-733-9212, fws.gov/refuge/national_elk_refuge.

Wyoming Game & Fish Department issues hunting, fishing, and trapping licenses. 420 N. Cache Drive, Jackson, WY; 307-733-2321; poaching hotline in Wyoming 800-442-4331; wgfd.wyo.gov.

Major Nonprofit Organizations

The Conservation Alliance: 541-389-2424, conservationalliance.com

Continental Divide Trail Coalition: 303-996-2759, continentaldividetrail.org

Grand Teton Association: 307-739-3606, grandtetonpark.org

Grand Teton National Park Foundation: 307-732-0629, gtnpf.org

Greater Yellowstone Coalition: 800-775-1834, greateryellowstone.org

The Murie Center: 307-739-2246, muriecenter.org

National Parks Conservation Association: 800-628-7275, npca.org

Teton Science Schools: 307-733-1313, tetonscience.org

Yellowstone Association: 406-848-2400, store orders 406-848-2400, yellowstoneassociation.org

Yellowstone Park Foundation: 406-586-6303, ypf.org

Yellowstone to Yukon (Y2Y) Conservation Initiative: 403-609-2666, 800-966-7920 in Canada, y2y.net

Outfitters, Guides, and Tour Operators

Yellowstone: Contact the NPS (nps.gov/yell/planyourvisit/guidedtours.htm) for a current list of outfitters permitted to lead guided day-hiking, backpacking, fishing, bicycling, llama- and horse-packing, cross-country-skiing, wildlife-watching, and photo-safari trips inside Yellowstone National Park.

Grand Teton: Contact the NPS (nps.gov/grte/planyourvisit/concessions. htm) for a current list of outfitters authorized to lead guided day-hiking, backpacking, climbing, fishing, rafting, kayaking, cross-country-skiing, snowshoeing, and equestrian trips within Grand Teton National Park.

Guided Hikes and Backpacking Trips

If you are nervous about organizing your own backpacking adventure, don't have the time, or just enjoy the companionship of other hikers in a group setting, the following regional companies specialize in guided hiking and backpacking trips in Yellowstone and Grand Teton:

Big Wild Adventures (bigwildadventures.com) Backpacking trips in Yellowstone and around, from Emigrant, Montana

The Hole Hiking Experience (holehike.com) Guided hiking and backpacking tours and winter snowshoeing, in Jackson, Wyoming

Llama Trips in Yellowstone (yellowstonellamatrips.com) Backpacking trips in Yellowstone with llamas, from Bozeman, Montana

Off the Beaten Path (offthebeatenpath.com) Top-end guided tours in the Yellowstone region, from Bozeman, Montana

Trail Guides Yellowstone (trailguidesyellowstone.com) Well-run operation in Bozeman, Montana

Wildland Trekking (wildlandtrekking.com) Treks throughout Greater Yellowstone, with an office in Bozeman, Montana

The Wild Side (wolftracker.com) Biologists Nathan Varley and Linda Thurston run spring wolf-watching hikes from Gardiner, Montana

Yellowstone Hiking Guides (yellowstonehikingguides.com) Guided nature hikes from Gardiner, Montana

Internet Resources

Visitor Information and Chambers of Commerce

Big Sky Chamber of Commerce (Montana): 406-995-3000, bigskychamber.com

Cody Country Chamber of Commerce (Wyoming): 307-587-2777, codychamber.org

Colter Pass, Cooke City & Silver Gate Chamber of Commerce (Montana): 406-838-2495, cookecitychamber.org

Destination Dubois (Wyoming): 307-455-2556, duboiswyoming.org

Gardiner, Montana, Chamber of Commerce: 406-848-7971, gardinerchamber.com

Jackson Hole Chamber (Wyoming): 307-733-3316, jacksonholechamber.com

Red Lodge Area Chamber of Commerce (Montana): 888-281-0625, redlodgechamber.org

Visit Idaho: 208-334-2470, visitidaho.org

West Yellowstone Chamber of Commerce (Montana): 406-646-7701, destinationyellowstone.com

Wyoming Office of Tourism: 800-225-5996, travelwyoming.com

Yellowstone Country Montana: 800-736-5276, yellowstonecountry.net

Miscellaneous

For hiking tips, visit hike734.com, trailguidesyellowstone.com, and teton hikingtrails.com. General hiking websites such as backpacker.com and alltrails.com also have excellent Yellowstone-related trail reports.

General websites such as yellowstonegeotourism.com, yellowstonepark .com, and yellowstone.net can answer most travel-related questions.

The website yellowstonereports.com is the best source of the latest wildlife-spotting data and reports, and is well worth the subscription price of $20 per year.

For a useful rundown of the park's main thermal features, visit geyser watch.com.

For up-to-date news on Yellowstone, visit the Yellowstone Insider (yellowstoneinsider.com), The Yellowstone Daily (theyellowstonedaily. com), and Yellowstone Gate (yellowstonegate.com).

For Grand Teton information, see Jackson Hole News & Guide (jhnews andguide.com) and Teton Valley News (tetonvalleynews.net).

Other sites include:

Old Faithful Geyser Streaming Webcam: tinyurl.com/oldfaithfulcam

Old Faithful Virtual Visitor Center: nps.gov/features/yell/ofvec/index2.htm

USGS Yellowstone Volcano Observatory: http://volcanoes.usgs.gov/yvo

Yellowstone's Webcams: tinyurl.com/yellowstonewebcams

Useful Books

Guidebooks

Adkison, Ron. *Exploring Beyond Yellowstone: Hiking, Camping, and Vacationing in the National Forests Surrounding Yellowstone and Grand Teton.* Out of print. Berkeley, CA: Wilderness Press, 1996.

Henry, Jeff. *Yellowstone Winter Guide.* Boulder, CO: Roberts Rinehart, 1998.

Mayhew, Bradley, and Carolyn McCarthy. *Lonely Planet Yellowstone & Grand Teton National Parks.* Oakland, CA: Lonely Planet, 2016.

Woods, Rebecca. *Jackson Hole Hikes.* Alpenbooks, 1999.

Geology

Bryan, Scott T. *The Geysers of Yellowstone.* Niwot, CO: University Press of Colorado, 2008.

Fritz, William J. *Roadside Geology of the Yellowstone Country.* Missoula, MT: Mountain Press Publishing, 1985.

Good, John M. and Kenneth L. Pierce. *Interpreting the Landscape: Recent and Ongoing Geology of Grand Teton and Yellowstone National Parks.* Jackson, WY: Grand Teton Natural History Association, 2016.

Love, David D., and John C. Reed, et al. *Creation of the Teton Landscape.* Grand Teton Association, 2016.

Smith, Robert B., and Lee J. Siegel. *Windows into the Earth: The Geologic Story of Yellowstone and Grand Teton National Parks.* New York: Oxford University Press, 2000.

Natural History

Craighead Jr., Frank C. *For Everything There Is a Season: The Sequence of Natural Events in the Grand Teton–Yellowstone Area.* Helena, MT: Falcon Press, 1994.

Halfpenny, James C. *Yellowstone Wolves in the Wild.* Helena, MT: Riverbend Publishing, 2003.

———. *Yellowstone Bears in the Wild.* Helena, MT: Riverbend Publishing, 2012.

———. *Tracks, Scats & Signs of Yellowstone and Grand Teton National Parks.* Quick Reference Publishing, 2012.

McEneaney, Terry. *Birds of Yellowstone: A Practical Habitat Guide to the Birds of Yellowstone National Park, and Where to Find Them.* Boulder, CO: Roberts Rinehart, 1988.

McNamee, Thomas. *The Return of the Wolf to Yellowstone.* New York: Owl Books, 1998.

Schreier, Carl. *A Field Guide to Wildflowers of the Rocky Mountains.* Moose, WY: Homestead Publishing, 1996.

Schullery, Paul. *The Bears of Yellowstone.* Worland, WY: High Plains Publishing, 1992.

Shaw, Richard J. *Plants of Yellowstone & Grand Teton National Parks.* Salt Lake City: Wheelwright Press, 2008.

Simpson, Ann, and Rob Simpson. *Yellowstone Wildlife: Nature Guide to Yellowstone National Park.* Falcon Press, 2015.

Smith, Douglas and Gary Ferguson. *Decade of the Wolf, Revised and Updated: Returning the Wild to Yellowstone.* Lyons Press, 2012.

Snow, Kathleen. *Taken by Bear in Yellowstone: More Than a Century of Harrowing Encounters between Grizzlies and Humans.* Lyons Press, 2016.

Varley, John D., and Paul Schullery. *Yellowstone Fishes: Ecology, History and Angling in the Park.* Mechanicsburg, PA: Stackpole Books, 1998.

History

Black, George. *Empire of Shadows: The Epic Story of Yellowstone.* St. Martin's Press, 2012.

Haines, Aubrey L. *The Yellowstone Story: A History of Our First National Park: Vols. 1 & 2.* Niwot, CO: University Press of Colorado, 1996.

Henry, Jeff, and Bob Barbee. *The Year Yellowstone Burned: A Twenty-Five-Year Perspective.* Taylor Trade Publishing, 2015.

Janetski, Joel C. *Indians in Yellowstone National Park.* Salt Lake City: University of Utah Press, 2002.

Miller, Mark M. *Adventures in Yellowstone: Early Travelers Tell Their Tales.* TwoDot, 2009.

Russell, Osborne. *Journal of a Trapper.* Crabtree, OR: Narrative Press, 2001.

Schullery, Paul. *Searching for Yellowstone: Ecology and Wonder in the Last Wilderness.* Helena, MT: Montana Historical Society Press, 2004.

Whittlesey, Lee H. *Yellowstone Place Names.* Yellowstone, WY: Wonderland Publishing Company, 2006.

Literature

Box, C.J. *Free Fire.* G.P. Putnam's Sons, 2007.

Cahill, Tim. *Lost in My Own Backyard: A Walk in Yellowstone National Park.* New York: Crown, 2004.

Ferguson, Gary. *Hawks Rest: A Season in the Remote Heart of Yellowstone.* Washington, D.C.: National Geographic Adventure Press, 2003.

Hoagland, Bill, ed. *Ring of Fire: Writers of the Yellowstone Region.* Cody, WY: Rocky Mountain Press, 2000.

Mernin, Jerry. *Yellowstone Ranger.* Riverbend Publishing, 2016.

Schullery, Paul. *Mountain Time: A Yellowstone Portrait.* Boulder, CO: Roberts Rinehart, 1995.

Turner, Jack. *Travels in the Greater Yellowstone.* St. Martin's Griffin, 2009.

———. *Teewinot: Climbing and Contemplating the Teton Range.* St. Martin's Griffin, 2001.

Yochim, Michael J. *A Week in Yellowstone's Thorofare: A Journey through the Remotest Place.* Oregon State University Press, 2016.

Photography

Adams, Ansel. *The Tetons and the Yellowstone.* Boston, MA: Little, Brown, 1970.

Holdsworth, Henry H. *Yellowstone & Grand Teton Wildlife Portfolio.* Helena, MT: Farcountry Press, 2003.

Lange, Joseph K. *Photographer's Guide to Yellowstone & the Tetons.* Mechanicsburg, PA: Stackpole Books, 2009.

Murphy, Tom. *The Light of Spring: The Seasons of Yellowstone.* Livingston, MT: Crystal Creek Press, 2003.

Quammen, David. *Yellowstone: A Journey through America's Wild Heart.* National Geographic, 2016.

Maps

The maps included in this book will be sufficient for on-trail navigation and following the hikes as they are described in this book. If you're planning off-trail exploration or longer overnight trips, you should pick up some of the following maps.

National Geographic's frequently revised *Trails Illustrated* topographic series are the most detailed and user-friendly maps of Yellowstone. The series covers the entire park with four waterproof, tear-resistant maps ($9.95 each) at a scale of 1:63,360, with a contour interval of 50 feet and selected GPS waypoints. The Grand Teton National Park map (no. 202) covers the entire park at 1:80,000 on one side, with UTM data for use with GPS units and a more detailed 1:31,680 inset covering many of the most popular backcountry camping zones on the reverse. 303-670-3457 or 800-962-1643, natgeomaps.com.

Bozeman's Beartooth Publishing also produces an excellent series of topo maps for both parks. The general 1:113,730 Yellowstone National Park map is a good overview; for more detail get the separate 1:80,000 Yellowstone North and Yellowstone South maps. The 2016 1:31,680 Teton Range Core Trails map is perfect for the most popular trails in the central Tetons and, unlike the Nat Geo map, has mileage distances between hiking junctions. Their Bozeman, Big Sky, West Yellowstone, and Absaroka Beartooth Wilderness maps are essential for explorations north of Yellowstone. All maps are $11.95. Visit beartoothpublishing.com.

The National Geographic Maps website also offers the 1:24,000 topographic quadrangle series published by the United States Geological Survey. The series covers all of Greater Yellowstone with 80 maps, but the level of detail (and number of maps required for a multiday hike) is a bit of overkill unless you plan to do some serious off-trail exploring.

Index

About the Authors

Andrew Dean Nystrom

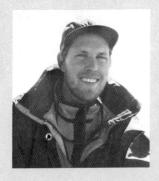

Andrew began exploring the wilderness of Denver, Colorado (creeks and prairie dog parks), straight out of the womb. After earning degrees in Geography and Education from the University of California, Berkeley, he contributed to two dozen Fodor's and Lonely Planet travel guidebooks, covering wildlands as varied as Antarctica, the Rocky Mountains, the US Southwest, Mexico, Bolivia, and Argentine and Chilean Patagonia and Tierra del Fuego. His essays about responsible, sustainable adventure and eco-travel have been translated into a dozen languages. His story about visiting Yellowstone's Thorofare patrol cabin, the most remote inhabited outpost in the Lower 48 United States, was featured in Lonely Planet's *Middle of Nowhere* pictorial book.

Over the past 15 years, Andrew has hiked the majority of trails in Yellowstone and Grand Teton, starting when he volunteered for the Yellowstone Center for Resources' Thermal Inventory project, via a Student Conservation Association (SCA) placement. In 2005 he won the National Outdoor Book Award for Best Outdoor Adventure Guidebook. He's also won several Webby Awards and Lowell Thomas Travel Journalism Gold Awards, often described as the "Pulitzer of travel writing," for his work editing, producing, and writing for the websites of Lonely Planet and the *Los Angeles Times*.

When not doing digital marketing for the world's leading sports brand, Andrew and his fine-art photographer wife, Morgan, and their two sons maintain a rapport with the wildlife in their backyard mini-farm in an untamed urban pocket of Portland, Oregon.

(Continued next page)

Bradley Mayhew

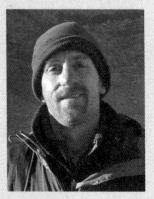

An expat Brit, Bradley has lived in Montana's Yellowstone County for the last decade and grabs every opportunity to backpack or mountain bike in the Beartooth, Absaroka, or Gallatin Ranges around Red Lodge, Livingston, and Bozeman. A frequent visitor to Yellowstone, he is the coauthor of four editions of Lonely Planet's *Yellowstone and Grand Teton National Parks* guidebook.

Bradley has been writing travel guidebooks to Asia for 20 years. His first guidebook was the *Odyssey Guidebook to Uzbekistan*, now in its eighth edition, and he has since written more than 20 guidebooks to countries across Asia. He is the coauthor of Lonely Planet guides to Tibet, Bhutan, Nepal, trekking in the Nepal Himalaya, China, Central Asia, and Bhutan, as well as previous editions of guidebooks to Mongolia, Morocco, and Jordan.

His great love is hiking in wild, remote places. He has trekked throughout the Himalaya, from Pakistan to Bhutan, and has updated trekking content for guidebooks to Tibet, Morocco, Bhutan, and Nepal. Bradley was featured in the 10-part TV series *Wanderlust: Europe's Ten Best Long-Distance Hiking Trails,* for French and German TV. When not writing or filming about trekking, he is doing it for fun, most recently in Zanskar, Ethiopia, and Kyrgyzstan.

Bradley studied Chinese at Oxford University and has since traveled to most corners of western and southwestern China, with a focus on China's ethnic borderlands. His other great love is central Asia; he has contributed to several books on the Silk Road and has been featured in a four-part Arte TV documentary retracing the route of Marco Polo from Venice to China via Afghanistan and Tajikistan.

Bradley was last spotted heading off to do a third kora (a type of pilgrimage) of Mount Kailash in Tibet. See what he's been up to recently at bradleymayhew.blogspot.com.